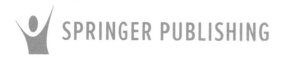

GET THE MOST FROM YOUR BOOK

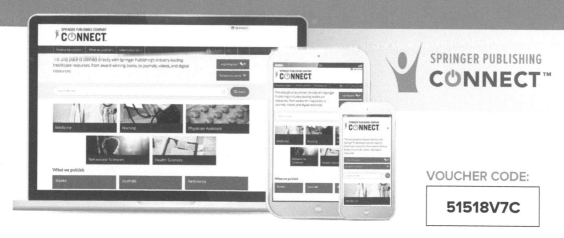

SPRINGER PUBLISHING
CONNECT™

VOUCHER CODE:

51518V7C

Online Access

Your print purchase of *Statistics and Data Analysis Literacy for Nurses*, includes **online access via Springer Publishing Connect**™ to increase accessibility, portability, and searchability.

Insert the code at http://connect.springerpub.com/content/book/978-0-8261-6582-4 today!

Having trouble? Contact our customer service department at cs@springerpub.com

Instructor Resource Access for Adopters

Let us do some of the heavy lifting to create an engaging classroom experience with a variety of instructor resources included in most textbooks SUCH AS:

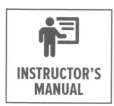

INSTRUCTOR'S MANUAL

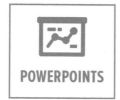

POWERPOINTS

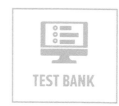

TEST BANK

Visit **https://connect.springerpub.com/** and look for the **"Show Supplementary"** button on your **book homepage** to see what is available to instructors! First time using Springer Publishing Connect?

Email **textbook@springerpub.com** to create an account and start unlocking valuable resources.

Statistics and Data Analysis Literacy for Nurses

James B. Schreiber, PhD, is a professor at the School of Nursing at Duquesne University and received his doctorate in learning and cognition from Indiana University Bloomington in 2000. He has published more than 100 articles in journals, such as *Journal of Educational Psychology, Semiotica, Clinical Simulation in Nursing, Aphasiology, Computational and Mathematical Organization Theory*, and *Research in Social and Administrative Pharmacy*, along with chapters and reviews. In addition, he has more than 130 national and international presentations. He is the former editor-in-chief of the *Journal of Educational Research, The Journal of Experimental Education*, and *Genetic, Social, and General Psychology Monographs*. He currently sits on multiple journal editorial boards. He is the also the author of a book on motivation with Springer Publishing.

He teaches courses in statistics, measurement, and human health and development along with specialty undergraduate courses concerning "Fake Data and What Counts." His statistics courses range from introduction to statistics to structural equations and quantitative modeling including artificial intelligence algorithms.

He has been an advisory board member for the Lemelson Center for the Study of Innovation and Invention, Collaborative Pediatric Critical Care Research Network within the National Institute of Child Health and Human Development, and a panel reviewer with the Institute of Education Sciences (IES) and the National Science Foundation (NSF). In addition, he held a research fellowship with the Smithsonian Institution from 2011 to 2012 and consulted for the education group at the United States Holocaust Memorial Museum and the Holocaust Center of Pittsburgh. He is currently an advisor on the Mars exhibit for the Carnegie Science Center. For the American Educational Research Association, he has been chair of the Semiotics in Education Special Interest Group, Chair of the Division D Early Career Award, member of the Division D Affirmative Action Committee, a Division C Mentor for over a decade, and currently is a member of the Working Group for Division D on Learning in Action Black Lives Matter working group.

Melanie T. Turk, PhD, RN, is an associate professor in the School of Nursing at Duquesne University. Dr. Turk received her PhD in nursing from the University of Pittsburgh in 2008. The focus of her research is body weight management for disease prevention, particularly among vulnerable populations, such as older adults, immigrants, and racial/ethnic minority groups. Her 75 published abstracts and manuscripts are in peer-reviewed journals, such as *Circulation, Journal of Cardiovascular Nursing, Obesity, International Journal of Behavioral Medicine, Nurse Educator*, and *Journal of Nursing Scholarship*. She has 35 regional, national, and international presentations and has written 6 book chapters. Dr. Turk serves as a peer reviewer for numerous journals and is an associate editor for the *Journal of Transcultural Nursing*. She has served as an invited reviewer for the National Institute of Health, National Institute of General Medical Sciences.

She teaches primarily graduate-level courses, including program analysis and evaluation and transcultural and global health perspectives in the DNP program, and methods of scientific inquiry and research and theory in health behavior in the PhD program. She has served as DNP project advisor and PhD dissertation chair for numerous doctoral students. She also teaches evidence-based practice to the MSN students and is the director of the Nursing Honors Program at the undergraduate level.

Dr. Turk is a member of the Society for Implementation Research Collaboration; the Transcultural Nursing Society, International; Sigma Theta Tau International Nursing Honor Society; and the American Heart Association, to name a few. She was inducted as a transcultural nursing scholar in the Transcultural Nursing Society, International, in 2021 and has received the Duquesne University Gaultier Teaching Fellowship and Duquesne University Creative Teaching Award.

Statistics and Data Analysis Literacy for Nurses

James B. Schreiber, PhD

Melanie T. Turk, PhD, RN

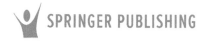 SPRINGER PUBLISHING

Springer Publishing Company, LLC
11 West 42nd Street, New York, NY 10036
www.springerpub.com
connect.springerpub.com/

Acquisitions Editor: Joseph Morita
Compositor: Amnet

ISBN: 978-0-8261-6581-7
ebook ISBN: 978-0-8261-6582-4
DOI: 10.1891/9780826165824

SUPPLEMENTS:

A robust set of instructor resources designed to supplement this text is located at http://connect.springerpub.com/content/book/978-0-8261-6582-4. Qualifying instructors may request access by emailing textbook@springerpub.com.

Instructor's Manual ISBN: 978-0-8261-6583-1
Instructor's PowerPoints ISBN: 978-0-8261-7605-9
Instructor's Test Bank ISBN: 978-0-8261-6584-8

22 23 24 25 / 5 4 3 2 1

The author and the publisher of this Work have made every effort to use sources believed to be reliable to provide information that is accurate and compatible with the standards generally accepted at the time of publication. Because medical science is continually advancing, our knowledge base continues to expand. Therefore, as new information becomes available, changes in procedures become necessary. We recommend that the reader always consult current research and specific institutional policies before performing any clinical procedure or delivering any medication. The author and publisher shall not be liable for any special, consequential, or exemplary damages resulting, in whole or in part, from the readers' use of, or reliance on, the information contained in this book. The publisher has no responsibility for the persistence or accuracy of URLs for external or third-party Internet websites referred to in this publication and does not guarantee that any content on such websites is, or will remain, accurate or appropriate.

Library of Congress Cataloging-in-Publication Data

Names: Schreiber, James, author. | Turk, Melanie T., author.
Title: Statistics and data analysis literacy for nurses / James B. Schreiber, Melanie T. Turk.
Description: New York, NY : Springer Publishing Company, [2023] | Includes
    bibliographical references and index.
Identifiers: LCCN 2022037134 (print) | LCCN 2022037135 (ebook) | ISBN
    9780826165817 (paperback) | ISBN 9780826165824 (ebook)
Subjects: MESH: Statistics as Topic | Nurses Instruction
Classification: LCC RT85.5 (print) | LCC RT85.5 (ebook) | NLM QA 276 |
    DDC 610.7302/1--dc23/eng/20220906
LC record available at https://lccn.loc.gov/2022037134
LC ebook record available at https://lccn.loc.gov/2022037135

Contact sales@springerpub.com to receive discount rates on bulk purchases.

Publisher's Note: **New and used products purchased from third-party sellers are not guaranteed for quality, authenticity, or access to any included digital components.**

Printed in the United States of America by Gasch Printing.

For,

Helene, Claudia, Annika, and Miles (the rescue dog).
– James B. Schreiber

For,

My husband, Ed. Thank you for your never-ending support.
–Melanie T. Turk

Contents

Foreword

Doctor of Nursing Practice (DNP) prepared practitioners and leaders are charged with engaging in and leading innovative and evidence-based practice that is reflective of the application of credible research findings. These new doctoral practitioners and leaders confront clinical problems on a daily basis that require analysis and interventions using their knowledge and expertise in quality improvement and evidence. Statistical literacy is another essential skill set for doctoral-level nurses as they evaluate evidence to tackle these significant clinical problems. Statistical acumen and confidence have evaded many nurses for multiple reasons requiring educators to find alternate ways to bridge this knowledge gap.

Drs. Schreiber and Turk's book, *Statistics and Data Analysis Literacy for Nurses*, fills a void and meets this need. Students and educators alike will benefit from its straightforward, pragmatic style in explaining applied statistical analysis. Chapters are replete with various quantitative methods including novel chapters on visual representation and humility, and examples to assist the reader in understanding what is generally complex content. Drawing on the deep expertise of its authors, the book should become a go-to reference for anyone looking to gain knowledge in applied statistics. The end-of-chapter review questions are an additional resource for readers to evaluate their mastery of the topic.

Rather than focus solely on mathematical statistics, this book's refreshing approach focuses on learning how to argue using research questions, methods, and aligned analyses. Utilizing Ableson's (1995) five points about statistics as argumentation as a premise for the book, the authors illustrate how MAGIC: Magnitude, Articulation, Generality, Interestingness, and Credibility are necessary to make a persuasive argument. In other words, nurses must critically evaluate a study and not just rely on a *p*-value, especially in single studies as a basis to support or refute findings. While most of the scientific world places a large emphasis on statistical significance, the authors argue that the focus of the results should be on the magnitude of the difference or the size of the association between variables and what those values mean.

DNP students with minimal statistical background will not be put off by this book's approach to statistics and data analysis. Well-written with a unique perspective, this book makes the case for placing the doctoral-level nurse in the mindset of being a good, applied statistician to refute incorrect claims and support claims with proper evidence.

Mary Ellen Smith Glasgow, PhD, RN, ACNS-BC, ANEF, FAAN
Dean and Professor
Duquesne University School of Nursing

Preface

This book was written for faculty who are teaching statistics to primarily Doctor of Nursing Practice students. The book can also be used with PhD students with the addition of some more technical and mathematical information. The DNP student was chosen as a focal point because of their need for statistical literacy.

THE SCOPE OF THE BOOK

Internally, the first 5 chapters are foundational for statistical analysis, measurement, descriptive statistics, visualization, and quantitative design. Chapter 1 is not the traditional introductory/history chapter. The content in the chapter is an immediate dive into important and problematic aspects of statistical analysis. We tackle the definition of p-values and null hypothesis significance testing (NHST) along with their problems. Additionally, we discuss how to reexamine data from published articles for correctness. Chapter 2 contains foundational topics in classical test theory and item response theory. We included this content because students are not seeing this information enough. And, no statistical analysis matters, no matter how fancy, if the data being analyzed are weak. We also discuss problems with current categorizations and metrics that are in almost every research study with human participants. Chapter 3 is a chapter only on descriptive statistics, another area we believe is not getting enough attention. A large proportion of time should be spent on the investigation of the data itself, and then after a thorough understanding of the data, the actual analyses to answer the research question. Chapter 4 stays in the descriptive arena but moves to visualizing the data. Visualization is seeing a massive rebirth from over 100 years ago due to technological advances and ease. Additionally, there is a new journal just on visualization, *Nightingale*, from the Data Visualization Society (https://nightingaledvs.com). Chapter 5 rounds off the foundational chapters with content on research designs.

Chapters 6 through 9 cover the traditional univariate analyses. Included are topics that are traditionally in multivariate books, such as ANCOVA, repeated measures, and multivariate traditional (OLS) and logistic regression. In all of these chapters, and the book in general, we do not focus on p-values at all, but on how large the differences or associations are, which is in alignment with the American Statistical Associations statements (see *The American Statistician, Volume 73*, March 19, 2019). This focus will also be observable in how we wrote the research questions. Chapters 6 through 9 are organized in stages. The first stage is conceptual knowledge about the analysis. Here, the reader will generally see more visual and narrative description of each analysis. Second, the technical components of each analysis are described with minimal mathematical symbol usage. Then there are core results for each analysis that should be included in publications or presentations.

Chapter 6 begins with between and within group designs covering t-tests through ANOVA along with their nonparametric partners. Again, we do not focus on p-values, but discuss a priori contrasts and post-hoc analyses as a way to examine how much and where. Chapter 7 is an extension of Chapter 6 with factorial ANOVA, repeated measures, and ANCOVA. Many instructors move from t-tests to correlation/regression. In actuality, you can choose any option of what to teach when because they are all part of the general linear model. Chapter 8 introduces correlation and regression. One component we focus on is the proper correlation for the types of data. We placed this as a focal point because we both see this error in many manuscripts we review. Chapter 9 extends regression to its logistic counterpart. In health sciences logistic regression is a common (and popular) choice for analysis due to the dichotomous nature of many outcome variables. Chapter 10 introduces Bayes analysis, which is becoming more and more popular as it is integrated into more and more software packages. JAMOVI, JASP, and SPSS all have easy implementable Bayes options for these analyses. Chapter 11 concerns quality improvement (QI). This content was chosen because it is a common topic for healthcare professionals. QI has grown in popularity over the past 20 years. It has its problems (e.g., over focus on quantitative metrics), but everyone should understand the basics. Chapter 12 is a rare event in a statistics book. Researchers and statisticians need to be more humble in the discussion of their results. Statistical analysis is not truth, but evidence for or against specific arguments. Thus, we wrote a chapter about being humble. Your results are not perfect or perfectly correct. Therefore, we all need to step back and be a bit less, "we have it right" and more "we think it works this way right now."

Finally, we are agnostic on statistical software. Thus, the book is not designed around a statistical package, but understanding statistical analyses and interpreting the results within the context of the data collected and the larger applied statistical framework (e.g., measurement and design). We do provide information about using different statistical packages.

James B. Schreiber, PhD
Melanie T. Turk, PhD, RN

Instructor Resources

 A robust set of instructor resources designed to supplement this text is located at http://connect.springerpub.com/content/book/978-0-8261-6582-4. Qualifying instructors may request access by emailing **textbook@springerpub.com**.

Instructor resources include:

- Instructor's Manual
  - Data Sets
  - Chapter Activities
  - Syllabus Package
  - Common Software Programs
- PowerPoint Presentations for Lectures
- Test Bank organized by chapter including a variety of true-false, multiple choice, matching, and short answer scenario problems.

CHAPTER 1

Statistical Understanding

CORE OBJECTIVES

- Explain the need for data literacy and statistics as argumentation
- Describe the problems with p-values
- Explain the different components of the null hypothesis statistical test system
- Explain techniques for examining results and arguments
- Describe causality and its three key features
- Discuss the concept of scholar before researcher

INTRODUCTION: THE NEED FOR QUANTITATIVE LITERACY

Data surrounds us whether we recognize it or not at our personal, community, regional, country, and global levels. Smart phones count our steps and track our location. Cookies track our web surfing. Smart watches track our heartbeats and are beginning to track our blood pressure. Communities have data on our library usage, taxes paid, mortgage amounts, size of our apartment; electronic health records can contain all of your medical records since birth; financial companies have data on all of our purchases and loans; and Facebook, Google, Tik Tok, Twitter have mountains of our personal data and images of what we find important or our activities and locations. Thus, the need for quantitative literacy is important to be a fully engaged citizen. To be fully engaged, knowledge is needed on the types of data that are collected, the processes of analysis, the decision made during those processes, and how to properly interpret them. This book is a start to becoming an engaged citizen and quantitatively literate practitioner.

BASIC STATISTICAL UNDERSTANDING

The first component of basic statistical understanding is to recognize that data come in many varieties. This book is focused on quantitative, that is, numerical analysis of, data. But data can come in any form—words, video, drawings, pictures and so on. With experience, it becomes easy to see how words are assigned numbers and numbers are assigned words. The separation between numeric and nonnumeric data is not as great as it might first appear. Essentially, anything is data. Data are gathered and analyzed, and results from those analyses are built into a narrative with a conclusion about what it all means. Therefore, a great deal of statistical analysis ends up being about argumentation, or producing reasoning to support your case.

Statistical Analysis Argumentation

Statistical analysis, and more explicitly, applied statistical analysis, which is where we focus, is about argumentation (Abelson, 1995). Many people focus on the mathematics or the mathematical equations that are the foundation of applied statistics. Mathematics is important, and it is hard, we will not lie or sugar coat it (Ellenberg, 2021). One of the authors used to teach Advanced Placement Calculus AB and Calculus II, and was honest with the students about the difficulty and cognitive strain associated with it. But, mathematics is not the central focus of applied statistical analysis in this book. The techniques in this book and their related mathematics are long established. There is ongoing research in new technical aspects of analyses, which are focused on mathematical statistics, but this book is focused on learning how to argue properly using research questions, methods, and aligned analyses.

Abelson (1995) has five points about statistics as argumentation, that is how to make a persuasive argument. He uses the acronym **MAGIC**. The M stands for **Magnitude** and focuses on the size of the results. This is commonly discussed with effect sizes, which express the strength of the relationship between two variables (Glass, 1976; Smith & Glass, 1977, see Chapter 6). The A stands for **Articulation**, which refers to how precisely the results are written. For example, a researcher has run multiple experiments with four different dosage groups (new drug), and writes, "there are differences among the mean scores." This is not precise. A more precise statement would be, "There are specific differences among the groups, where participants who received doses over 10 mgs recovered faster across multiple experiments." Writing for academic literature needs to be as precise as possible. The G stands for **Generality** and is how widely are the results applicable. Most studies' results are actually quite narrow due to a variety of issues (e.g., convenience sample, low reliability of scores, data collected), but during the design phase, a range of variations should be planned. One such variation is to collect the data a second time, i.e., replication with a second sample. I, **Interestingness**, is the study that has the potential to change what people believe or observe; something that is contradictory to current thought. Many studies only provide observations of what is already established. This is great if the focus is simply replication, but new work should extend the current work or provide more nuanced understanding of what is currently known. The last is C, **Credibility**, and means that the results must be seen as credible, which includes the sample of participants, the measures or tools, how the data were collected, the design, and analysis. The combination of the five is what is most powerful, especially if the researcher has consistent credible results that are interesting and generalize to the larger population.

The Need to Focus on the Amount of Difference or Association

While most of the scientific world places a large emphasis on statistical significance, we argue that the focus of the results should be on the magnitude of the difference or the size of the association between variables and what those values mean (see Ziliak & McCloskey, 2008). More than 100 years ago, at the beginning of the modern age of applied statistics, the focus was on the values and especially the values over time or across studies. During the past 80 years, the focus has turned from trying to get very exact measures and figure out how much of a difference or effect there is, to what is the sample size needed so that the results will be below 0.05, the p-value most commonly assigned as revealing statistically significant results.

p-Value Definition

Most textbooks do not start with p-values, but given their dominance over the past 80 years, it is important to discuss them now and then move past them. The **p-value** is defined as the probability of the evidence given that the null hypothesis is true $(P(E|H)$. The null hypothesis can be thought of as simply no difference between groups or no association between the variables being studied. Thus, the researcher wants to say the evidence he or she has collected is different enough that the null hypothesis does not work. The p-value, more specifically defined, is the probability of the observed result or a more extreme result, given the null hypothesis is true, there was random sampling of participants or observations, and all the statistical assumptions were met (Kline, 2016). Thus, it is not just a probability, but a special kind of probability called conditional. Conditional probabilities mean certain conditions must be met in order to interpret the probability.

The observed p-value is the value the researcher gets after performing statistical testing in comparison to a mathematical distribution of scores. There are several different mathematical distributions of scores, such as, z-distribution, F-distribution, and Chi-Square. This book covers a few. If a researcher has an average resting heart rate value from a sample in her community and knows the average for the state, a z-value can be calculated and compared to the z-distribution. The z-value provides a spot on the distribution that is aligned to the probability; the z-value observed is equal or greater than the value on the z-distribution. From there, the p-value is determined. A full description and an example are at the end of this chapter. Historically, the most common, desirable threshold is a p-value of less than 0.05. Yes, this is difficult and confusing at first to understand, but with practice, it is easy to understand and then realize that p-values do not provide much information or help with understanding a study completely and what decisions to make from the study's results.

The Problem With p-Values

Although they are a very common statistical convention used when reporting the results of quantitative studies, p-values are actually quite problematic. There are really two correct interpretations of p-values (Kline, 2016). The first is, a researcher repeatedly randomly samples participants from the same population, and the null hypothesis is true, which means every result occurred by chance. With this repeated study set up, less than 5% of these results would be more inconsistent with the null hypothesis (no difference or association) than the observed result. The second is less than 5% of the statistics from many random samples are farther away from the mean on the sampling distribution under the null hypothesis than the one for the actual result. Yet, researchers do not repeatedly sample due to logistical and financial constraints. The p-value can only tell us whether the null hypothesis is supported.

How did statistical analysis get to this point, that a probability at 0.05 or less means the results are important? The answer is a bit shocking. R. A. Fisher made it up in the 1920s. Yes, there is an amazing group of other individuals involved, but its central focus in analysis is due to Fisher. Specifically, in his classic statistical methods book (Fisher, 1925), Fisher evolved the 5% rule within a few sentences (Ziliak, 2008). Fisher started out with stating 2 standard deviations was a convenient cutoff, and by the end of the next sentence states that they are "regarded as significant" (Fisher, 1925, pg. 42). The change from being *convenient* to *significant* is enormous and there is no justification, mathematical or otherwise, for this choice. The choice is simply personal preference. Fisher clearly shows where he is headed in the future. In 1926 he writes, "Personally, the writer prefers to set a low standard of significance at the 5% point and ignore entirely all the results which fail to reach this level" (Fisher, 1926, pg. 504). It is ironic that he did not always follow his own rule (Schreiber, 2020). The p-value cut-off has always been an artificial rule on whether something is significant, but more importantly the researcher should focus on the degree of accuracy the experiment allows and how important the issues at stake are (Gosset, 1904).

As many in data analyses will argue, the smaller the p-value, the more unusual the data would be, given that every single assumption of the data and the analysis were met (Greenland et al., 2016) This rarely happens and, for example, we have never actually seen a perfectly normally distributed outcome variable, which is one of the assumptions of many statistical tests. The p-value also does not allow a researcher to know which assumption or assumptions are incorrect. Researchers can obtain small p-values for a variety of reasons, such as the study design procedures were not followed (Greenland et al., 2016), or just a large sample size. A large p-value, which to some just means greater than 0.05, indicates the data are not unusual but does not mean the model is correct or incorrect for that matter. And, the p-value assumes the long-run result, as if the study was replicated many times. Most studies are never replicated by the researcher, nor was replication developed in the design phase of the study. When all of this is put together, p-values are not being used correctly. Even, if everyone started using them correctly, the 0.05 cut-off is still an arbitrary choice and dichotomy for statistically significant or nonsignificant results. The p-value has become such a dominant metric that people cheat with it and use it to misrepresent their research findings.

p-Hacking the Easy Way

P-hacking is cheating with p-values. It is a problem in quantitative research because the focus on p-values at 0.05 or below is all encompassing. *P*-hacking occurs when multiple statistical tests are run and only those less than 0.05 are presented. This can be intentional or unintentional—some people do not realize this selective presentation of results is a problem. But it is all an abuse of the p-values. The applied analysis field has attempted to try to deal with this issue over the years, such as all analyses and p-values must be reported, prior registration of studies where specific tests to be run are stated, p-values are adjusted for the number of tests (Chapter 6), or arguments for replication. These are all small band-aids on the larger problem of a hyper-focus on p-values, versus a focus on accuracy.

Power Versus Accuracy

A **power analysis** is used to estimate the minimum size of the sample of participants or observations needed to detect a difference or effect between groups or variables. Power analyses are usually focused on obtaining a sample size under certain conditions in order to "make sure" the results will reach the 0.05 criterion. This emphasis has become the focal point for decades and most likely hurt or slowed down a great deal of research (Szucs & Ioannidis, 2017). We believe one of the most damaging aspects of the power focus has been an almost complete disregard for the need for accurate measures (Chapter 2) to arrive at accurate results. What power, and really just sample size, does is reduce the sampling error value, which represents the error that occurs as the result of using a sample from the population and not the entire population. As sample size increases, the sampling error value will get smaller because the sample size is in the denominator of the equation used. For example, $1/3$ is smaller than $½$. As you increase the denominator, the error value will get smaller. This does not mean you have an accurate measure or that the value you have is correct for the population of people in which you are interested. It just indicates you had a large sample size compared to a small one. One way to try to focus on accuracy is to think about sample size in terms of how close to the population do you want to be and at what probability level are you willing to accept (Trafimow & MacDonald, 2017). For example, do you want to be really close to the population mean and be very certain that your value is close to the population mean? Then you need to plan for that in your study design, sampling procedures, and measurement of variables. Trafimow and MacDonald (2017) have been working in this area and provide tables and graphs that help with this decision-making process.

Null-Hypothesis Statistical Test (NHST)

There are several definitions that are important to understanding null hypothesis statistical testing (NHST) system from its historical roots to current form and the associated problems with this system. They are:

- **Null Hypothesis (H_0):** A hypothesis set up with the actual intention of showing it is incorrect, thus nullifying it. In most NHST studies, H_0 is historically set so that there is no effect or no association. For example, the relationship between weight and blood pressure would have a null hypothesis indicating no association between the two (see Appendix 1.1).

- **Alternative Hypothesis (H_A):** The generic alternative hypothesis argues there is an effect or association traditionally described as a nonzero difference between treatment levels and/or groups or a nonzero relationship. H_A is the supposed to be the complement of H_O. Most researchers have more than a generic alternative hypothesis, they typically have a directional specific hypothesis in mind (see Chapter 2), such as the experimental group will outperform the control by at least 10 points. It has been argued that the alternative is almost useless in practice (Hubbard & Bayarri, 2003; Hubbard et al., 2003; Jaynes, 2003).

- **Type I error:** This is also known as the False Positive error, which is the error of mistakenly rejecting the null hypothesis and stating a "statistically significant" observation exists when the null is actually true. Researchers never really know for sure if their single study has this error because there is very little replication. The research argument is that Type I error rate can be controlled by a fixed α level set by the experimenter. But alpha was originally designed to be a control rate for long-term repeated testing (Neyman & Pearson, 1933).

- **Alpha (α) level:** Alpha is the *long run* probability of committing a Type I error (rejecting a null hypothesis this is true). Alpha and p have historically been confused as the same thing, or one occurs before the other—they are not—they are very different. Specifically, alpha is a fixed value for repeated measurement. P-values are a data-based random variable. They have been merged as a pair, where in the design phase-you set the arbitrary cut-off with your alpha value. At the end of the study after the analysis, if the p-value is less than or equal to the originally set alpha value, then the researchers argues that the observed result is "statistically significant." This is actually incorrect. Alpha is an error rate, p-values are a test of significance. Related to only p-values, Gossett actually thought this was wrong and told Fisher. Gosset stated that one should try to see the exact same results 20 out of 20 times, and if the result was seen only 19 out of 20 times, then one should spend time figuring out why it failed that one time (Ziliak & Mcloskey, 2008). As a reminder, the p-value that is used is completely arbitrary, and no mathematical proof or justification exists for 0.05 versus any other cut-off.

- **Type II error:** This is the False Negative error and occurs when the researcher does not reject the null hypothesis when the *alternative* hypothesis is true. This error, again, is never truly known because most researchers only run the study once. To control for Type II error, it is argued that if the researchers knows the expected effect size, then adjusting the sample size will control for the error.

- **Beta (β):** Beta is also a long-run probability, but concerns committing a Type II error. Beta also has the assumption that the alternative hypothesis based on an effect size and probability distribution is true. Mathematically, $\beta = 1 - \text{Power}$.

- **Power:** The power of a study is the *long-run* probability of detecting true positive findings if they really exist given that H_A has a particular probability distribution and a particular effect size. Power is a function of the sample size and effect size. Typically, power ≥ 0.80 is considered optimal. This means that if an experimental effect equal to or larger than the expected effect size (H_A) is true, then using a given sample size, researchers would have 80% chance to identify this true effect in a *long-run* of experiments. If power is 0.80, beta is 0.20.

Original NHST

The alternative hypothesis, alpha, beta, power, Type I and Type II errors system was designed by Neyman and Pearson (N-P) (1933) to be a decision process in the world of quality control. Fisher did not use an alternative hypothesis, argued against the N-P model, and thought it was bad for science (Fisher, 1960; Szucs & Ioannidis, 2017). For N-P, the goal was to minimize Type II or false negative error rates to an acceptable level and maximize power. Also, alpha was a set fixed *error-rate* value. The central key in this system assumes (expects) long repeated testing, or what we would call exact replications focusing on *the replications,* and not be wrong too often. Thus, setting alpha and beta was about assuring efficient long-term decision making by setting error rates. Over the decades, this has been made into a simple 2 x 2 table and stripped of all its original meaning. These were two completely separate systems—Fisher with *p*-values and a null hypothesis and N-P with alpha, beta, null, and alternative hypotheses.

Current Problems With NHST

At some point, seemingly in the 1950s or early 1960s, Fisher and Neyman and Pearson were merged, probably in a textbook, and this merger is where the current system is today. The implementation of this merger has been described as the "mindless" and the "null ritual" (Gigerenzer, 2004). Additionally, researchers do not actually quantitatively define the alternative hypothesis; thus, power cannot actually be calculated before the experiment (Szucs & Ioannidis, 2017). This is a major part of this married framework. The fact is, these are two incompatible systems, technically and philosophically. As noted earlier, alpha is an error rate, and *p*-values are a test of statistical significance. Fisher specifically discussed the nonequivalence of the two (Fisher, 1960).

Where the Focus Should Be and What to Do

After all of these problems with *p*-values, and NHST, where should the practitioner or researchers focus? In this book, we will provide the *p*-values as is customary. Because of the well-engrained focus on *p*-values in the scientific community, they cannot be completely disregarded. However, the focus will be on the size of the difference between groups or the size of the association between variables, along with issues of reliability and validity in interpreting the results. These aspects of analysis are where the focus should. Normally, these topics are briefly put in the methods section or the limitations sections, but they should be integrated into the results and conclusions, not simply a separate section or at the very end. We will discuss other options that should also be a focus, such as compatibility (confidence) intervals, effect sizes, and other ways to think about the p-value (See Chapter 6).

AM I BEING LIED TO?

One of the reasons data literacy and the need to be an engaged citizen, especially in applied statistical analysis, is so important is the fact that people inadvertently make claims from data that simply do not make sense. There are also cases where the results are generalized much further than the sample, design, or analysis allows. We admit many of these mistakes are inadvertent and not lies, but they seem to persist. Alberto Brandolini is known for his asymmetry principle about the amount of energy it takes to refute a false or incorrect claim versus the amount of energy it takes to make the claim (Bergstrom & West, 2020). This is not new. Charles Spurgeon's is quoted as saying "a lie will go round the world while truth is pulling its boots on" (1859, pg 155), which is similar to Jonathan Swift's "falsehood flies, and the truth comes limping after it" (1710, pg 2, column1).

Becoming comfortable with data analysis and data in general will help to stop incorrect claims and will assist in refuting them. There are some useful skill sets for examining data claims and putting the researcher in the mindset of being a good applied statistician.

Fermi Estimation

A story told by Carl Sagan (2007) has Enrico Fermi, the Italian physicist, talking to military officers during the development of the Manhattan nuclear weapons project. Fermi is told that one general is a great general. He asks, what is the definition of a great general? Fermi is told that a great general is one who has won many consecutive battles. And Fermi asks, how many? The two discuss this and settle on five battles. Then he asks what fraction of American generals are great. After a few discussions, they settle on a few percent are great. Sagan extends the story and asks the reader to think about if all armies are equally matched, then winning a battle is purely chance. The chance of winning one battle is 50/50, the chance of winning both battles of two battles is 25%, the chance of winning three battles is 12.5%, and so on. The chance of winning five consecutive battles would be 3.125%, which is just over 3%. Thus, a few percent, as discussed, and winning could be just by luck, and maybe not a great general. Fermi estimation is a quick way to really look at what a long run probability will be if you have the starting probabilities.

GRIM

The GRIM (Granularity Related Inconsistent Means) test (Brown & Heathers, 2016) is a simple method for evaluating the accuracy of published research. The researcher just needs the mean values and the sample sizes. In social sciences, we collect samples of scores that are generally made up of whole numbers. Age,

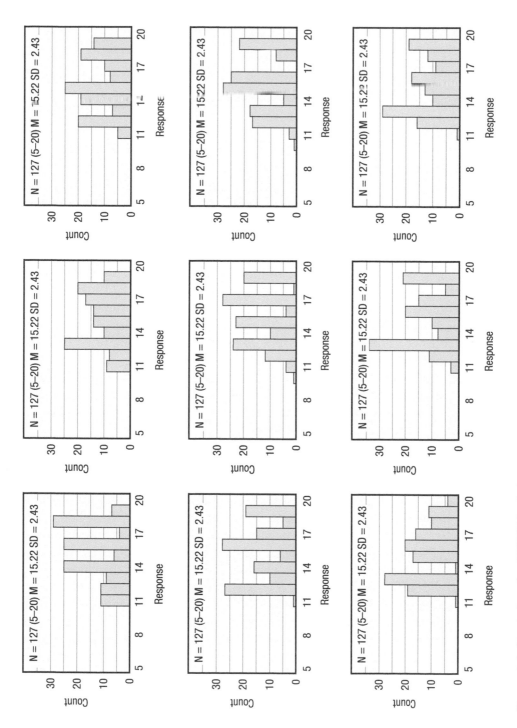

Figure 1.1. Simulations for SPRITE Analysis.

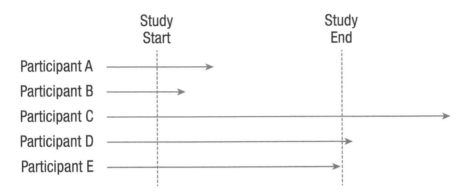

Figure 1.2. Right Censored Example.

scores on a survey using a Likert-type scale (Chapter 2), and weight in pounds are three common ones. A nurse gathers weight on 10 people: 104, 111, 125, 137, 143, 152, 167, 189, 191, 200. The average is 151.9. If the person with the lowest weight were to gain a pound, the average would increase to 152. The change is 0.1, or 1/10, and this is the minimum amount by which the average can change. Now, imagine the surprise when the average weight was 151.73, which is not possible. Whole numbers and the average have to make sense. What can occur is sample sizes change because of missing values, and the difference in sample sizes is not reported, which can be inadvertent, yet still very problematic. If there is a consistent problem across a study or studies when the sample size is known or reported, then that is red flag. There are several websites that have GRIM set up where you just need the information (e.g., http://www.prepubmed.org/grim_test/). Heathers has also set up an open source site where a spreadsheet can be downloaded and used (https://osf.io/qcvx9/).

An extension of the GRIM test is Sample Parameter Reconstruction via Iterative Techniques (SPRITE) (Heathers et al., 2018). SPRITE takes GRIM a step further by adding in the standard deviation (Chapter 3) and possible maximum and minimum of a variable. The researcher inputs the mean, standard deviation, possible maximum and minimum values and the sample size. The results provide up to 100 different possible distributions. Figure 1.1 has nine simulated data sets in SPRITE based on a scale that has a range from 5 to 25. There are five items, and the scale is 1 to 5 Likert-type. Notice none of the distributions look normally distributed (bell-shaped curve); the pattern of the distributions is key, not just a single distribution. The lowest value of the scores is 10 when you have this sample size, mean, and standard deviation. SPRITE lets a researcher examine or re-examine plausible distributions along with plausible analytic results such as an ANOVA (Chapter 6). It is also a great exercise with data the researcher is using!

Right Censoring

Right censoring occurs when data are missing because the event did not occur (David & Johnson, 1952, 1956). For example, researchers are studying medicine noncompletion (aka noncompliance), and some people are still taking their medicine at the end of the study time period. **Figure 1.2** displays five patients who were tracked taking their heart medication. Patients A and B stopped taking their medication just after the study started. Participant C kept taking the medication throughout the study and quite some time beyond. D stopped just after the study time period ended, and E stopped near the end of the study. Participants C and D are right-censored because the event the researcher was interested in happened after the study ended. Imagine another participant (F) who stops taking the medicine before the study starts but is already enrolled, this would be a case of left censoring.

There are ways to handle censored data in some multivariate analyses. The key is to understand when censoring affects the conclusions. When data are censored, the inferences made from the results can be interpreted incorrectly. Bergstrom and West (2020) have an excellent example of right censoring with a fictional study about the life span of chameleons. Some of the chameleons lived past the span of the study, though most died during the study. Thus, how to account for every chameleon given the study was about life-span of a chameleon? What happens, many times in research, is the chameleons who were living at the end of the study are removed from the analysis, right censoring, thereby biasing the actual life span average. In the medication example, if this were to happen 100% of the participants would be noncompliant because they stopped before the end of the study, when only 3/5 had actually stopped.

Causality

Causality, like *p*-values, is a problematic area in research and is a rich area of thought and research in philosophy. For this book, we will use a basic definition of causality as the process of one thing causing another. For example, if a person threw a rock at a window and it breaks, people generally would state throwing the rock caused the broken window. Proving this from a philosophical standpoint is actually quite difficult, but people generally agree that the rock broke the window. If someone threw hundreds of rocks at hundreds of windows and many of them broke, people would generally make the same claim. But in this instant, what exists is a relationship between thrown rocks and windows that is not 100% nor is it zero. That relationship is commonly referred to as a correlation. Correlations do not generally imply causation, but they can in specific situations.

Causality can feel exact in some domains, such as, mortality in medical research. There is a cause of death on the death certificate. Jim's father's death certificate states immediate cause of death is cardiac arrhythmia. This appears straightforward and is observable. Now, arguing about what caused the arrhthmia is another part of the causality chain—one could argue his rheumatic fever as a child in the 1930s and slow degradation of the heart since that time period is the cause. Another example with many causal claims associated with it is weight. Weight is correlated with heart disease, but does higher weight cause heart disease? Well, no not exactly, and that is where it gets tricky proving causality. Maybe it is just coincidence, or there are other variables that are involved (i.e., confounding variables). In many research disciplines, causality is difficult to show, and researchers tend to argue for causality and about which variables are causal. Thus, the plausibility of the relationship becomes the focal point based on current and past data and, hopefully, future data.

For researchers and the general purpose of this book, a causal argument has two features: a cause and an effect (Kenny, 2000). One way to discuss arguing for causality is through three defining attributes around a claim that A causes B:

1. *Time precedence*: For A to cause B, A must precede B.

2. *Relationship*: There is a functional relationship between A and B.

3. *Nonspuriousness*: A third variable (C), or more variables (D, E, F, and so on), do not explain the relationship of A to B.

Returning to the cardiac arrhythmia and death, the time precedence is able to be argued because the arrythmia happened before death, so A precedes B. There is a functional relationship between the two based on a great deal of medical research is in this area. Where the tenuousness of the causality claim occurs is at the nonspuriousness attribute. The rheumatic fever is one other variable that could be involved, the fact he was 83 and had been losing a great deal weight before death are two more. These could all be associated with the death. Thus, when we talk about A causing B, most of the time we are making a censored type of statement (Kenny, 2000) that, all things being equal, cardiac arrythmias cause death.

In daily life, people have many causal assumptions that seem to make the day move easily; water comes out if we open the faucet, friends say hello if we say hello, and so on. In research, assumptions are crucial and must be examined in sometimes painstaking detail. Unexamined assumptions can lead to incorrect inferences about the results, bad policy decisions, and endanger people's lives.

BAYES FORMULA

This book, and most applied statistics courses over the past decades, focuses on Fisher, aka Frequentist, based statistics, and really that means a focus on p-values. Bayesian analyses are philosophically and technically different than Fisher based statistics. Thomas Bayes (1702–1761) was an English Presbyterian minister, and after his death, a manuscript was found. This manuscript was a probability-based theorem and was published by the Royal Society (Bayes, 1763).

Bayes Theorem is a conditional probability, meaning the probability you are interested in is based on knowledge of something else. When a die is rolled, the probability is just based on the number of sides. If the die has six sides, then the probability of any one side coming up on top is $1/6$ or 16.67% before the die is rolled. Mathematically, the probability of rolling a six is written as $P(6) = 1/6$. An example of a conditional probability is "the probability a BSN nursing student passes the NCLEX given the student has all A grades in the clinical courses." This is traditionally written as P (Passing NCLEX | All As). The vertical line is the indicator for "given," that is, a condition that must have occurred first.

There is another distinction for understanding the differences between the traditional statistical analysis (Fisher) and Bayesian analyses (Chapter 10). Fisher argued one should only use data that had been collected for the study. Bayesian analyses want prior information in the analysis. There is a wonderful example of Bayes vs. Fisher from the Royal Society (see a Visual Version in Chapter 10). Sir David Spiegelhalter uses a billiard table from Bayes' thought experiment to highlight this difference. A ball is randomly rolled, but Spiegelhalter cannot see where it stops. The ball is removed, and only the host Dr. Bryan Cox knows where the ball stopped. And Spiegelhalter wants to guess where that ball stopped. Cox then rolls 5 balls and tells Speigelhalter that 2 of the 5 were to the right of the line and 3 were to the left. Spiegelhalter then states that Fisher would argue the line where the original ball stopped is 2/5ths along the table, whereas Bayes would add in the information from the roll of the first ball (1/2) and the probability would be 3/7ths. The key is the addition of prior knowledge. Most of the technologies affecting life are probably a Bayesian based system, such as searching for pictures of a dog through thousands of pictures on a smart phone, or deciding if an email is spam.

SCHOLAR BEFORE RESEARCHER

To conduct research well, you have to be a scholar first (Boote & Beile, 2005). By this we mean, you have to be a scholar of every component of your study or project. We want you to know the literature in-depth for the content area you are interested in because that detailed knowledge leads to strong research and evidence-based practice questions. Researchers and practitioners cannot write questions without having a deep understanding of the area of interest. For example, the researcher might start with the construct motivation and students in clinical rotations, but there are multiple models of motivation and thousands upon thousands of articles. And the researcher decides that, within motivation, the Expectancy-Value theory is the closest to the area of interest for the researcher (Wigfield, 1994). Now, the researcher cannot just ignore the other models, the researcher should be knowledgeable about the other models and how those models might explain the results from the future study.

With the choice of Expectancy Value theory, the researcher needs to read all articles related to student learning, performance, clinical success, and so on, that discuss this model. This will provide the researcher with a deep understanding and the ability to write excellent research questions. This is just the beginning because the researcher needs to read about different sampling methods and determine which is *needed* for this study, *not* which is possible. Sampling processes are a common weak spot in studies because sampling does not get enough scholarly time to understand the real strengths and weaknesses of different sampling processes and how they are related to the research questions. Additionally, the data to be gathered and how to gather that data has to be researched, whether it is numeric-based data or not, there is a large literature base that needs to be understood. For quantitative studies, there are important concepts and technical issues to understand about measurement (Chapter 2).

Interacting with both sampling and data gathering is the actual design of the study. Each study design has strengths and weaknesses and, obviously, affects what can be said at the end of the study (Chapter 5). Once sampling, data gathering, and design have been solidified, then the planned analysis can be studied. Again, there is a large literature base that should be understood. Researchers and doctorally-prepared nurses in advanced practice should have a core plan for the analysis and a back-up data analysis plan if the assumptions of the planned analysis cannot be met.

There is not a "single" checklist that can be simply followed, and then the study will be wonderful. Changes in any part propagate through the rest of the study. If the sample gathered is not representative of the population, and that was desired, then the ability to generalize the results is greatly weakened. Additionally, planned analyses may not be able to be fully completed. An investigator cannot do any of this without being a scholar first.

Finally, when an investigator is the study lead, all aspects of the study must be understood and be able to be explained to others. We have described this akin to being the CEO of a small company or the project manager of something being built. Both people in these jobs must fully understand what is occurring, what needs to be done, the time frames, the issues and concerns, and so on. Therefore, be a scholar before a researcher because it will allow you to fully run and analyze a study or project.

SUMMARY

There are foundational components of applied statistical analysis that should be understood. The first is understanding that investigators are making arguments based on the evidence that is gathered. Because these are probability-based analyses, there is no such thing as proof. There is evidence that supports or does not support a claim along a continuum of the arguments being made. Science also does not age well. As time goes on, new research and methods begin to find cracks and problems with previous research. This is a normal process and a good one. Our understanding of a phenomenon of interest should change over time. The p-value is not the value most researchers are actually interested in; most want a very accurate understanding of an association or difference. P-values will not provide that information. The NHST system also suffers from problems because it was originally designed for long-term, repeated data collection. Therefore, researchers must critically evaluate the full study and not just rely on a p-value or rejection of the null, especially in single studies. Techniques such as GRIM or the FERMI thought experiment are good ways to keep a critical eye at all times. One easy path to keeping that critical eye is to focus on being a scholar first.

END-OF-CHAPTER RESOURCES

REVIEW QUESTIONS

Answers and rationales for the review questions are located in the Appendix at the end of the book.

1. TRUE or FALSE?

   Applied statistical analysis involves learning how to properly build an argument using research questions, methods, and appropriate analyses.

2. TRUE or FALSE?

   A researcher is presenting the results of her study precisely by stating, "The treatment resulted in a statistically significant difference between the control group and the intervention group."

3. TRUE or FALSE?

   Most studies' results are very generalizable because of a variety of factors, such as the manner in which the sample of participants was recruited and the way the data were collected.

4. Which of the following is a correct interpretation of a $p < 0.05$?
   a. There is a 5% probability that the test parameter observed occurred by chance alone.
   b. Statistical testing for an association between variables has revealed the null hypothesis has only a 5% chance of being true.
   c. The relationship observed between the variables under study would occur only 5% of the time under the alternate hypothesis.
   d. Less than 5% of the statistical test parameters from many random samples are farther away from the mean on the sampling distribution for the null hypothesis than the test parameter for the result observed.

5. Which of the following areas do the authors recommend shifting the focus to in research design and statistical analysis, in lieu of a hyper-focus on p-values?
   a. alpha and beta
   b. accuracy and measurement precision
   c. multiple testing and type II error
   d. power and sample size

6. A DNP is evaluating a quality improvement program she implemented to decrease central-line-associated blood stream infections (CLABSIs) in the cardiac intensive care unit. In analyzing the data on CLABSI rates from before the program was implemented to 3 months after it was implemented, she incorrectly notes that there was no significant change in infection rates. What type of error has she committed?

7. The power of a study is directly dependent on which two factors?

   a. sample size and effect size

   b. null hypothesis and alternate hypothesis

   c. probability distribution and effect size

   d. type I error and sample size

8. A publication about a 6-month study discussed the effect of wearing a face mask in crowded public places on the prevention of COVID-19 infection in adults. Researchers found that there was not a statistically significant difference, at a p-value of <0.05, between the face mask group and the control group, but during the study, the face mask group experienced 4 infections while the control group had 10 infections. What should the reader focus on and examine closely in this study?

9. An investigator is trying to make an argument that variable A causes variable B to occur. He has demonstrated that variable A occurs prior to variable B, and there is an operational relationship between variable A and variable B. What else must this researcher demonstrate in the argument that variable A causes variable B?

10. Discuss some essential elements needed to conduct and interpret research well.

A robust set of instructor resources designed to supplement this text is located at http://connect.springerpub.com/content/book/978-0-8261-6582-4. Qualifying instructors may request access by emailing textbook@springerpub.com.

REFERENCES

Abelson, R. P. (1995). *Statistics as principled argument*. Psychology Press.

Bayes, T. (1763). An essay towards solving a problem in the doctrine of chances. *Philosophical Transactions of the Royal Society, 53*, 370–418. Reprinted in *Biometrika, 45*(1958), 296–315, and in this volume as Appendix, pp. 122–149.

Bergstrom, C. T., & West, J. D. (2020). *Calling bullshit: The art of skepticism in a data-driven world*. Random House.

Boote, D. N., & Beile, P. (2005). Scholars before researchers: On the centrality of the dissertation literature review in research preparation. *Educational Researcher, 34*(6), 3–15. https://doi.org/10.3102/0013189X034006003

Brown, N. J. L., & Heathers, J. A. J. (2016). The GRIM test: A simple technique detects numerous anomalies in the reporting of results in psychology. *PeerJ Preprints, 4*, e2064v1. https://doi.org/10.7287/peerj.preprints.2064v1

David, F. N., & Johnson, N. L. (1952). The truncated poisson. *Biometrics, 8*(4), 275–285. https://doi.org/10.2307/3001863

David, F. N., & Johnson, N. L. (1956). Some tests of significance with ordered variables. *Journal of the Royal Statistical Society. Series B (Methodological), 18*(1), 1–31.

Ellenberg, J. (2021, June 25). Editorial: Want kids to learn math? Level with them that it's hard. *The Washington Post.* https://www.washingtonpost.com/outlook/math-hard-easy-teaching-instruction/2021/06/25/4fbec7ac-d46b-11eb-ae54-515e2f63d37d_story.html

Fisher, R. A. (1925). *Statistical methods for research workers.* Oliver and Boyd.

Fisher, R. A. (1926). The arrangement of field experiments. *Journal of the Ministry of Agriculture, 33,* 503–513. https://doi.org/10.23637/rothamsted.8v61q

Fisher, R. A. (1960). Scientific thought and the refinement of human reasoning. *Journal of the Operations Research Society of Japan, 3,* 1–10.

Gigerenzer, G. (2004). Mindless statistics. *The Journal of Socio-Economics, 33*(5), 587–606. https://doi.org/10.1016/j.socec.2004.09.033

Glass, G. V. (1976). Primary, secondary, and meta-analysis of research. *Educational Researcher, 5*(10), 3–8. https://doi.org/10.2307/1174772

Gosset, W. S. (1904). *The Application of the 'Law of Error' to the Work of the Brewery.* Laboratory Report, 8, Arthur Guinness & Son, Ltd., Diageo, Guinness Archives, 3–16 and unnumbered appendix.

Greenland, S., Senn, S. J., Rothman, K. J., Carlin, J. B., Poole, C., Goodman, S. N., & Altman, D. G. (2016). Statistical tests, P values, confidence intervals, and power: A guide to misinterpretations. *European Journal of Epidemiology, 31*(4), 337–350. https://doi.org/10.1007/s10654-016-0149-3

Heathers, J. A., Anaya, J., van der Zee, T., & Brown, N. J. (2018). Recovering data from summary statistics: Sample Parameter Reconstruction via Iterative Techniques (SPRITE). *PeerJ Preprints, 6,* e26968v1. https://doi.org/10.7287/peerj.preprints.26968v1

Hubbard, R., & Bayarri, M. J. (2003). P values are not error probabilities. *Institute of statistics and decision sciences, Working Paper,* (03-26), 27708–0251.

Hubbard, R., Bayarri, M. J., Berk, K. N., & Carlton, M. A. (2003). Confusion over measures of evidence (p's) versus errors (α's) in classical statistical testing. *The American Statistician, 57*(3), 171–178.

Jaynes, E. T. (2003). *Probability theory: The logic of science.* Cambridge Cap University Press.

Kenny, D. A. (2000). *Correlation causation: Revised.* http://davidakenny.net/doc/cc_v1.pdf

Kline, R. B. (2016). *Practice of principles of structural equation modeling* (4th ed.). Guilford.

Neyman, J., & Pearson, E. S. (1933). On the problem of the most efficient tests of statistical hypotheses. *Philosophical Transactions of the Royal Society of London. Series A, Containing Papers of a Mathematical or Physical Character, 231,* 289–337. https://doi.org/10.1098/rsta.1933.0009

Sagan, C. (2007). The fine art of baloney detection. In *Paranormal claims: A critical analysis,* 1, Sagan Publishing House: University Press of America.

Schreiber, J. B. (2020). New Paradigms for Considering Statistical Significance: A Way Forward for Biomedical Journals, their Authors, and their Readership. *Research in Social and Administrative Pharmacy, 16*(4), 591-594. 10.1016/j.sapharm.2019.05.023

Smith, M. L., & Glass, G. V. (1977). Meta-analysis of psychotherapy outcome studies. *American Psychologist, 32*(9), 752. https://doi.org/10.1037/0003-066X.32.9.752

Spurgeon, C. H. (1859). *Spurgeon's gems: Being brilliant passages from the discourses of the rev. CH Spurgeon.* Sheldon, Blakeman & Company.

Swift, J. (1710). The Examiner, November 2 to November 9, Number 15, Quote Page 2, Column 1. Printed for John Morphew, near Stationers-Hall, London.

Szucs, D., & Ioannidis, J. (2017). When null hypothesis significance testing is unsuitable for research: A reassessment. *Frontiers in Human Neuroscience, 11,* 390, 1–21. https://doi.org/10.3389/fnhum.2017.00390

Trafimow, D., & MacDonald, J. A. (2017). Performing inferential statistics prior to data collection. *Educational and Psychological Measurement, 77*(2), 204–219. https://doi.org/10.1177/0013164416659745

Wigfield, A. (1994). Expectancy-value theory of achievement motivation: A developmental perspective. *Educational Psychology Review, 6*(1), 49–78. https://doi.org/10.1007/BF02209024

Ziliak, S., & McCloskey, D. N. (2008). *The cult of statistical significance: How the standard error costs us jobs, justice, and lives.* University of Michigan Press.

Ziliak, S. T. (2008). Retrospectives: Guinnessometrics: The Economic Foundation of "Student's" t. *Journal of Economic Perspectives, 22*(4), 199–216. https://doi.org/10.1257/jep.22.4.199

APPENDIX 1.1: BLOOD PRESSURE NULL HYPOTHESIS EXAMPLE

A community nurse researcher has collected a sample of 100 residents' resting heart rates in her community, and the average resting heart rate is 71. She also knows the average heart rate for the state is 74. Thus, she has a sample mean (71) and a population mean of 74. A traditional research question asks, "Is the sample mean different than population mean?" The equation to answer this question is

$$t = \frac{(\bar{x} - \mu)}{\sqrt{\frac{s^2}{n}}}$$

eq. 1.1

where,

t is the t-ratio that is compared to critical values on a t-distribution table,

$\bar{x}$ is the sample mean (new information),

μ is the population mean (prior information),

s^2 is the sample variance, and

n is the sample size.

This is a one sample test. The sample mean is 71, the population mean is 74, the sample variance for this example is 49, and the sample size is 100. Putting the values into the equation

$$t = \frac{(71 - 74)}{\sqrt{\frac{49}{100}}}$$

$$t = \frac{(-3)}{\sqrt{0.49}}$$

$$t = \frac{(-3)}{0.7} = -4.29$$

The result is a t-value of −4.29. The negative in this case is an artifact of the subtraction. The value 4.29 is the most important part. We can look at the t-distribution table to see if it would be greater than a critical value cut off. The critical cut-off is based on the traditional value of 0.05 and the degrees of freedom. Degrees of freedom can be thought of as how much extra space do you have. Planning seating for dinner for the family at holiday time is one way to think about this. If there are 10 seats and 10 relatives, it looks fine, until a problem occurs, such as Auntie Barb cannot sit next to Uncle Ray and adjustments must occur. If there were 11 seats, that extra seat provides some flexibility. Degrees of freedom work in a similar matter.

In general, most t-values over 2.00 will exceed the critical t-value to reach the "magic 05" value. Any t-ratio over 2.00 will be greater than the traditional critical value. In the table below there appears to be a list of numbers in columns. These numbers follow a pattern. The first is degrees of freedom. The degrees of freedom for a single test is the sample size minus 1, (n-1). In this example, that is 100-1, or 99. Next, move over to the column for 0.05, two tails, which is the traditional one to use. Notice the values move from 30 to 120, that is because the values do not change that much. Extrapolating a value between the two, 30 and 120, which is closer to 120, the critical value, is approximately 1.99. Since 4.29 > 1.99 the observed t-value is greater that the critical t-value and the conclusion would be the results are less than 0.05. Looking at the column to the left, 0.01, critical value is about 2.61 and, therefore, the results would be less than 0.01. Because the t-value is quite large, most statistical packages would print out $p < 0.001$ for this result.

t-table, traditional two tailed 05 cut offs in **bold**.

	t-distribution			
One Tailed	0.005	0.025	0.05	0.1
Two Tailed	0.01	**0.05**	0.1	0.2
df				
1	63.66	**12.71**	6.31	3.08
2	9.92	**4.30**	2.92	1.89
3	5.84	**3.18**	2.35	1.64
4	4.60	**2.78**	2.13	1.53
5	4.03	**2.57**	2.02	1.48
6	3.71	**2.45**	1.94	1.44
7	3.50	**2.36**	1.89	1.41
8	3.36	**2.31**	1.86	1.40
9	3.25	**2.26**	1.83	1.38
10	3.17	**2.23**	1.81	1.37
11	3.11	**2.20**	1.80	1.36
12	3.05	**2.18**	1.78	1.36
13	3.01	**2.16**	1.77	1.35
14	2.98	**2.14**	1.76	1.35
15	2.95	**2.13**	1.75	1.34
16	2.92	**2.12**	1.75	1.34
17	2.90	**2.11**	1.74	1.33
18	2.88	**2.10**	1.73	1.33
19	2.86	**2.09**	1.73	1.33
20	2.85	**2.09**	1.72	1.33
21	2.83	**2.08**	1.72	1.32

(continued)

	t-distribution			
22	2.82	**2.07**	1.72	1.32
23	2.81	**2.07**	1.71	1.32
24	2.80	**2.06**	1.71	1.32
25	2.79	**2.06**	1.71	1.32
26	2.78	**2.06**	1.71	1.31
27	2.77	**2.05**	1.70	1.31
28	2.76	**2.05**	1.70	1.31
29	2.76	**2.05**	1.70	1.31
30	2.75	**2.04**	1.70	1.31
120	2.62	**1.98**	1.66	1.29

CHAPTER 2

Background of Design, Measurement, and Analysis

CORE OBJECTIVES

- Define traditional hypotheses
- Explain differences between independent and dependent variables
- Describe levels of measurement
- Explain core measurement concepts (reliability, validity) and how they are estimated
- Discuss problems with metrics and issues in measurement

INTRODUCTION: RESEARCH AND QUALITY IMPROVEMENT QUESTIONS

Best practices in healthcare rely on evidence generated from research as well as the evaluation of the application of that evidence to clinical practice to determine whether practice changes have improved patient outcomes. Research questions are answered by conducting original research studies, whereas quality improvement (QI) and evidence-based practice questions are answered by collecting and analyzing data on patient outcomes after the research evidence has been applied to practice. Distinguishing between original research and QI can sometimes be challenging. Both original research and QI projects involve a problem, often a treatment or intervention to improve the problem, and measurement of outcomes to evaluate the effect of the intervention on the problem. However, knowledge generated from research is intended to be generalizable, or applicable to, the broader population at large. Information gleaned from a QI project is used to enhance the quality of care and applicable to the specific healthcare setting where the project was conducted (Gregory, 2015). Projects addressing research and QI questions require careful measurement of data to adequately answer the questions posed.

Important Quality Issues

Top ranking patient quality issues are driven by the landmark publication of the Institute of Medicine, *Crossing the Quality Chasm* (Institute of Medicine, 2002), and the areas of safety, effectiveness, efficiency, timeliness, patient-centeredness, and equitability. QI questions to address these areas may include:

What bundle of interventions will help decrease the number of falls on the orthopedic unit?

Which dressing change protocol is most effective in reducing the number of catheter-associated central line infections?

Is an antibiotic-infused portal cap a cost-effective method of preventing blood stream infections among patients receiving chemotherapy for breast cancer?

Which call-bell system improves the timeliness with which patient requests for assistance are addressed?

Does the new process for ordering food trays improve patient satisfaction with dietary services during their hospital stay?

Does performing a cultural assessment enhance the quality of care that post-partum patients who are immigrants receive?

TRADITIONAL HYPOTHESES

While patient quality and safety issues are addressed by QI questions, research studies use research questions and traditional hypotheses to investigate and generate new knowledge about the problem. Though we discussed the problems with the null hypothesis (H_O) model in Chapter 1, we provide examples here because it is what you will read as you are examining the literature base. Evaluation of study outcomes is often determined by formulating a research question with a research hypothesis (also known as the alternate hypothesis, or H_A) and statistically testing the H_O. The research hypothesis specifies the expected relationship between the variables being studied; the H_O states that no relationship between the variables exists, and the aim in statistical testing is to reject this H_O (Polit & Beck, 2020). For example, a **nondirectional research hypothesis** would state,

"Compared to usual care (uc), a virtual reality (vr) game will affect ratings of pain during dressing changes among pediatric burn patients."

$$H_A: \mu_{vr} \neq \mu_{uc}$$

This nondirectional research (or alternate) hypothesis states that the mean population pain scores will be different for those receiving a virtual reality game (μ_{vr}) compared to those receiving usual care (μ_{uc}).

A **directional hypothesis** (indicates the direction of the relationship between the variables) would be,

"Compared to usual care, a virtual reality game will decrease ratings of pain during dressing changes among pediatric burn patients."

$$H_A: \mu_{vr} < \mu_{uc}$$

This directional research (or alternate) hypothesis states that the mean population pain scores will be lower for those receiving a virtual reality game (μ_{vr}) compared to those receiving usual care (μ_{uc}).

The null hypothesis for both of these research hypotheses would then be,

"Compared to usual care, there is no effect of a virtual reality game on ratings of pain during dressing changes among pediatric burn patients."

$$H_O: \mu_{vr} = \mu_{uc}$$

This H_O states that the mean population pain scores will be the same for those receiving a virtual reality game (μ_{vr}) compared to those receiving usual care (μ_{uc}). Hypothesis testing is conducted via statistical analysis to show that the H_O, no difference or association, is not tenable with this data.

Research Questions

After a problem has been identified and the literature has been consulted, if no definitive answer to the problem is identified, a research question is formulated, which will be answered by the study. The question is answered through an analysis of the data collected. Attributes of a good research question have been outlined by (Hulley et al., 2013), and consist of assessing whether the question is *feasible* to answer, *interesting* to the researcher and scientific community, *novel* to the topic area, *ethical* to answer, and *relevant* to science and the public. Important components of a research question include, at a minimum, the population of interest, the independent variable, and the dependent variable. Often, the research question describes a potential relationship between the independent and dependent variable.

VARIABLES

Variables are the concepts of interest being studied and, as the name suggests, are things that can vary or change. Investigators are often interested in learning how variations or changes in one variable are associated with variations in another variable. Variables need a conceptual definition associated with the how the concept is defined theoretically and an operational definition that specifies how the variable will be measured (Polit & Beck, 2020). For example, for the question, "Does performing a cultural assessment enhance the quality of care that post-partum patients who are immigrants receive?" Theoretical and operational definitions for *cultural assessment* and *quality of care* would need to be established. The two major types of variables associated with research and QI projects are independent and dependent variables. Whether a variable is an independent variable or a dependent variable depends upon the question being asked.

Independent and Dependent Variables

Independent variables are concepts that are being examined for their effect on or association with the dependent variable, also known as the outcome of interest. In intervention projects, the independent variable is the intervention itself, and we are looking for its effect on the outcome of interest (dependent variable). The investigator is manipulating the independent variable (administering or not administering the intervention) to see its impact on the dependent variable. Using the question above where a cultural assessment intervention is being administered to see its effect on quality of care, the cultural assessment is the independent variable and quality of care is the dependent variable. Changes in the outcome might be said to "depend on" the influence of the independent variable, hence the term dependent variable (Polit & Beck, 2020).

In projects that are descriptive or explanatory rather than interventional in nature, variables are not manipulated; they are simply observed and measured. Thus, it is sometimes challenging to distinguish which is the independent variable and which is the dependent variable. As noted above, the independent variable could be being examined for its association with the dependent variable and may be known as the explanatory variable. For example, consider a project to describe the association of environmental variables, such as smoking in the home, living near a busy highway, and city of residence air quality index score, with prevalence of childhood asthma. The independent variables in this example are smoking in the home, living near a busy highway, and air quality index score while the dependent variable is prevalence of childhood asthma. Variables have a range of values and are classified according to a system known as levels of measurement.

TYPES OF DATA AND LEVELS OF MEASUREMENT

The level of measurement associated with a variable is important because it dictates the manner in which the data can be analyzed, and the level of measurement is driven by the nature of the data (Table 2.1). Data collected to measure a variable may be continuous or categorical in nature, which means data are measured on a numerical scale and values exist along a continuum, for example, birth weight, or data describe a quality or attribute of a person or thing, for example, blood type, respectively. The four most commonly agreed upon levels of measurement are found in Table 2.1 and can be considered a hierarchy, with nominal level variables being the lowest level of measurement and ratio level variables the highest. The hierarchy is only important in the context of analysis. Nominal-level variables are not necessarily less valuable than interval-level variables, but more sophisticated statistical analyses can be performed the further up the hierarchy you go.

Variables that fall into categories are measured on a nominal or ordinal scale. Nominal data for categorical variables simply capture traits, attributes, or characteristics, and categories must be mutually exclusive, for example, employment status (employed or unemployed). Variables measured on a nominal scale

Table 2.1. Expanded Steven's (1946) Table: Nominal, Ordinal, Ratio, Interval.

Scale Name	Stevens' Statement	Characteristic	Measures	Descriptive Statistics	Inferential Statistics	Generic RQ
Nominal—Categorical	Determination of a quality	You can tell objects apart. Discrete units of categories. e.g., gender, political affiliation	Measures in terms of names	Number of cases Mode Contingency Correlation	Contingency Correlation (aka Chi-Square)	Which is the most common?
Ordinal—Ordered Categorical	Determination of greater or less	You can tell if one object is better or smaller for example, hospital rankings.	Measures in terms of more or less than	Median Percentiles	Rank Correlation	Which is first? What is the middle?
Interval—Continuous	Determination of equality of intervals or differences	You can tell how far apart objects are, for example, test scores, or temperature.	Measure in terms of equal distances	Mean, median, Standard Deviation	Pearson Product moment correlation	What is the average? Are these different?
Ratio—Continuous	Determination of equality of ratios	You can tell how big one object is in comparison to another, for example, velocity.	Measures in terms of equal distances with an absolute zero point	Geometric Mean, median, mode, standard deviation,	Coefficient of Variation	Same as above.

Source: Adapted from Schreiber, J. B. (2021). Issues and recommendations for exploratory factor analysis and principal component analysis. *Research in Social and Administrative Pharmacy, 17*(5), 1004-1011.

can only be determined to be equivalent or not, and although categories are frequently coded with a number, these numbers have no mathematical meaning. Descriptive data such as frequency counts and percentages can be calculated, for example, of 200 participants, 110 (55%) were female and 90 (45%) were male. The measure of central tendency that can be reported is the mode (Chapter 3), for example, most frequently occurring admitting diagnosis for a medical-surgical unit in February is pneumonia.

Rank-ordering categories of data to indicate incremental amounts of a trait or characteristic puts the data on an ordinal scale. While ordinal measurements specify an order for the data, they do not indicate the degree of difference between the rankings, and individual rankings cannot be assumed to be equidistant. Examples of variables measured on this type of scale include the finishing place in a race (1st, 2nd, 3rd, etc.) and staging of severity in lung cancer (stage 1 to stage 4); the first-place winner was faster than the third-place winner, but we cannot say the person was three times as fast. A Likert scale is a type of ordinal scale, with labels such as "very happy," "happy," "neutral," "unhappy," or "very unhappy." However, for analysis purposes, Likert scales are often treated as interval level data (see below). With an ordinal scale, the central tendency of a variable (Chapter 3) can be described by the mode (or most common response) or the median (response ranked in the middle).

Quantitative characteristics that have an order and an equal distance between the points of measurement, but there is no actual (true) zero point to indicate the absence of the characteristic, are measured on interval scales. A common example of interval scale measurement is temperature using the Fahrenheit scale; the difference between 40°F and 50°F is the same as the difference between 50°F and 60°F, but 0°F does not indicate the complete absence of warmth. The zero point on an interval scale is arbitrary. Some argue a Likert scale, when well-designed with a clear equidistance between each value, can be considered an interval scale, especially if there are a larger number of response points, for example, choices from 0 to 10 (Wu & Leung, 2017). The central tendency of an interval-level variable can be represented by its mode, median, or mean.

The highest level of measurement on which a variable can be measured is a ratio scale. Variables measured using this scale type have a nonarbitrary zero value that is meaningful and an equal distance between the points of measurement. The Kelvin temperature scale is a popular example because it has a nonarbitrary zero point of absolute zero (0K) where particles that compose matter at this temperature have zero kinetic energy (Crocker & Algina, 1986). A clinical example could be measuring chest tube output in cubic centimeters per hour; a zero value is possible if there was no chest tube output in a given hour. Since ratio scales have a meaningful zero, data points can be added, subtracted, multiplied and divided. As with interval-level variable, the central tendency of a ratio-level variable measured can be denoted by its mode, median, or mean. More advanced statistical analysis options exist for ratio-level variables.

CORE MEASUREMENT CONCEPTS (BELIEVABILITY)

Earlier in this chapter, we discussed how variables must have a conceptual or theoretical definition in order to be measured and evaluated. There are two main measurement theories that serve as frameworks for how the scores generated by questions (items) on a measurement tool (questionnaire or instrument) represent the unobserved theoretical constructs they are attempting to measure. Measurement theories give us information about the statistical relationships between questionnaire items and the theoretical construct being measured (Polit & Yang, 2016). The two theories that will be briefly presented here are **classical test theory** and **item response theory**.

Classical Test Theory

Classical test theory (CTT) (Novick, 1966) is a traditional quantitative measurement approach that assumes each observed score (X) on a questionnaire/tool can be seen as a combination of an underlying "true" score (T) on the concept of interest plus or minus random error (E). This idea is depicted in the following equation:

$$X = T \pm E$$

or

Observed score = True Score ± Error

With CTT, we assume that each person has a true score (T) that we would obtain if there were no errors in how the variable was measured. One's true score is the expected score obtained over an infinite number of administrations of the questionnaire, but it is a hypothetical value that can never be obtained because no measurement tool is perfect. Therefore, we never actually obtain one's true score; we only estimate it using an observed score (X). We assume that the observed score (X) = true score (T) plus (or minus) some error (E).

Several assumptions are associated with CTT. Each item on the tool or questionnaire is assumed to signify the theoretical construct it is measuring, and the construct is driving responses to each of the items. For example, a person who has a high level of anxiety will answer "strongly agree" to the item "I am often restless." Another assumption is that the construct being measured has one dimension and that the items in totality are measuring the same thing. CTT also has a few assumptions about error—the amount associated with an item will vary randomly, error terms will have a mean of zero and be normally distributed across an infinitely large number of people, and error terms are not correlated with each other or the true score (Novick, 1966). Measurement tools developed using CTT include items that are distinct yet intentionally redundant because the tool is trying to collectively measure the construct in slightly different ways in order to arrive at the true score, and balance out measurement errors that may have been introduced with the items.

Item Response Theory

Item response theory (IRT) can be thought of as a group of measurement models that try to explain the link between observed item responses on a tool and an underlying theoretical construct (Lord & Novick, 1969). IRT models are probabilistic and describe the relationship between a person's level on a latent characteristic or trait and the probability of the person's specific response to an item. Items for the tool are selected to represent different levels of the characteristic or trait; the difficulty of an item and the amount of the trait a person possesses are connected in IRT models. For example, items that are "easier" to agree with are linked to lower levels of the trait. Figure 2.1 displays a Wright Map which provides information on the difficulty or endorsement ease of an item and what a normal distribution of scores (the latent trait being measured like anxiety). Notice that items 2 and 3 are easiest to endorse and 4 is hardest to endorse. The left side of the display shows the distribution of the latent trait where most of the people are in the center.

The amount of a trait is indicated on a standardized continuum that can be used to determine where people fall in terms of how much of the trait they have and how difficult it is to endorse an item. As with CTT, IRT expects that each item is separate from the other items yet should be similar and consistent with them in representing all important elements of the underlying trait. Whereas items for a tool developed using CTT are created to assess the underlying trait in a similar way (hence some redundancy), items on an IRT tool are specifically selected and polished to evaluate different degrees of the trait.

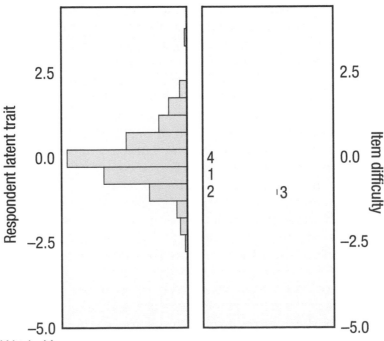

Figure 2.1. Wright Map.

IRT is a more complicated approach to developing and assessing items for a measurement tool, and it requires more advanced statistical techniques to accomplish, which are beyond the scope of this text. Therefore, we offer only a brief overview here.

Reliability and Stability

Reliability is one of the major core measurement concepts used to determine if a questionnaire or tool is of quality, but what we are really judging is whether the tool's scores are reliable, not the actual tool itself. This notion is logical because a tool can be used in different settings with different people and for different purposes and could very well show different levels of reliability among those different circumstances. Reliability is the feature of a tool's scores that indicates consistency; it represents lack of variation in measuring a characteristic that is truly stable. A classic example of reliability is a scale that measures an item at the same weight time and time again, for example, the item weighs 50 pounds each time it is placed on the scale. We are not able to determine if that weight is accurate, only that the scale measures it consistently at the same weight. In estimating reliability, replication is needed to assess the extent to which scores for a stable characteristic remain the same. Reliability cannot be estimated directly because that would require one to know the true scores, which according to CTT is not possible. However, estimates of reliability can be obtained by several methods, and expressed as a reliability coefficient between 0 and 1; 0 indicates no reliability while 1 represents perfect reliability. A new reliability estimate should be determined each time a tool is administered. We discuss a few popular methods below.

KR-20/KR-21

KR-20, also known as Kuder-Richardson 20, is an evaluation of the **internal consistency** reliability for tools with responses that are binary, for example, yes/no, true/false (Kruder & Richardson, 1937). Internal consistency measures whether items on a tool are measuring the same theoretical construct; it is frequently determined by whether items on the same tool are correlated with each other. For example, a tool intended to measure anxiety would need to contain items that are all assessing anxiety, not some that measure anxiety and some that measure depression. KR-20 is for tools that have items with various degrees of difficulty; KR-21 should be used when the items have similar degrees of difficulty. Most statistical software packages will have the ability to calculate KR-20, but the formula to use is:

$$\text{KR-20} = [n/n - 1] \times [1 - (\Sigma_{\text{item variances}}) / \text{Var}]$$

where:

n = sample size for the tool, that is, number of items
Σ = sum (add up)
Var = variance for the whole tool

The closer the score is to 1, the more reliable the tool is. What is considered an acceptable KR-20 scores varies depending on the tool, and KR-20 can vary based on the length of the tool, item difficulty, and the range of scores. A general rule of thumb for a minimally acceptable value is 0.70.

Cronbach Alpha Versus Guttman Lambda 4

Cronbach alpha (Cronbach, 1951) (also known as coefficient alpha) is also a measure of the internal consistency of a tool when there are more than two response options; it signifies the extent to which response on one item of a tool is an indicator of response on any other item from the same tool. A tool's Cronbach alpha is frequently reported in the literature because it can be calculated from one administration of the tool and is commonly recognized. The formula to use is similar to KR-20:

$$\text{Alpha} = [n/n-1] \times [1-(\Sigma_{\text{standard deviation for each item}})/\text{Var}]$$

where:

n = sample size for the tool, that is, number of items

Σ = sum (add up)

Var = variance for the whole tool

A high Cronbach alpha value suggests the tool's items are highly correlated with each other. A common misconception is that high alpha values indicate the items are measuring the same theoretical construct, for example, anxiety. This is not necessarily correct (Schmitt, 1996). A researcher can observe a high alpha value and still be measuring multiple constructs (Schmitt, 1996). Additionally, alpha is dependent on more than just the magnitude of the correlation among the data from tool's items; it is also a product of how long the tool is, that is, the number of items it has. The more items a tool has, the higher its Cronbach alpha will be; thus, we should not automatically assume that a high alpha value indicates good internal consistency. Moreover, an overly high alpha (e.g., ≥ 0.95) may indicate the tool's items are overly redundant and ask the same thing in slightly different ways (Boyle, 1991; Hattie, 1985), which suggests the tool could be shortened. A commonly noted minimum value for an acceptable Cronbach alpha is 0.70 (Nunnally, 1978). However, some suggest that researchers be cautious when using arbitrary cutoffs for Cronbach alpha values, and choose the appropriate level of reliability according to the precise research purpose and importance of the decision connected with the scale's use (Cortina, 1993).

Guttman lambda 4 (Guttman, 1945) is an alternate index for internal consistency reliability some consider better than Cronbach alpha (Benton, 2015). While Cronbach alpha may underestimate reliability, Guttman reliability may overestimate reliability if the sample size is small or the tool has a large number of items (Benton, 2015). Guttman lambda 4 is calculated by dividing the items in a tool into two halves such that the covariance between scores on the two halves (a nonstandardized measure of the linear relationship between the scores) is as high as possible. Because it is more difficult to compute, Guttman lambda 4 is less commonly performed or reported in the literature (McNeish, 2018).

Test-Retest Reliability

Test-retest reliability measures the stability of a tool over repeat administrations; it is only applicable when measuring characteristics or traits that are not expected to change. For example, it would not be appropriate to assess test-retest reliability in a pre-test/post-test project design with an intervention because one would expect the scores to change. To assess test-retest reliability for a tool that measures a stable characteristic, such as conscientiousness, one would administer the tool to the same group of people twice over a relatively short period of time, for example, 2 weeks. The timeframe for readministration should be carefully considered to avoid any carryover effects from the first administration, for example, too short of an interval may result in participants simply remembering their initial response. If scores on the tool are consistent on both occasions, then stability reliability is demonstrated. If the scores are not similar and the characteristic is indeed stable, differences may be the result of measurement error. When scores are of a continuous nature, test-retest reliability is often reflected using an intraclass correlation (ICC) for which there are multiple formulas (McGraw & Wong, 1996; Shrout & Fleiss, 1979), but as with other correlation coefficients, the closer to 1 the ICC is, the stronger the relationship is between the scores.

Inter-Rater and Intra-Rater Reliability

Some measurements of variables require the use of observers (or raters) to make observations and then judgments about the scores. In this circumstance, it is important to determine how reliably the scores reflect the characteristics of the person being rated rather than characteristics of the person doing the rating. This type of reliability is frequently relevant for clinical variables, such as tools to measure hyperactivity in children or physiological measures such as waist circumference. Inter-rater reliability is used assess the extent to which two or more raters use the tool in the same manner with the same individuals they are rating. An inter-rater reliability assessment examines if the raters' scores are comparable. If the same rater is making observations and ratings on more than one occasion, intra-rater reliability needs to be assessed to determine if the person is consistently using the tool at each administration. Both inter-rater and intra-rater reliability can be enhanced with careful training of the observers using detailed instructions, specific scoring guidelines and unambiguous examples (Polit & Yang, 2016). If scores are continuous, an ICC can be calculated as with test-retest reliability. If scores are measured on a nominal scale, a kappa coefficient can be determined, as discussed below.

Cohen's Kappa

Cohen's Kappa (Cohen, 1960) is a frequently used as an indicator of the reliability of repeated measurements when scores are categorical (nominal) in nature, and may be used to evaluate inter-rater reliability, intra-rater reliability, and test-retest reliability. Kappa is commonly used to reflect the proportion of agreement between rater scores, but it corrects for how often the rater scores

Rater 2

		Correct	Incorrect
Rater 1	Correct	W	X
	Incorrect	Y	Z

Figure 2.2. Two Raters' Agreement Table.

W = Total number of times that both raters were correct, representing agreement.

X = Total number of times Rater 2 was incorrect, but Rater 1 was correct, representing a disagreement.

Y = Total number of times Rater 1 was incorrect, but Rater 2 was correct, representing a disagreement.

Z = Total number of times both Raters were incorrect, representing agreement.

may be in agreement by chance alone. Computing a kappa value necessitates the some understanding of probability of agreement between raters. **Figure 2.2** provides an example.

To obtain the kappa value, one must determine the probability of agreement (P_o), which is indicated by the diagonal boxes for W and Z (number of scores in agreement) divided by the total number of scores. Using **Figure 2.2**, this would be:

$$P_o = (W + Z)/ (W + X + Y + Z)$$

Probability of random agreement (P_e) also needs to be known, which is more complicated and requires calculating the following: total number of times that Rater 1 was correct divided by the total number of ratings, then multiplying this by the total number of times that Rater 2 was correct divided by the total number of ratings ($P_{correct}$), added to the total number of times that Rater 1 was incorrect, then multiplying by the total number of times that Rater 2 was incorrect ($P_{incorrect}$). With **Figure 2.2**, this looks like the following three steps:

$$P_{correct} = (W + X / W + X + Y + Z) \times (W + Y / W + X + Y + Z)$$

$$P_{incorrect} = (Y + Z / W + X + Y + Z) \times (X + Z / W + X + Y + Z)$$

$$P_e = P_{correct} + P_{incorrect}$$

Finally, the formula for Cohen's Kappa is the probability of agreement minus the probability of random agreement divided by 1 minus the probability of random agreement, which looks like:

$$Kappa = P_o - P_e / 1 - P_e$$

Values can range from −1 to +1, but are nearly always positive, and a kappa of 1.0 means that all ratings are in agreement. Cut points for various interpretations of agreement represented by kappa are frequently cited as: <0.20 = poor, 0.21 − 0.40 = fair, 0.41 − 0.60 = moderate, 0.61 − 0.80 = substantial, ≥0.81 = almost perfect (Landis & Koch, 1977).

Validity

Validity is another major core measurement concept used to determine if a questionnaire or tool is of quality and is defined as the degree to which a tool measures the theoretical construct it is intended to measure. Can we say the data from the tool supports the *inference* that this tool is actually measuring the target construct? For example, the scores from a tool designed to measure intrinsic motivation should actually reflect intrinsic motivation and not something similar, such as perseverance. Because validity is driven by the underlying theoretical construct, the construct must be clearly defined as to what it is exactly, and what it is not. For concrete concepts, such as height, validity is easier to establish, but for more abstract theoretical constructs, one must collect different sources of evidence according to the different types of validity to support the inference that a tool is measuring its intended construct. There are no straight-forward formulas to apply to the assessment of validity and expert input is needed.

Types of Validity

The three main types of validity include 1) face and content validity, 2) criterion validity, which has two sub-components of predictive and concurrent validity, and 3) construct validity.

Face and Content Validity

Face validity is the lowest type of validity and essentially answers the question, "Does the tool *appear* to measure the construct is intended to measure? Face validity does not offer much in terms of substantiating the validity of the data for use of a tool but may have merit when it comes to the population and individuals completing the tool. The appearance of a tool should not discourage people from completing it or contain potentially offensive questions; thus, face validity should be assessed by experts in the construct as well as persons who would potentially complete the tool. Content validity is somewhat related to face validity and assessments of these two types of validity may overlap.

Content validity is defined as the extent to which a tool's content adequately represents the construct being measured, thus an inference is being made that the content represents the construct. Three main components—relevance, comprehensiveness, balance—are thought to make up content validity and require input from experts in the theoretical construct. Relevance must be evaluated for each individual item as well as the total set of items, for example, the item must be relevant to a specific aspect of the construct. Comprehensive tool should encompass all elements of the construct, and a balanced tool measures the various aspects of the construct in an equal manner. A content validity ratio (CVR) can be used to assess content validity at the item level. Using at least three experts, a common method of calculating a CVR is for each expert to rate each item on a 4-point scale (not relevant, somewhat relevant, quite relevant, highly relevant). Then, an item CVR is determined by the proportion of the experts who agree that the item is quite relevant or highly relevant, for example, an item rated as quite relevant or highly relevant by five out of six experts would have an item CVR of 0.83. An item with a CVR <0.78 should be revised or removed (Polit et al., 2007). The content validity index (CVI) for the entire tool can be calculated by determining the mean CVR using all items (DeVon et al., 2007); a CVI greater than 0.80 is preferable (Davis, 1992).

Criterion Validity

The extent to which scores on a tool correlate with an existing "gold standard" tool is known as criterion validity, and there are two types of criterion validity—predictive and concurrent. To evaluate criterion validity, there must be an existing tool to which this new tool can be compared, but if there is already a gold standard, why create a new one? Reasons that have been put forward include that the gold standard is too expensive to administer on a routine basis, the new tool is more efficient, or the gold standard is too difficult to access (Polit & Yang, 2016). Predictive validity reflects the degree to which the data from a tool is a good predictor of a future indicator of the construct. For example, a screening tool for depression could be correlated with symptoms of depression assessed in 3 months, such as loss of appetite or excessive sleeping. Concurrent validity is the degree to which a tool's scores correlate with scores on the gold standard at the present time. Statistical methods to assess predictive and concurrent validity often use correlation coefficients (Chapter 3) if the two tools are measured on a continuous scale, but the precise method is driven by the level of measurement. A discussion of each analysis method is beyond the scope of this text, but commonly used parameters include sensitivity/specificity, area under the curve, Spearman's rho, Pearson's r, and ICC (Polit & Yang, 2016).

Construct Validity

Construct validity is most concerned with the abstract theoretical construct and whether data from the items on a tool are consistent with the theoretical construct. A strong conceptualization of the construct is needed and particularly important if the construct is multi-dimensional in nature. Supporting evidence for construct validity comes from convergent validity, known-groups validity (also known as discriminative), divergent validity (also known as discriminant), and via the multitrait-multimethod approach. Convergent validity means that scores on the tool being evaluated correlate with scores on another tool measuring a similar construct or a construct with which it would be expected to be related. For example, according to Self-Determination Theory (Ryan & Deci, 2019), a tool measuring autonomy might be expected to correlate with a tool measuring competence. To demonstrate known-groups validity, the tool is administered to two groups of individuals who are known to be possess very different levels of the construct being measured; thus, the scores for each group should significantly differ. For example, a tool measuring self-care behaviors among patients with type 2 diabetes should display different scores for a group of patients with high hemoglobin A1c levels compared to a group with low A1c levels. Divergent, or discriminant, validity is concerned with evidence that a tool's scores are different from scores on another tool measuring a different construct. Thus, a tool measuring self-confidence should be not correlated or very weakly correlated with a tool measuring anxiety, for example. The multitrait-multimethod approach is essentially a combination of efforts to demonstrate convergent validity and efforts to demonstrate divergent (discriminant) validity but with two or more constructs (hence multitrait) and using two or more measuring tools or methods (multimethod).

Consequential Validity

Consequential validity fits into a broad definition of validity as a whole and refers to the unintended social consequences of administering a tool or test (Messick, 1989). It includes the assessment of whether a tool is used for its intended purpose. If, for example, a tool is intended to produce some common good, then consequential validity is relevant. Evidence supporting consequential validity usually shows how intended outcomes have been accomplished, no disparate effect among subgroups of people, and the existence of positive and lack of negative systemic results from the delivering the tool or test. Some questions associated with this type of validity may include: How does society view one's performance on this tool? What ramifications exist if one scores above or below an established cut point? In administering this tool, is there any evidence of bias associated with underserved groups?

NORM GROUPS

For a standardized tool, a norm refers to data that characterizes the scores produced by members of a specific reference group to which we can compare a score produced by a certain individual (Nunnally & Bernstein, 1994). Norms are useful for determining how an individual's score aligns with scores from a representative sample of people measured in the same manner using the same tool. The reference group is known as a norm group. Because the scores of persons selected for the norm group are compared to future scores on the tool, individuals comprising the norm group must correctly reflect the larger population for whom the tool was intended. Based on the purpose and specific applicability of the tool, members of the norm group for a tool should represent, for example, the age group, cultural group, educational level, and precise circumstances/experiences associated with the construct the tool is measuring, such as a cognitive functioning test for older adults with mild cognitive impairment. Norms may be categorized according to the scope of the population from which scores were generated, for example, national or regional. A national norm group would have considerable heterogeneity, however, and sub-categories of norm groups may also be useful for comparative purposes, for example, age group-specific norms or identified gender-specific norms.

CRITERION

Different than norm groups are criterion levels. Criterion levels are present standards for performance. In essence, did you meet the criterion or not. Thus, the comparison, is not against a norm group, or any group for that matter, but to a pre-determined cut-off. For example, a grade of A in a course would be set before the class starts, such as gaining 90% of the points possible. There is a criterion for passing a driving test. The new driver is compared to the criterion, not to other drivers.

MEASUREMENT, CATEGORIZATION, AND METRICS: THE GOOD, BAD, AND UGLY

There are many measurement and inference concerns with numbers whether they are "simple" demographics or metrics. Gender and Race/Ethnicity are two specific variables that are pervasive in research and are inherently problematic from instrument development to interpreting the results. Gender is culturally labeled at birth, a girl or a boy; yet, biological sex is vastly more complicated, dynamic (Montañez, 2017) and on a spectrum. But, researchers commonly mix sex and gender terminology in research reports (Westbrook & Saperstein, 2015). More recently, researchers have argued that sex and gender are nonbinary, and that binary (male and female) is not completely accurate based on research in multiple fields (Hyde et al., 2019). Relatedly, sexuality also has a history of being equated to gender and/or biological sex, but it is a different construct. If any one of these variables is being considered for research, first thoroughly answer, "Why is including this important as a variable?" Then answer, "What are the analytic goals of this variable?"

Gender, sex, and sexuality are rich research areas, and we recommend that time be spent reading, that is, scholar before researcher, the current issues and how and why these variables are being collected in the literature. When considering developing questions related to these topics, the researcher needs to think specifically and clearly. As Westbrook and Saperstein wrote (2015), "A hyper-gendered world of 'males' and 'females,' 'brothers' and 'sisters,' and 'husbands' and 'wives' shapes what we can see in survey data. If not altered, surveys will continue to reproduce statistical representations that erase important dimensions of variation and likely limit understanding of the processes that perpetuate social inequality" (p. 534).

Here are two examples that allow for more than the traditional binary categories. These are obviously not meant to be the only option but are provided to open thinking about how to collect these data if the need is warranted.

A generic open example:

A simple option is to use an open-ended item such as,

To which Gender do you most identify?_____

If categories are desired, then use a more inclusive set such as,

To which Gender do you most identify?

Female

Male

Transgender Female

Transgender Male

GenderQueer

Not Listed: _____

Prefer not to say.

Other categories that are currently being used for gender are nonbinary and gender fluid. The key is to be inclusive, provide options, and not intentionally or unintentionally leave anyone out.

Race and Ethnicity are also problematic variables, not just from their racist beginnings, but they, like gender, are social constructs often used to subordinate and superordinate groups of people (Cox, 1948; Zuberi, 2001). There is an evolutionary history to Race and Ethnicity categories. The conceptual beginning with the racial classification is based on the Great Chain of Being where all creation is ranked hierarchically from animals, to women, to men to God (Zuberi, 2001). The highest animal was the ape and therefore the lowest humans would be apelike. This allowed for racial stratification and laid the groundwork for enslavement (Zuberi, 2001). The first U.S. Census was taken in 1790, which had three categories, Free white males & females, All other free persons, and Slaves. In 1859, Darwin's work was published, and people used his work to push the racial classification argument further, which led into social statistics, eugenics, and social Darwinism. The focus on social statistics led to the rise of racial statistics that were used to explicitly to argue for differences among races (Zuberi, 2001).

Examining the changes in the U.S. Census is an interesting way to see the implementation of changes in arguments and culture over time. The U.S. Census in 1890, used eight categories with persons of African descent separated into Black, Mulatto (Black and one other race), Quadroon (one-fourth Black) and Octoroon (1/8 or any trace of black blood) (Census Bulletin, No., 199 July 14, 1892). Indian, Chinese, and Japanese categories were also added. In 1930, The U.S. Census added the category Mexican to the "color or race" categories but removed it in 1940. In 1970, it comes back as person origin or descent, but as six categories as Central or South American, Mexican, Puerto Rican, Cuban, Other Spanish, and No, none of these (Census, 2021). For 2020, there are 15 categories for Race and four classifications for Ethnicity along with some write-in options to explain the choice. Clearly, Race/Ethnicity is a social construct (Zuberi, 2001).

It is imperative to understand that the inferences made on limited conceptions of gender or race/ethnicity, especially from older articles, are probably misleading and most likely wrong. For example, differences in health and wellness when examined based on Race/Ethnicity are common in research studies, and simply indicate a difference exists, but why the difference exists is not discussed or examined. Most importantly, how the data were collected could be driving the observations, leading to incorrect inferences. In many instances, it is systematic racism that drives differences in care or simply access to care (Feagin & Bennefield, 2014).

Metrics

Problems with the use of and inferences from numbers are not limited to nominal data, such gender and race/ethnicity. First, when we speak about the problems with metrics, it is not just the number but *how* the number was obtained. How the number was obtained is called data provenance (D'Ignazio & Klein, 2020). The data that are gathered, how they are gathered, why they are gathered, why some data are not gathered, and so on are all decisions that are made by someone. Thus, there is a provenance to it, and a power component that should be more widely recognized. Because of this provenance and power, data cannot speak for themselves, and researchers should not let them (D'Ignazio & Klein, 2020). Context is necessary and a well written data user guide can be helpful. The Western Pennsylvania Regional Data Center is one example of incredible data user guides. For example, the data guide on Diabetes and Hypertension is very explicit about the problems with the data and interpretation, along with how the data is gathered and updated. Contextual information is important in making inferences from the data. We expect at some point, ethical implications for data sets (D'Ignazio & Klein, 2020) will be included in data user guides as the expectations change for what must be included.

Metrics affect every aspect of our lives, and as we just stated, someone made the decision about what metrics to collect, how to collect, and so on. There are merit metrics, quality metrics, rankings, indicators, essentially hundreds in every industry. They are hailed as a way to improve or be more efficient, but they are just numbers that have a provenance. Additionally, the collected data are embedded and created within a system (context) which is also rarely discussed. A common metric in healthcare is the body mass index (BMI). Most individuals have no idea where this came from or its original purpose. The BMI was developed by Quetelet (1796–1894), and interestingly he began a great deal of human health research, standardization, and growth rates. The ICD codes so common today can be traced to his work. In 1832, he developed the Quetelet index to try to understand the average man and understand the distribution of weight—not to measure obesity. In 1972, Ancel Keys and colleagues named it the BMI (Keys et al., 1972). Like most metrics, and the main problem with many metrics, BMI is a blunt indicator and does not accurately assess health risk consistently across gender, race/ethnicity, or many healthy individuals. BMI has been associated with adverse outcomes, but there is also a wide variance of outcomes and obesity-related outcomes among people with similar BMI values (Blüher, 2012).

Another common metric is performance, which is used for compensation or as report cards. The argument for pay-for-performance metrics in healthcare is, by attaching payment to the performance of the doctor, patient care and patient outcomes will increase. Patient care and outcomes for report cards are typically operationalized with easy to collect data such as readmittance, complications, or death. Given the wide use of this system, there should be consistent evidence that it works, but that is not what has been observed (Muller, 2018). What seems to be clear is a mix of results most likely due to a mix of issues, such as poor operationalization of the metrics and the complexity of performance measurement, which occurs in every industry. For example, teaching—a massively complex performance—when evaluated at many institutions just boils down to course evaluations. Students are asked a series of questions or provided statements to which they respond. The research has been quite clear on the problems with measuring teaching this way, such as student lack of knowledge of pedagogical techniques, assessment, and design, along with biases toward instructors (Flaherty, 2020; Hoorens et al., 2021). Yet, with all these problems, the course evaluation data are still used to make high stakes decisions (e.g., tenure or continuing contract).

In addition to the problems of the metrics, there is the fixation on the metric itself. The obsessive fixation occurs even if there is a strong theoretical definition, clear operational definition, and stable and useable scores. Once that fixation has occurred, the true limitations of the metric are bypassed, the context in which the metric is collected, and its provenance are ignored. It is now just a number that must go up or go down. At this stage, the metric ceases to work and it has reached Goodhart's law stage. Goodhart's law states, "Any observed statistical regularity will tend to collapse once pressure is placed upon it for control purposes" (pg. 96–1984) (Goodhart, 1984). Luckily, anthropologist Dame Ann Margaret Strathern broadened the topic with the quote "When a measure becomes a target, it ceases to be a good measure (pg. 308)" (Strathern, 1997) when discussing measurement in higher education. If you are going to use or develop metrics, we suggest being a scholar and reading deeply about the metric or area of interest, and for development of a metric a good place to start is Muller's (2018) checklist on when and how to use metrics.

SUMMARY

To answer research and QI questions of clinical importance, investigators must carefully define and measure the independent and dependent variables of interest. The type of data collected for each variable, for example continuous or categorical, determines to which of the four levels of measurement a variable belongs; that level of measurement drives the data analysis decisions. Valid and reliable measurement of variables is essential to establish the believability and trustworthiness of the data collected to answer the question. While measurement is an imperfect process, and problems with measuring variables appropriately sometimes exist, several approaches can be undertaken to document the validity and reliability of the data collected.

END-OF-CHAPTER RESOURCES

REVIEW QUESTIONS

Answers and rationales for the review questions are located in the Appendix at the end of the book.

1. You are assessing the internal validity of a tool's scores for the project you have just conducted. The tool's items have five possible responses, for example, 1 to 5. What test would you use to determine the internal consistency, and what is a generally agreed upon acceptable minimum score?

2. TRUE or FALSE?

   A main difference between CTT and IRT is that items for a questionnaire developed using CTT are intended to similarly assess the underlying attribute being measured, while items developed using IRT are explicitly chosen to evaluate different degrees of that attribute.

3. TRUE or FALSE?

   Reliability is the measurement concept that indicates whether the scores obtained from a tool are consistent when measuring a variable that is truly stable.

4. TRUE or FALSE?

   Measurement practices and the resulting metrics must carefully take into consideration how and why data are collected, why some data are not collected, and the power differential under which data are collected in order to avoid incorrect inferences and conclusions.

5. TRUE or FALSE?

   Test-retest reliability measures the stability of a tool's scores over time and should be calculated for a variable such as self-efficacy during a project that is aiming to increase the participants' self-efficacy from baseline to 12 weeks.

6. Comparing the scores of a new tool to measure the characteristic grit to the gold standard tool that has been used for several years would be a method of establishing which type of validity?

   a. construct validity

   b. content validity

c. criterion-related validity

d. predictive validity

7. A nurse manager is interested in determining if the program she has implemented to improve sleep quality for patients on the cardiac continuous care unit has enhanced patients' sleep. She asks patients to complete a questionnaire on their sleep quality and wear a device on their wrist that measures hours of sleep. If the scores on the questionnaire are highly correlated with the scores on the wrist device, this demonstrates which type of construct validity?

8. Which of the following features distinguish between original research studies and QI projects?

a. research results can be applied to the larger population of patients

b. quality improvement projects are performed to increase scientific knowledge

c. data from a QI project is used to improve care outside of the setting where the project took place

d. QI projects are intended to be generalizable beyond the people in the project

9. Which of the following is an example of a nondirectional hypothesis?

a. The investigational drug will not affect heart rate compared to digoxin.

b. The investigational drug will decrease stomach acid compared to the proton pump inhibitor.

c. The investigational drug will have no effect on blood clot prevention compared to warfarin.

d. The investigational drug will change blood pressure compared to the standard of care.

10. A patient with prostate cancer receives information on the grading of his disease progression. He learns that his cancer is Gleason Grade 3, and there are Grades 1 to 5. The Gleason Grade is an example of what type of variable?

a. nominal

b. ordinal

c. interval

d. ratio

11. Identify the independent and dependent variables in the following purpose statement:

The purpose of this project is to determine the association between nutritional status, degree of subdural moisture, skin pigmentation and pressure ulcer development.

A robust set of instructor resources designed to supplement this text is located at http://connect.springerpub.com/content/book/978-0-8261-6582-4. Qualifying instructors may request access by emailing **textbook@springerpub.com.**

REFERENCES

Benton, T. (2015). *An empirical assessment of Guttman's lambda 4 reliability coefficient* (Vol. 89). Springer Proceedings in Mathematics & Statistics. https://doi.org/10.1007/978-3-319-07503-7_19

Blüher, M. (2012). Are there still healthy obese patients? *Current Opinion in Endocrinology, Diabetes and Obesity, 19*(5), 341–346.

Boyle, G. J. (1991). Does item homogeneity indicate internal consistency or item redundancy in psychometric scales? *Personality and Individual Differences, 12,* 291–294. https://doi.org/10.1016/0191-8869(91)90115-R

Census Bulletin, No., 199 July 14, 1892. https://www.census.gov/library/publications/1890/dec/bulletins.Demographics.html. ftp://ftp2.census.gov/library/publications/decennial/1890/bulletins/demographics/199-colored-population-african-chinese-japanese-indians.pdf

Census. (2020). *About race.* https://www.census.gov/topics/population/race/about.html

Census. (2021). History. https://www.census.gov/history/www/through_the_decades/questionnaires/1970_1.html

Cohen, J. (1960). A coefficient of agreement for nominal scales. *Educational and Psychological Measurement, 20,* 37–46.

Cortina, J. M. (1993). What is coefficient alpha? An examination of theory and applications. *Journal of Applied Psychology, 1,* 98. https://doi.org/10.1037/0021-9010.78.1.98

Cox, O. C. (1948). *Caste, class, & race: A study in social dynamics.* Doubleday.

Crocker, L., & Algina, J. (1986). *Introduction to classical and modern test theory.* Holt, Rinehart and Winston.

Cronbach, L. J. (1951). Coefficient alpha and the internal structure of tests. *Psychometrika, 16,* 297–334. https://doi.org/10.1007/BF02310555

Davis, L. L. (1992). Instrument review: Getting the most from a panel of experts. *Applied Nursing Research, 5*(4), 194–197. https://doi.org/10.1016/S0897-1897(05)80008-4

DeVon, H. A., Block, M. E., Moyle-Wright, P., Ernst, D. M., Hayden, S. J., Lazzara, D. J., Savoy, S. M., & Kostas-Polston, E. (2007). A psychometric toolbox for testing validity and reliability. *Journal of Nursing Scholarship, 39*(2), 155–164. https://doi.org/10.1111/j.1547-5069.2007.00161.x

D'ignazio, C., & Klein, L. F. (2020). *Data feminism.* MIT press.

Feagin, J., & Bennefield, Z. (2014). Systemic racism and US healthcare. *Social Science & Medicine, 103,* 7–14.

Flaherty, C. (2020, February 27). *Even "Valid" student evaluations are unfair.* Inside Higher Education. https://www.insidehighered.com/news/2020/02/27/study-student-evaluations-teaching-are-deeply-flawed

Goodhart, C. A. E. (1984). Problems of monetary management: The UK experience. *Monetary theory and practice.* MacMillan Press. https://doi.org/10.1007/978-1-349-17295-5_4

Gregory, K. E. (2015). Differentiating between research and quality improvement. *Journal of Perinatal and Neonatal Nursing, 29*(2), 100–102. https://doi.org/10.1097/JPN.0000000000000107

Guttman, L. (1945). A basis for analysing test-retest reliability. *Psychometrika, 10*, 255–282. https://doi.org/10.1007/BF02288892

Hattie, J. (1985). Methodology review: Assessing unidimensionality of tests and items. *Applied Psychological Measurement, 9*(2), 139–164. https://doi.org/10.1177/014662168500900204

Hoorens, V., Dekkers, G., & Deschrijver, E. (2021). Gender bias in student evaluations of teaching: Students' self-affirmation reduces the bias by lowering evaluations of male professors. *Sex Roles, 84*(1), 34–48. https://doi.org/10.1007/s11199-020-01148-8

Hulley, S. B., Cummings, S. R., Browner, W. S., Grady, D. G., & Newman, T. B. (2013). *Designing clinical research* (4th ed.). Wolters Kluwer | Lippincott, Williams & Wilkins.

Hyde, J. S., Bigler, R. S., Joel, D., Tate, C. C., & van Anders, S. M. (2019). The future of sex and gender in psychology: Five challenges to the gender binary. *American Psychologist, 74*(2), 171–193. https://doi.org/10.1037/amp0000307

Institute of Medicine. (2002). *Crossing the quality chasm: A new health system for the 21st century*. National Academies Press.

Keys, A., Fidanza, F., Karvonen, M. J., Kimura, N., & Taylor, H. L. (1972). Indices of relative weight and obesity. *Journal of Chronic Diseases, 25*(6–7), 329–343. https://doi.org/10.1016/0021-9681(72)90027-6

Kruder, G. F., & Richardson, M. W. (1937). The theory of estimation of test reliabilty. *Psychometrika, 2*, 151–160.

Landis, J. R., & Koch, G. G. (1977). The measurement of observer agreement for categorical data. *Biometrics, 33*, 159–174. https://doi.org/10.2307/2529310

Lord, F. M., & Novick, M. R. (1969). *Statistical theories of mental test scores*. Addison-Wesley.

Messick, S. (1989). Meaning and values in test validation: The science and ethics of assessment. *Educational Researcher*, 18, 2, pp. 5-11.

McGraw, K. O., & Wong, S. P. (1996). Forming inferences about some intraclass correlation coefficients. *Psychological Methods, 1*, 30–46. https://doi.org/10.1037/1082-989X.1.4.390

McNeish, D. (2018). Thanks coefficient alpha, we'll take it from here. *Psychological Methods, 23*(3), 41–63. https://doi.org/10.1037/met0000144

Montañez, A. (2017). Beyond XX and XY. *Scientific American, 317*(3), 50–51. https://doi.org/10.1038/scientificamerican0917-50

Muller, J. (2018). *The tyranny of metrics*. Princeton University Press.

Novick, M. R. (1966). The axioms and principal results of classical test theory. *Journal of Mathematical Psychology, 3*, 1–18. https://doi.org/10.1016/0022-2496(66)90002-2

Nunnally, J. C. (1978). *Psychometric theory* (2nd ed.). McGraw-Hill.

Nunnally, J. C., & Bernstein, I. H. (1994). *Psychometric theory* (3rd ed.). McGraw- Hill.

Polit, D. F., & Beck, C. T. (2020). *Nursing research: Generating and assessing evidence for nursing practice* (11th ed.). Wolters Kluwer.

Polit, D. F., Beck, C. T., & Owen, S. V. (2007). Is the CVI an acceptable indicator of content validity? Appraisal and recommendations. *Research in Nursing & Health, 30*(4), 459–467. https://doi.org/10.1002/nur.20199

Polit, D. F., & Yang, F. M. (2016). *Measurement and the measurement of change*. Wolters Kluwer.

Ryan, R. M., & Deci, E. L. (2019). Supporting autonomy, competence, and relatedness: The coaching process from a self-determination theory perspective. In P. Brownell, S. English, & J. Sabatine (Eds.), *Professional coaching: Principles and practice*. Springer Publishing Company.

Schmitt, N. (1996). Uses and abuses of coefficient alpha. *Psychological assessment, 8*(4), 350-353

Shrout, P. E., & Fleiss, J. L. (1979). Intraclass correlations: Uses in assessing rater reliability. *Psychological Bulletin, 36*, 420–428. https://doi.org/10.1037//0033-2909.86.2.420

Strathern, M. (1997). Improving ratings: Audit in the British University system. *European Review, 5*(3), 305–321. https://doi.org/10.1002/(SICI)1234-981X(199707)5:3<305::AID-EURO184>3.0.CO;2-4

Westbrook, L., & Saperstein, A. (2015). New categories are not enough: Rethinking the measurement of sex and gender in social surveys. *Gender & Society, 29*(4), 534–560.

Wu, H., & Leung, S.-O. (2017). Can Likert scales be treated as interval scales?—A simulation study. *Journal of Social Service Research, 43*(4), 527–532. https://doi.org/10.1080/01488376.2017.1329775

Zuberi, T. (2001). *Thicker than blood: How racial statistics lie*. University of Minnesota Press.

FURTHER READING

Blumenbach, J. F. (1795:1969). *On the natural varieties of mankind*. Bergman Publishers.

Census. (1970). https://www.census.gov/history/www/through_the_decades/questionnaires/1930_2.html

Darwin, C. (2004). *On the origin of species, 1859*. Routledge

Dobson, R., Burgess, M. I., Sprung, V. S., Irwin, A., Hamer, M., Jones, J., Daousi, C., Adams, V., Kemp, G. J., Shojaee-Moradie, F., Umpleby, M., & Cuthbertson, D. J. (2016). Metabolically healthy and unhealthy obesity: Differential effects on myocardial function according to metabolic syndrome, rather than obesity. *International Journal of Obesity, 40*(1), 153–161. https://doi.org/10.1038/ijo.2015.151

Linnaeus, C. V. (1758). *Systema naturae* (Vol. 1).

Malthus, T. (2013). *An essay on the principle of population (1798)* (pp. 15–30). Yale University Press.

Quetelet, L. A. J. (2013). *A treatise on man and the development of his faculties*. (R. Knox, Ed., T. Wimbert, Trans.). Cambridge University Press. (English Edition Originally printed 1842).

Time Magazine. (1961, January 13). *Medicine: The Fat of the land* (Vol. LXXVII; No. 3). http://content.time.com/time/subscriber/article/0,33009,828721-1,00.html

CHAPTER 3

Descriptive Analyses

CORE OBJECTIVES

- Understand the role and importance of descriptive analysis
- Write descriptive types of research questions
- Describe the shapes of data, for example, normal, skewed, kurtotic
- Describe mean, median, mode, standard deviation, skewness, and kurtosis
- Explain differences between continuous and noncontinuous data
- Explain when to use cross-tabulation tables
- Explain a correlation value

INTRODUCTION: DESCRIPTIVE ANALYSES AND INVESTIGATIVE JOURNALISM

Descriptive analyses of data have not had the level of discussion they deserve. If there is one area of analysis where we spend most of our time, it is on exploring and understanding what is in the dataset and what the data look like in a variety of tables and graphs (Tukey, 1977). One way to approach descriptive work is to think of it as investigative journalism (Houston et al., 2002). Investigative journalism is one form of journalism where the reporter dives deeply into a topic where they spend sometimes months or years on a story. We are not recommending that months be spent on descriptive information, but we are stating that a dedicated focus on describing the data in a variety of ways is imperative. The time and work dedicated to the descriptive analysis phase will save analytic resources later and, in some cases, stop an inferential statistical analysis that will obviously not work. Finally, it is helpful to think about descriptive analysis as the foundation for the story or narrative that will told in the rest of the study.

QUESTION FOCUS

Not commonly discussed in research methods or statistics books, descriptive statistics do have questions associated with the analyses. For example,

What is the mean on the distribution of scores?

How much variance or spread is there in the distribution of scores?

What is the mean score for female respondents on survey Q?

Is the overall shape (distribution) of the scores for survey Q normal?

Is the overall shape bi-modal? Or skewed?

Do respondents who chose Y also choose Z?

How many blue candies are in a 16 oz bag on average?

Does height and weight appear linearly related?

How many people chose X?

How many people chose X and Y?

These questions are not asking for a probability or to make a statistical inference, they are focused more on "how much?" or "how many?" Answering these questions is just as important as getting results from a *t*-test (Chapter 6) or a regression analysis (Chapter 8). Now it is time to look at different types of data (Chapter 2) and how to descriptively deal with them.

ANALYSIS OF CONTINUOUS DATA

Mean, Median, Mode, Standard Deviation, Variance, Skewness, Kurtosis

Continuous data (interval and ratio) are described using the mean, median, mode, standard deviation, skewness, kurtosis, range, and interquartile range. In research articles, mean and standard deviation are the two most commonly presented, but you should examine all of these when working to describe your continuous data. The descriptive statistics values obtained are estimates. The reason the values are estimates is due to the fact the values are based on a sample from the population and not the whole population.

Estimation has existed in some form for quite some time, and one early written estimation is from Herodutus dated to (485–420 BC) (Rubin, 1968). Let us look at a distribution of values (e.g., scores) from a single variable (e.g., quiz). Here are twenty scores in numeric order from a 20-point quiz, 11, 12, 12, 13, 13, 14, 14, 14, 15, 15, 15, 15, 16, 16, 16, 17, 17, 18, 18, 19. Each score is an individual data-point, and the group quiz scores are the variable. Figure 3.1 displays these data graphically.

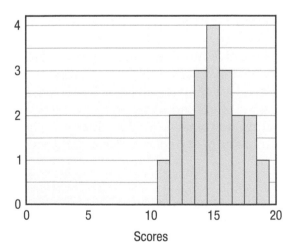

Figure 3.1. Distribution of Quiz Scores in a Histogram.

Notice the range of scores are 11 to 19 (Figure 3.1). The scale in the figure goes down to 0 for Scores because the possible range of the quiz is 0 to 20. Including the full possible range allows the researcher to locate the distribution of actual scores. The **mean**, the average score, is a continuous variable. Early versions of the concept of the mean by Thucydides (460–400 BC) by (Rubin, 1968). Examining the distribution of the quiz scores in Figure 3.1, a researcher can infer the average value might be around 15. To obtain the mean, sum the individual scores (11, 12, 12, 13, 13, 14, 14, 14, 15, 15, 15, 15, 16, 16, 16, 17, 17, 18, 18, 19 = 300) and divide by the number of scores, in this case 20. This process produces a mean of 15 (i.e., 300 / 20). The mathematical equation can be found in Appendix 3.1.

The **median** is the middle score in the distribution of values and appears to have been developed sometime after 1600 (Eisenhart, 1974). The median can be thought of as the median in a road-half the road is on the right side of the median, the other half is on the left side. There are two key questions that must be answered before calculating the median by hand, 1) are the data in order?, and 2) are there an even or odd number of values? The quiz data are in order lowest to highest and there are an even number of values, 20 scores. With even number of values for the quiz scores, there is no exact middle value. Therefore, take the two middle values, the 10th and 11th values, add them together and divide by two. In this case, the two middle values are 15 and 15.

11, 12, 12, 13, 13, 14, 14, 14, **15, 15, 15, 15**, 16, 16, 16, 17, 17, 18, 18, 19.

The median of this variable is (15 + 15) / 2 = 15. If the variable had 19 values, then the exact middle value would be the median. Removing the lowest score of fourteen, leaving 19 values, the median value would be 15.

12, 12, 13, 13, 14, 14, 14, 15, 15, 15, 15, 16, 16, 16, 17, 17, 18, 18, 19.

There are nine scores lower than 15 and nine scores higher than fifteen, each side is balanced.

The **mode** was potentially discussed by Thucydides (460–400 BC) (Rubin, 1968) and is the most common score. A distribution can have no mode, one mode, and more than one mode. In this variable, the value 15 is the mode because it appears four times, the most of any value. If there are two modes, it is called **bimodal**, and three or more are termed **multimodal**.

Quick review!

Here is a set of data (or vector of data): 5, 6, 2, 4, 1, 8, 6, 9, 2. Find the mean, median, and mode. Write them down here: _____

_____

The **variance** and **standard deviation** are mathematically related and extremely important to the analyses that follow analysis chapters. The variance is a numeric description of the variability or variance of the data. The variability can also be described as the dispersion or spread of the data. If the scores are all the same, the variance is 0. The standard deviation is the standardized view of the variance and is easily interpretable, which is why researchers report and discuss the standard deviation. The phrase and development of the standard deviation was from Karl Pearson (around 1893) and probably first appeared in his lecture syllabus (Plackett, 1983). The standard deviation and variance values *must* be positive due to the calculation of each one. The standard deviation mathematically describes the spread of the scores from the mean and is the square root of the variance. In **Figure 3.2**, there is a normal curve with the standard deviations marked above and below the mean of 0. The positive three to the far right indicates the proportion of the curve where scores are "three standard deviations above the mean." In the figure, the standard deviation value is equal to 1.

The **normal curve** has some interesting properties, but for our purpose here, the key property is the area underneath the curve is set equal to 1. The area between −1 and 1 standard deviations is just over 0.68 or 68% of the total area. The area between −1 and −2 (also 1 and 2) is approximately 0.13 or 13% for each. The final areas underneath the curve, between −2 and −3 and 2 and 3 are 0.25 or 2.5% percent each. Notice, the curve does not touch the x-axis in **Figure 3.3** because mathematically the normal curve never actually touches the x-axis. Historically, the curve and its description have been stopped at +/−3 or +/−4 standard deviations.

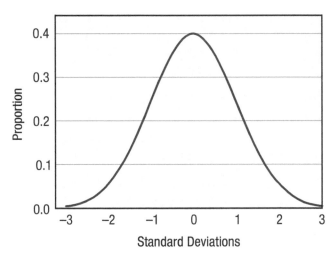

Figure 3.2. Normal Curve With Standard Deviations.

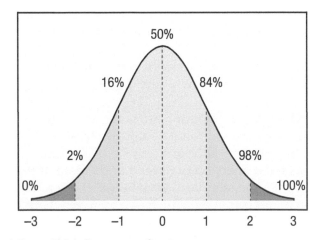

Figure 3.3. Normal Curve With Percentage Sections.

The range of the data also provides information related to the variability. The **range** is simply the lowest value subtracted from the highest value. For example, if the tallest student during a school wellness check is 6′1″ (73 inches) tall, and the shortest student is 5′3″ (63 inches) tall, the range would be 10 inches.

There is no one normal curve shape. A normal curve may have a large variance and be spread out or a small variance and be closer together- each is considered a normal curve because it follows the mathematical properties of the normal distribution. In **Figure 3.4** there are two simulated normal distributions (N= 10,000) both with a mean of zero using a histogram. **Histograms** display the frequency of the different values of a single variable in numeric order. The first histogram in **Figure 3.4** has a standard deviation of 5 and the second one, a standard deviation of 10. They are both normal distributions, but their shapes appear very different.

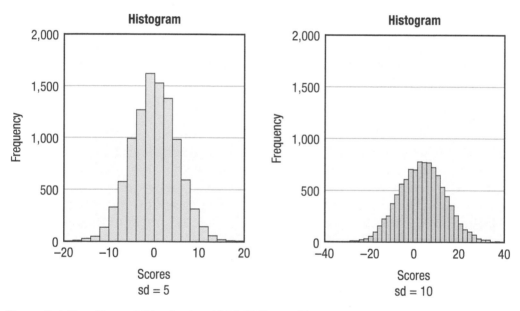

Figure 3.4. Two Normal Distributions With Different Shapes.

The standard deviation value can be confusing because it is affected by the raw data and essentially the shape of the distributions. The standard deviation can take on any positive value; therefore, it could be one, or it could be 23.68. The histogram in **Figure 3.5** has a mean of 21.4 and a standard deviation of 5.31. In **Figure 3.2** and 3.3, with a mean of 0 and standard deviation of 1, one standard deviation above the mean, is just 1. But, what is one standard deviation above the mean for the data in **Figure 3.5**? One standard deviation above the mean would be a score of 26.71 (21.40 + 5.31). One standard deviation below the mean would be 16.09 (21.40 − 5.31). Therefore, approximately 68% of the scores will be between 16.09 and 26.71.

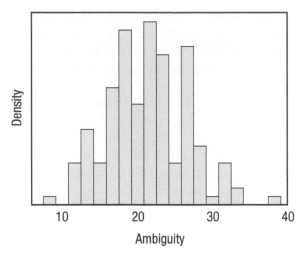

Figure 3.5. Histogram of Simulated Ambiguity Score Data.

Mathematically, squaring the standard deviation provides the variance value. Or, if you have the variance, the standard deviation is equal to the square root of the variance. For the example with **Figure 3.5**, the standard deviation is 5.31, so the variance is $(5.31^2) = 28.20$, rounded.

Skewness and Kurtosis concern the shape of the distribution. Distribution of the data can have a positive skew, negative skew, or be symmetrical (no skew) (**Figure 3.6**). In a perfectly normal distribution, the skewness value would be zero and the mean, median, and mode values would be equal. When skewness of a distribution occurs the location of the mean, median, and mode are different (**Figure 3.6**). The larger to positive skew, the more the mean is "pulled" to the right or toward higher values. The larger the negative skew, the more the mean is "pulled" to the left or toward lower values. The skewness of the distribution can affect the results from many statistical analyses. In **Figure 3.6**, the first distribution is normal, and the mean, median, mode are 0.50. The second distribution is a positive or right skewed and notice the mean and median are not the same. The mean is 0.28 (green line) and the median is 0.26 (red line) because the higher

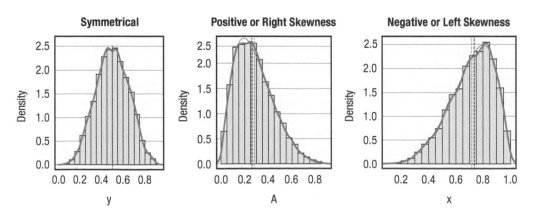

Figure 3.6. Symmetrical and Skewed Distributions.

values are pulling the mean toward the right end of the distribution. The skewness value of the second distribution is 0.57, indicating slight positive skewness. The third distribution has a skewness values of −0.59, with a mean of 0.71 (green line) and a median of 0.74 (red line). The lower scores are pulling the distribution to the left. In reality, normality is somewhat of a mythical creature, fantasized about, desired, but not real in applied settings. As Geary (1947) stated, "Normality is a myth; there never was, and never will be, a normal distribution"(pg. 241), and went on to say about the myth statement, "This is an over-statement from the practical point of view, but it represents a safer initial mental attitude than any in fashion during the past two decades" (pg. 241).

Kurtosis describes the flatness or peakedness of a distribution. Therefore, "Is it pointy like a mountain peak or flat more like a brick?" The statistical terms for these are *leptokurtic (pointy)* and *platykurtic (flat)*. A leptokurtic distribution has a positive kurtosis value, whereas a flat distribution is platykurtic and has a negative kurtosis value (**Figure 3.7**).

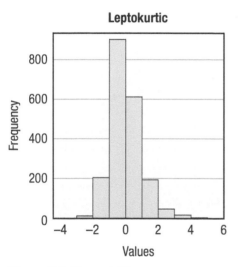
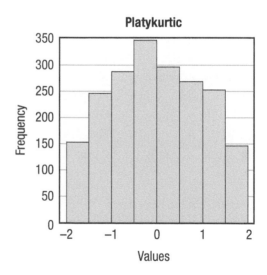

Figure 3.7. Kurtosis Types.

The simulated examples in **Figure 3.7** were designed to have has a kurtosis of −1 and 3, respectively.

How much skewness and kurtosis are problematic? Historically, skewness greater than +/−1 has been used as a cut-off for transforming the distribution so that it approximates normality, and 7 for kurtosis. Skewness and kurtosis will also be discussed in future chapters, but there are techniques for testing the normality of a distribution. With these tests though, as sample sizes increase (over 100), small deviations from normality start to look problematic. Once the size is over 200, much of the kurtosis problems disappear (Tabachnick et al., 2007; Waternaux, 1976). Kurtosis and skewness interact in many analyses, so it is important to examine both during the descriptive phase of your data analysis.

ANALYSIS OF CATEGORICAL DATA

Categorical data, nominal or ordinal, are easily presented in frequency tables. Frequency tables are considered a univariate display of data because there is only one variable that is the focus. For example, the number of patients (Table 3.1) on any a specific day. Research articles and other data-based documents commonly present categorical variables such as gender identification, employed (yes/no), vaccinated (yes/no), and medication compliance are presented in table form with frequency counts and sometimes percentages. There are also continuous data that have been grouped, such as age, that will be presented in a table with the percentage or frequency count of participants in each age grouping.

Table 3.1. Frequency Count Example of Hospital Units.

Unit	Frequency (Patient Count)
NICU	12
PICU	8
SICU	21
Pediatric	14
Oncology	20
Post-Surgery	10
Rehabilitation	27

Cross-Tabulations

Cross-tabulations are a special type of frequency table where two (or more) categorical variables are examined simultaneously, and it is considered a multivariate display of data because the focus is on more than one variable. In Table 3.2, the individuals are categorized by their medical school training and current role in the hospital system. From this cross-tabulation, two Residents have a Doctor of Osteopathy (DO) degree and were educated in the United States. Each box is referred to as a cell, thus DO with Residents is one cell. Cross-tabulations provide a richer display of categorical information for the readers than

Table 3.2. Cross-Tabulation of Medical School Training by Role.

	Role			
Training	Attending Physician	Fellow	Resident	Medical Student
US MD	57	43	1	2
US DO	7	1	2	0
Foreign Med. Graduate	2	3	1	0

the typical frequency tables. Cross-tabulation of categorical data is extremely important because many analyses cannot be completed properly if cell counts of the frequency counts are below five.

Analysis of Mixed Continuous and Categorical Data

Data can also be presented in cross-tab like charts when the variables are mixed between continuous and categorical data, and even between categorical types of nominal and ordinal. A common example are means and standard deviations split by experimental groups or other demographic characteristics (e.g., year in school). Table 3.3 provides an example of continuous and categorical data for students with year in school and sleep grouping categories with confidence scores as the continuous variable. Third year students with excellent sleep have the highest mean academic confidence scores of all groups.

Table 3.3. Academic Confidence Scores According to Year in School and Sleep Quality Category.

Year/Sleep Quality Group	Poor	Moderate	Good	Excellent
First Year	10.87	12.14	16.56	19.83
Second Year	9.48	11.79	17.21	20.62
Third Year	11.59	14.37	20.45	23.77

Correlation

Correlations are a numeric representation of the association between two variables. If both variables are continuous in nature (e.g., height and weight) and normally distributed, the correlation value will be an estimate of the linear relationship between the two variables. This is commonly referred to as Pearson Correlation (Pearson, 1895). Correlation tables allow you to examine two or more variables in the table at once. Table 3.4 has three health related variables.

Correlations have two components, the direction and the magnitude. The direction can be positive or negative. Positive correlations indicate as one variable increases so does the other. If the value is negative, as one variable increases the second decreases. The magnitude describes the size of the correlation. Values closer to 0 indicate a weak relationship, and values closer to 1 indicate a strong relationship. Chapter 8 will discuss several types of correlations in depth.

Table 3.4. Correlation Table Example.

Health	Social	Mental	Physical
Social	1.00		
Mental	0.85	1.00	
Physical	0.71	0.87	1.00

DATA WRANGLING

Descriptive statistics analysis is also the time when researchers begin "data wrangling" (O'Neill & Schutt, 2014). **Data wrangling** is the process of understanding what is actually in the data set and getting the data set into usable fashion. This usually occurs first, before calculating any values. In addition to understanding the basics of the data, it also provides the opportunity to identify what is missing and where the potential problems for later analyses exist. Thus, data wrangling allows the researcher to obtain a detailed understanding of the data and deal with potential problems and issues. Small data sets are quite easy to wrangle and understand what is there and not there, but as the data sets increase to a few hundred cases and 10 or 20 variables, the wrangling of the data becomes more difficult because it is not easy to examine what is going on with the data.

Missing Data

In small data sets, missing data can be a serious problem because with a few lost cases a small data set can become a very small data set. In larger data sets, it is not always as serious of an issue but can become one with more advanced analyses. Formally, there are three types of missing data, **missing completely at random, missing at random, and nonignorable missing data** (Dong & Peng, 2013; Little & Rubin, 2002). If the data are missing completely at random (MCAR) then the missing data from a one variable has no relationship to any other variables *in the data set*. For example, a researcher has data on individuals' weight but some of the cases are missing the weight value. The cases that are complete with the cases that are missing need to be compared to other variables, such as age, gender identification, height, or socio-economic status to demonstrate there is no systemic pattern to the missing data. Specifically, with MCAR, if the researcher could obtain the missing values, the distribution of weight would look exactly like the distribution of weight for the variable with the missing data. There is one warning though; the data could still not be MCAR because the variable associated with the missing data was not collected.

With **MCAR** status, data can be imputed, that is, fill in values for those that are missing. For example, multiple imputation and maximum likelihood are two techniques for filling in the data (Dong & Peng, 2013). There is also the option of listwise delete, which is removing cases from the analysis that are missing data. We recommend imputation if there is access to software to do that. For listwise deletion, the amount of data missing becomes an issue and researchers need to think about it from two perspectives. How much actual missing data is there? How many cases will it affect? If there are 100 participants with 20 variables, there are 2,000 data points. If there are 30 data points missing, that is a missing rate of 0.015 and may look random. But, if those 30 data points are missing across 20 people, a listwise deletion would remove 20 participants or 20% of the cases, which could drastically alter the results. Listwise deletion has been shown to produce unbiased estimates (i.e, results) if the data are truly MCAR (Allison, 1987, 2001).

Missing at random (MAR) indicates there is some level of relationship between the missing data and another variable and the researcher can, therefore, account for the missingness. For example, those who identify as male may be less inclined to fill out a survey on personal anxiety. There are analytic techniques that can be used to impute data with MAR data, such as maximum likelihood, but that is out of the scope of this book. MAR is impossible to test statistically, which is another indicator why good analysis is about argumentation (Abelson, 1995) and not about proof.

Missing not at random/nonignorable (MNAR) is when the relationship between the missing data and another variable has a strong causal link. For example, males do not fully complete an anxiety survey because of their anxiety level. A continuous variable with missing not at random data could also be truncated if a specific range of cases is missing. In the weight example, the researcher might notice that weights over 220 are missing values in the variable when that should not happen because the population of interest has 25% of participants over 220. Missing not at random cannot be easily solved with imputation.

Outliers and Nonnormal Distributions

Outliers and **nonnormal distributions** of continuous variables can cause problems with analyses as discussed previously. An outlier is a possible value on a continuous variable, but in the data set being examined, it appears to be much farther away from the mean than the other data. Thus, outliers are sample dependent. This means that an outlier in one collected data set, may not be an outlier if the researcher collects the data a second or third time and so on. The same scenario applies for nonnormal distributions. There are several options to deal with outliers. The first is to not remove and examine if the outlier or outliers causes a residual analysis problem (see Chapter 8 on Regression). A second option is to run the descriptive analyses with and without the outliers and see if there are differences in mean, median, mode, skewness and kurtosis. If there is not much of a difference, running the analysis with and without the outliers would occur next along with a residual analysis. In large data sets, for example, $n > 500$, one univariate outlier will typically not be a problem.

A third option is to remove any cases that are $+/-3$ standard deviations away from the mean. This is quite common in practice with smaller data sets ($n < 100$) because it removes the outlier and typically helps the data be normally distributed. The downside is that data point is a possible value and removing it could provide a false sense of accuracy of later analyses. For example, if you remove an outlier and the mean value of the variable decreases, any inferences made about that mean could be incorrect because it could be lower than the actual population mean value. As the data is being wrangled so that it can be analyzed, it is important to be thoughtful about removing outliers, how it helps, but also how it can detract from the research questions being asked.

Transformations

Transformations are a technique used in order to turn nonnormally distributed continuous variables into normally distributed variables. More accurately, the researcher is "re-expressing" (Tukey, 1977) the data. Transformations are mathematically legal moves, but the issues occur with the proper interpretation of the results of the re-expressed data. For this reason, we do not recommend transforming variables unless it is absolutely necessary to run the analysis, or the nonnormal data is creating severe residual problems (Chapter 8). Grissom (2000) noted the means obtained from transformed variables may reverse the difference of means compared to the original variables. Thus, it is imperative that the researcher pay attention to what occurs and what that means for conclusions and interpretations. Tabachnick and Fidell (2019) point out that, although data transformations are recommended as a remedy for outliers and for failures of normality, linearity, and homoscedasticity, they are not universally recommended. Howell (2007) argues that the data should examined with both, re-expressed data and the original data. The results should provide the same basic conclusion. As suggested by Tabachnick and Fidell (2019) the following guidelines are in Table 3.5, if you choose to transform data for positively and negatively skewed distributions.

Table 3.5. Distributions and Appropriate Transformation Skewness and Mathematical Generic Visual of Skewness and Direction Adjustment Direction.

Mathematical Transformation x is the variable	Shape of Raw Data	Description of Skewness	Basic Change to Raw Variable
$1/x$		Heavy positive skew	Inverts the relationship with the raw variable. High values now low values and "shrinks" the range.
Log10(X)		Substantial positive skew	"Shrinks" the range such that values are much closer together.
Log10(X + C)		Substantial skew with 0 values in data	"Shrinks" the range such that values are much closer together while dealing with zero values.
$\sqrt{X}$		Moderate positive	"Shrinks" the range such that values are closer together

Table 3.5. Distributions and Appropriate Transformation Skewness and Mathematical Generic Visual of Skewness and Direction Adjustment Direction. (*Continued*)

Mathematical Transformation x is the variable	Shape of Raw Data	Description of Skewness	Basic Change to Raw Variable
$\sqrt{K - X}$		Moderate negative	"Shrinks" the range such that values are much closer together and inverts the relationship
$Log10(K - X)$		Substantial negative skew	"Shrinks" the range such that values are much closer together and inverts the relationship.
$1 / (K - X)$		Heavy negative skew	"Shrinks" the range such that values are much closer together but does not invert the relationship.

C is a constant added to each score so that the smallest score is 1.

K is a constant from which each score is subtracted so that the smallest score is 1; usually equal to the largest score + 1. Note you cannot have a 0 when using log10, mathematically log10 of 0 is undefined. X represent values of the variable.

Once the transformation is completed, the correlation between the re-expressed and the original variable needs to be computed along with descriptive statistics to examine what has happened and how to properly interpret the re-expressed values. Scatterplots (Chapter 4) are also helpful here to examine the change. Re-expressions for negatively skewed distributions change the direction of the relationships with other variables.

Examples of Transformations

The variable for this example is age, measured in years and days, and then converted to years with a decimal for days. The ages range from 11.25 to 36.75 with a mean of 16.66 and a standard deviation of 3.71. The skewness is 1.46 (positively skewed) with a kurtosis of 2.833 (a bit peaked). With this skewness level, starting with a transformation using the square root of the raw variable (moderate skewness) is a good starting point. The new skewness value is 1.138 for the transformed variable (Table 3.6). Historically, when skewness was over 1, the rule of thumb was to transform, but that is just a rule of thumb. The transformed distribution still has a skewness over 1. Using a log10 transformation, the skewness is now less than 1. Table 3.6 displays the changes to the descriptive statistics from the original and the two transformations. The correlation between the original Age and Age(Square root) is 0.998 and between Age and Age(log 10) is 0.991.

Table 3.6. Raw and Transformed Descriptive Statistics for Age.

	Range	Min	Max	Mean	sd	Skew	Kurtosis
Age	25.50	11.25	36.75	19.65	3.71	1.45	2.83
Age (Square root)	2.71	3.35	6.06	4.41	0.39	1.13	1.73
Age (log10)	0.51	1.05	1.57	1.28	0.08	0.83	0.97

The next example uses an overall health score that ranges from 13.45 to 66.06 with a mean of 45.28 and standard deviation of 10.80. The skewness is −0.78 and kurtosis is −0.25. Though the skewness value is not over 1, the shape of the distribution resembles a moderately skewed variable. To re-express a moderate negative skew transformation, use $\sqrt{(K - X)}$, with a K value of 67.06, such that the smallest new value will be 1 (67.06 − 66.06). The new skewness is 0.35. But more importantly, the correlation between the transformed health score and the original is −0.99, indicating that the transformed scores are reversed. Thus, for the original variable the higher the score, the higher the overall health of the participant. For the transformed variable, the higher the score, the worse the health. The transformation reverses the score pattern (high becomes low and vice versa) and therefore reverses the inference. This can be confusing, so taking time to understand this is important.

Multivariate Normality

Previously, the focus has been on examining one variable for normality and for a few analyses, this works. But, for more complicated analyses, for example, multiple regression, structural equation models, and factor analysis, **multivariate normality** of continuous variables is another assumption that must be examined. Multivariate normality is the test of the normality of two or more variables simultaneously. Researchers commonly use the Mahalanobis (1936) distance for examining multivariate outliers during the data examination phase by running a regression analysis (Chapter 8) with the participant number as the dependent variable and the independent variable of interest. This will be discussed in detail later in the book.

Finally, if you make transformations of the data, it is imperative that you go back and look at multivariate normality for those analyses that have this assumption. Interestingly, we have read too many manuscripts where a post-transformation multivariate normality examination did not occur and there were multivariate outliers affecting the results. The lack of examination became apparent through a deep examination of the results and the provided descriptive statistics.

Scaling and Z-Scores

In some analyses, the scales of the variables can cause problems due the size difference. For example, one variable has a 1 to 10 scale and another has a 50 to 200 scale. Those are very different sized scales. Thus, some researchers will re-scale some normally distributed variables as part of the data wrangling process and describe it as a z-scale transformation or other adjustment such as dividing each value by 10. A z-scale transformation is completed by taking each value subtracting the mean, and then dividing that value by the standard deviation. The new variable will have a mean of 0 and a standard deviation of 1. This transformation allows the scales of the variables in the analysis to be closer together (Kline, 2016).

SUMMARY

Descriptive analysis of the data is an important process in research. It deserves more time and care than it currently receives. We recommend researchers or anyone completing analyses of data to specifically dedicate time for this in order to deeply understand the data individually and their interrelationships. Researchers should focus on understanding the data, not just a simple checklist in an attempt to reach a desired outcome. The diligent examination of descriptive statistics, that is the hours of work on the front end, will provide a level of confidence in the results at the very end. An upside effect of this is the researcher's ability to explain the data in excruciating detail to anyone who asks, and that is priceless.

END-OF-CHAPTER RESOURCES

REVIEW QUESTIONS

Answers and rationales for the review questions are located in the Appendix at the end of the book.

1. You are assisting with a study where third-year undergraduate nursing students are receiving an intervention to improve their clinical judgment skills in the practice setting. State a research question that could be answered using descriptive statistics.

2. TRUE or FALSE?

   When reading research articles, it is common to see the median and interquartile range reported.

3. TRUE or FALSE?

   After running a descriptive analysis of the variables, the resulting values are considered estimates.

4. TRUE or FALSE?

   The average score for a variable measured on a continuous scale is known as the mean.

5. Determine the median for the total cholesterol levels below:

   185 210 145 290 170 238 290 166 222 199 139 248 125 264 277

6. Review the histogram in the figure below. What is the height of a person who is two standard deviations below the mean?

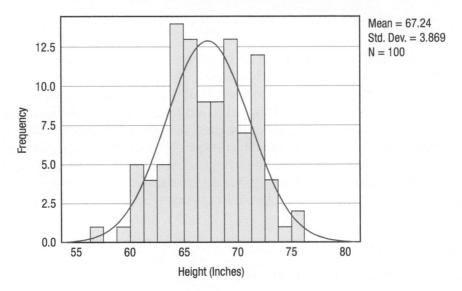

Mean = 67.24
Std. Dev. = 3.869
N = 100

7. Among a set of fasting blood glucose levels, the mean is 99 and the variance is 16.04. What is the standard deviation?

8. A nurse performs an analysis examining the distribution of body weight (x-axis) versus prostate specific antigen (y-axis) and produces the graph below. What is the correct description of the distribution?

   a. normal
   b. positively skewed
   c. negatively skewed
   d. bimodal

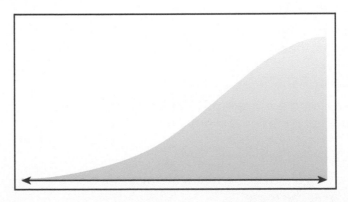

9. A researcher is examining the relationship between systolic blood pressure and level of education in a sample of cardiac rehab patients. The results indicate a correlation of −0.04. Which of the following accurately describes the direction and magnitude of this correlation?

    a. positive and strong

    b. negative and strong

    c. positive and weak

    d. negative and weak

10. An investigator notices that the missing values for depression scores are correlated with the age of the participants, such that the missing scores are among the participants who are younger than 50. In this case, the missing data can be said to be:

    a. missing not at random

    b. missing completely at random

    c. missing repeatedly

    d. missing at random

11. The distribution of the scores for the outcome variable of interest is moderately positively skewed, and a square root transformation is applied to the data. What should the researcher do next to aid in interpretation?

12. TRUE or FALSE?

    Multivariate normality must be established before conducting a correlation between two variables.

 SPRINGER PUBLISHING CONNECT™ | A robust set of instructor resources designed to supplement this text is located at http://connect.springerpub.com/content/book/978-0-8261-6582-4. Qualifying instructors may request access by emailing textbook@springerpub.com.

REFERENCES

Abelson, R. P. (1995). *Statistics as principled argument*. Psychology Press.

Allison, P. D. (1987). Estimation of linear models with incomplete data. In C. Clogg (Ed.), *Sociological methodology 1987* (pp. 71–103). American Sociological Association.

Allison, P. D. (2001). *Missing data*. Sage.

Dong, Y., & Peng, C. Y. J. (2013). Principled missing data methods for researchers. *SpringerPlus, 2*(1), 222. https://doi.org/10.1186/2193-1801-2-222

Eisenhart, C.: 1974, 'The development of the concept of the best mean of a set of measurements from antiquity to the present day', 1971 ASA Presidential Address. Unpublished manuscript.

Geary, R. C. (1947). Testing for normality. Biometrika, 34(3/4), 209-242.

Grissom, R. J. (2000). Heterogeneity of variance in clinical data. *Journal of Consulting and Clinical Psychology, 68,* 155–165. https://doi.org/10.1037//0022-006x.68.1.155

Houston, B., Bruzesse, L., & Weinberg, S. (2002). *The investigative reporter's handbook: A guide to documents, databases and techniques.* Bedford/St. Martin's.

Howell, D. C. (2007). *Statistical methods for psychology* (6th ed.). Thomson Wadsworth.

Kline, R. B. (2016). *Principles and practice of structural equation modeling* (4th Ed.). Guilford Press.

Little, R. J., & Rubin, D. B. (2002). *Statistical analysis with missing data.* John Wiley & Sons.

Mahalanobis, P. C. (1936). Mahalanobis distance. In *Proceedings National Institute of Science of India* (Vol. 49, No. 2, pp. 234–256).

O'Neill, C., & Schutt, R. (2014). *Doing data science: Straight talk from the frontline.* O'Reilly.

Pearson, K. (1895). Correlation coefficient. In *Royal Society Proceedings* (Vol. 58, p. 214).

Plackett, R. L. (1983). Karl Pearson and the chi-squared test. *International Statistical Review/Revue Internationale de Statistique, 51*(1) 59–72.

Rubin, E. (1968). The Statistical World of Herodotus. *The American Statistician, 22*(1), 31–33.

Tabachnick, B. G., Fidell, L. S., & Ullman, J. B. (2007). *Using multivariate statistics* (Vol. 5). Pearson.

Tabachnick, B. G., & Fidell, L. S. (2019). *Using multivariate statistics* (7th ed.). Allyn and Bacon.

Tukey, J. W. (1977). *Exploratory data analysis* . Pearson.

Tukey, J. W. (1988). *The Collected Works of John W. Tukey: Graphics: 1965–1985* (Vol. 5). Chapman & Hall.

Waternaux, C. M. (1976). Asymptotic distribution of the sample roots for a nonnormal population. *Biometrika, 63*(3), 639–645. https://doi.org/10.1093/biomet/63.3.639

FURTHER READING

Bühler, W. K. (1987). *Gauss: Eine biographische Studie.* Springer Publishing Company.

Gravetter, F. J., & Wallnau, L. B. (2007). Statistics for the behavioral sciences. Thomson Learning.

Rubin, E. (1971). Quantitative Commentary on Thucydides. *The American Statistician, 25*(4), 52–54.

Tukey, J. W. (1970). Exploratory data analysis. Addison-Wesley.

APPENDIX 3.1

$$Mean = \overline{X} = \frac{\sum_1^n x_i}{n}$$

CHAPTER 4

Visual Representations

CORE OBJECTIVES

- Understand that the data drive the narrative, not the other way around
- Describe the basic rules and questions related to visualization design
- Describe the difference between univariate and multivariate visualizations (MVs)
- Explain differences between visualizations types (e.g., histogram) and when to use each one
- Explain how to use visualizations for data wrangling
- Discuss data in their daily lives and ways to visualize it
- Describe two famous visualizations

INTRODUCTION: THE IMPORTANCE OF VISUAL REPRESENTATION

Visual representations have seen a resurgence over the past 20 years with the change in computing power and software programs. In the history of graphing data, there have been several waves and one golden age of visualization (1850–1900) according to Friendly (2008) along with several milestones (Friendly & Denis, 2001). In a similar vein as descriptive statistics, visually representing data is a crucial process to understanding, wrangling, and describing the data. Visual representation allows for the early exploratory work of the data (Tukey, 1970, 1988) and will save time later during the inferential analysis stage. Finally, data visualization is a key component of analysis because it can highlight outlying cases and unique issues typically hidden when using the normal aggregations such as, mean, skewness, or a single correlation value.

Figure of the Day

In several of our classes, figures of the day are presented to students without labeled axes or legends. The purpose of this exercise is to learn to carefully examine the visualization without immediately trying to interpret it. Visualization interpretation is a continual problem for individuals, especially students (Cronin et al., 2009; Invanjek et al., 2017; Shah & Hoeffner, 2002), but it is important to really see what is presented and think about it first. In **Figure 4.1**, there is a partial visualization—no labels. The full visualization is at the end of the chapter but wait to look at it. In **Figure 4.1**, what do you notice? Look for details. After you have exhausted the details, then try to figure out what this might be.

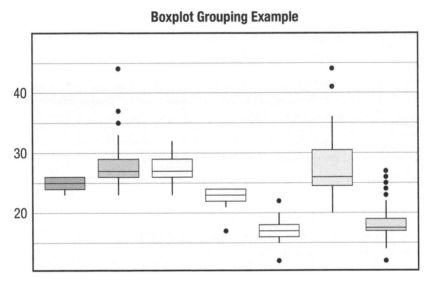

Boxplot Grouping Example

Figure 4.1. Visualization Without Labels.

Narratives

Each visualization should be a narrative on its own and the data drive that narrative. The designer should not drive the narrative but work to find the best visualization to illuminate the data. The data cannot speak for themselves (D'Ignazio & Klein, 2020), but in general, the less verbal explanation needed for the visualization the better the visualization is. There are some basic rules to follow and questions to guide the design. The information below is a conglomeration of years of working in this area and information from Tufte (1983), The United Kingdom government style guide, Friendly (2008), Mulbrandon (2013), Yau (2011), D'Ignazio and Klein (2020), and the Data Visualization Society (https://www.datavisualizationsociety .org).

Basic Questions: What is the overall goal?

To understand the shape of the data? Histograms are excellent to see the distribution shape.

To compare? Bar charts and grouped bar charts work well here.

To find a trend? Time is the typical component in a trend analysis, and line charts and boxplots are common in trend analysis.

To examine a relationship or connection? Scatterplots, heatmaps, and tree diagrams are used when looking for relationships or connections.

To examine part of something? Pie charts, stacked bars, and donuts are useful for parts.

Basic Rules:

Publication rules: Read any formatting or rules for the publication you are submitting to. Many publications and even government agencies have rules for visualizations.

Audience: Focus on who the audience is for the visualization.

Let the data speak: The data should tell the story; the designer should not be trying to force the story with the data. The data cannot speak for themselves, though, because every data set has a context in which it was collected and that context matters.

Data type: Align the graphic to the type of data being used, and within each graphic there are choices. Thus, a few versions should be created.

Provide appropriate context: The graphic should provide the narrative and be able to stand on its own, but important contextual information should be added around into the graphic. The graphic should not be deceptive in any manner.

Less can be more: Visualizations can become heavy with too much information. Thus, a focus on keeping it simple can be helpful.

Correct size: The chart or graphic should not take over the surrounding narrative or be too small to be useful.

Limit the number of lines: Time series charts become quite heavy when there are too many lines. Additionally, the time series chart can be separated into several charts with one line highlighted in each.

Color: Color is not always needed and grayscale can be quite useful. Additionally, try to use colors or color palettes that are sensitive to those who are color blind.

Interval lines: Interval lines run across the interior portion of a graph. There can be too few or too many. Here is where a few versions will help determine the right balance.

Axes: Axes are a constant argument. One side argues for 0 being in visualizations all the time, and others argue only if it is appropriate. We believe that if 0 is not included the designer must make it clear in the narrative why 0 is not included and how the graphic should be interpreted properly.

Annotate: Annotate the axes and the data points so that reader understands what has been done.

Ink coverage: Makes sure the size of the differences in the numbers matches the actual area in the charts. Bubble charts are notorious for having area much larger than the numeric differences. It biases the interpretation.

Ink coverage 2: Less ink more data is a good motto. Maximize the data displayed.

Remove: Remove unnecessary design features or text. 3D graphs or pseudo 3-D graphics do not let the data speak and can be confusing to interpret.

Consistency: Keep charts, fonts, and so on consistent. If you have multiple charts where comparisons are desired, consistency of axes and labeling are even more important.

SINGLE VARIABLE-UNIVARIATE

Common visualizations in research are the histogram, boxplot, bar chart, pie chart, and line graph. These five visualizations are called univariate visualizations because there is only one variable of focus. The histogram is a visualization of a continuous variable's distribution across the full range of values. The x-axis displays the range of values and the y-axis shows the frequency of the values (Figure 4.2). The values range from −33.96 to +36.18, with a mean of zero, a standard deviation of 10 (sd = 10). The data is grouped into "bins" for this example, 40-cut points, or bins were used.

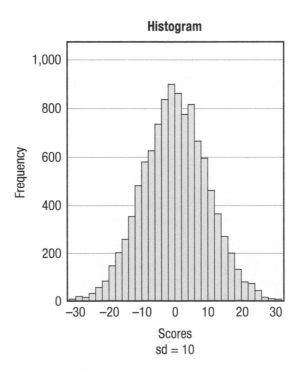

Figure 4.2. Generic Example of a Histogram.

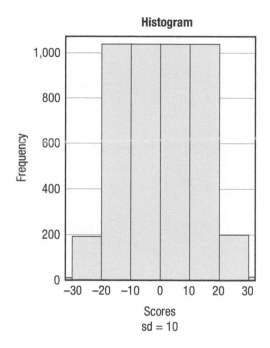

Histogram

Figure 4.3. Figure 4.2 Data With 10 Cut-Points.

The number and size of the bins affects how the histogram looks. In general, the wider the range and the larger the sample, the more bins are needed. **Figure 4.3** displays the same data with only 10 cut-points. The fewer number of bins makes it difficult to understand the actual distribution of scores. Histograms are an excellent visualization for examining the shape of the distribution (e.g., skewness or kurtosis) and identifying potential outliers.

Box plots can be used with one continuous variable or one continuous variable with one categorical variable or more. Boxplots are continuous data separated into quartiles. Each quartile has 25% of the data, hence the name. There are several key attributes to the boxplot (**Figure 4.4**). The main attribute is the box, which covers the middle 50% of the data and is **the inter-quartile range** (IQR). The blue horizontal line is the median. The IQR value is derived from subtracting the Quartile 1 value from the Quartile 3. There are two arms (dashed lines), Quartile 1 and Quartile 4 respectively, that extend out from the box and each contains 25% of the data.

In this example, the third quartile value is 56.36 and the first quartile value is 42.06. These values are the maximum value in each of the respective quartiles. The IQR in **Figure 4.4** is 14.30 (56.36 − 42.06). The maximum value is 74.08 and the minimum value is 18.96. Notice that the minimum value is a univariate outlier indicated by an open blue circle. This **outlier** was determined by taking the Quartile 1 value and subtracting the quantity of the IQR multiplied by 1.5.

Lower outliers: Q1 − (IQR × 1.5)
42.06 − (14.30 × 1.5)
42.06 − 21.45 = 20.61

Any value below 20.61 would be considered a lower outlier and in this example that is 18.96. For the upper outliers, Quartile 3 value is used along with adding the quantity:

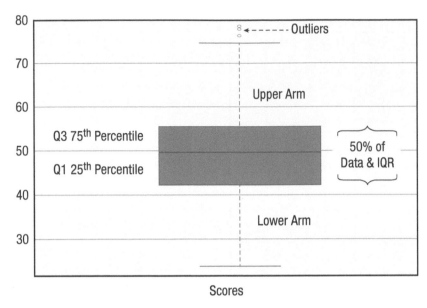

Figure 4.4. Boxplot With Annotation.

Upper outliers: Q3 + (IQR × 1.5)
56.36 + × (14.30 × 1.5)
56.36 + 21.45 = 77.81

Thus, any value above 77.81 would be considered a univariate outlier. The maximum value was 74.08, thus no potential outliers. Outliers are values that appear deviant or outside of the bounds for a sample of data. The values are possible values and not a miscoded or typo data point in the data set. Outliers might also indicate that the sample data is not fully representative of the population data.

Details in box plots can also be added to include the mean and the individual data values In **Figure 4.5**, each solid blue dot is an individual data point. Data points with the same value are stacked upon each other, so you only see them once.

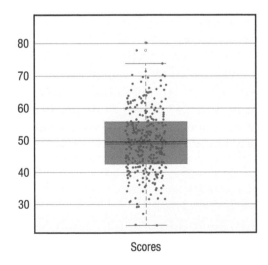

Figure 4.5. Boxplot With Data Points and Mean.

The mean is the black line, and the one outlier is the solid blue dot. The mean is slightly to the left of the median, indicating slightly negatively skewed data.

Bar charts are used when the focus is on the how much within categories, such as frequency or percentage. Bar charts can look multivariate, but the focus is on the categories (e.g., categorical data). **Figure 4.6** displays a bar chart of faculty by academic unit. Interpretation is relatively straight forward with a bar chart. In **Figure 4.6**, the School of Medicine has 89 faculty members, and the School of Music has 25.

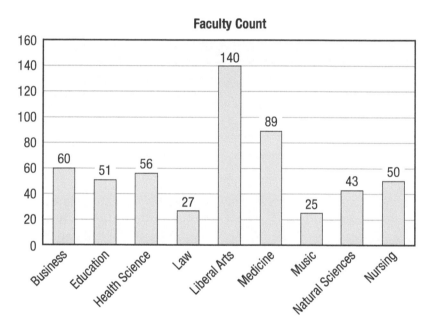

Figure 4.6. Bar Chart Example Faculty Count Within Academic Unit.

Pie charts, first used by William Playfair in the early 1800s, are circle shaped graphics that are commonly used to display proportions and sometimes counts of categorical data. But pie charts are also severely abused and many times incorrect. The most common mistake is to have percentages not equal to 1 or the counts for each slice not equal to the total number. **Figure 4.7** is a pie chart of the faculty data from **Figure 4.6** with percentages and a note of total sample size. When percentages are used, the total sample size should be included so individuals can determine the number in each slice.

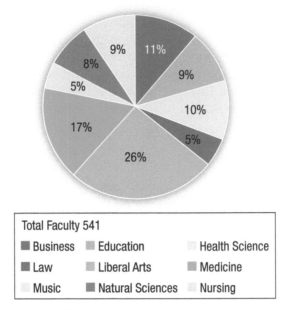

Figure 4.7. Pie Chart of Faculty Percentages.

Times series graphs (repeated measures) have one variable of interest that has been observed or collected over a span of time. In research, this generally defaults to a minimum of three time points of collection, but can included hundreds, if not thousands, of time points.

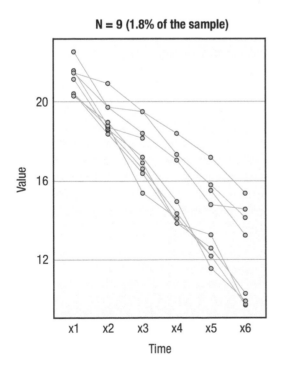

Figure 4.8. Time Series Graph.

Time is traditionally put on the x-axis and the values are placed on the y-axis. **Figure 4.8** follows this pattern with time in years of a moving average value. The values are decreasing over time, such as individuals stress levels over time.

MULTIVARIATE VISUALIZATION (MV)

Analysis of Mixed Continuous and Categorical

MV occurs when two or more variables are used in one visualization. MVs are simply the best aspect of visualization because complex narratives can be created in a small space with minimal word counts. Basic MVs are those that combine continuous and categorical data to provide richer visualizations using both types of data. **Figure 4.9** displays two histograms from two groups of respondents from a simulated experiment using a wellness survey as the outcome variable. The mean value for each group on the wellness survey is also provided in this display along with an orange section where the two distributions overlap.

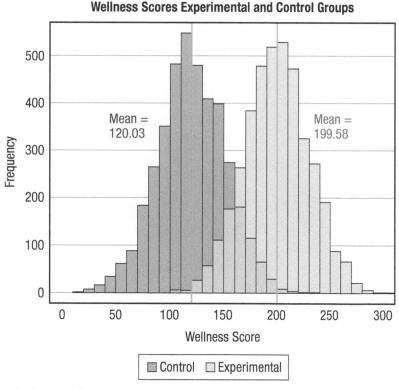

Figure 4.9. Multigroup Histograms.

Multigroup boxplots also use one continuous variable and one categorical variable. In **Figure 4.10** four different experimental groups and mental health scores are displayed. Sleep + Meditation participants have the highest median value, just under 20, and Sleep participants have the largest dispersion of scores, from 0 to 59. The control group has the lowest mean, smallest dispersion, and the only one with no outliers.

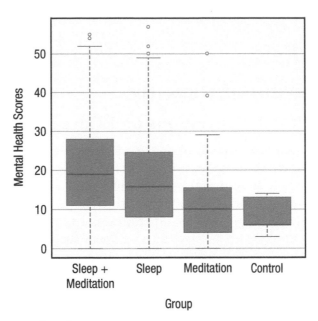

Figure 4.10. Multigroup Boxplot.

Heat maps are one multivariable visualization, which use continuous variables to highlight the range of the values (i.e., the hot/cold range) along with other variables such as geographic location. Geographic based heat maps use one or more variables, which are situated geographically—such as a county.

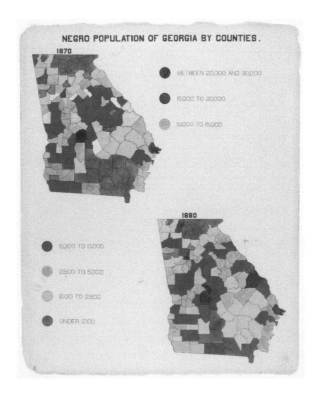

Figure 4.11. W. E. B. Du Bois Heat Map https://www.loc.gov/pictures/item/2013650425/

This heat map of Georgia in **Figure 4.11** is one of more than 60 visualizations designed and created by W. E. B. Dubois and students at Atlanta University in the late 1800s for the *1900 Paris Exposition*. All of the images can be obtained from the Library of Congress and an incredible volume with contextual information is also available (Battle-Baptiste & Rusert, 2018). In **Figure 4.11**, the population of African-Americans in Georgia by county is displayed for 1870 and 1880. In the visual, at the very bottom left is Decatur County (now split into Seminole and Decatur) and in 1870 the color is red, indicating a population of 5,000 to 10,000 and in 1880 it has changed color, grey, indicating a population of 10,000 to 20,000.

Heat maps can also be used to help identify patterns more easily, such as in correlation tables. **Figure 4.12** has a general heat map of correlations for health and wellness variables. The darker the green, the larger the positive correlation. Notice the darkest green, also numerically 1, are the variables correlated with themselves.

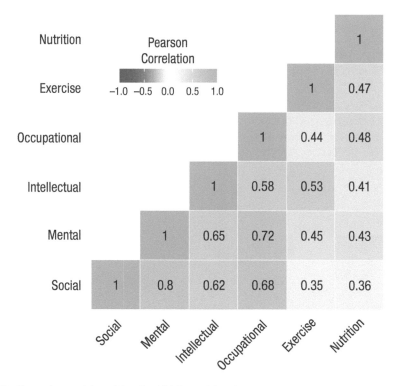

Figure 4.12. Correlation Heat Map for Wellness Variables.

A different version of the heatmap using circles, circle size, and color to indicate magnitude and direction of the correlation is in **Figure 4.13**.

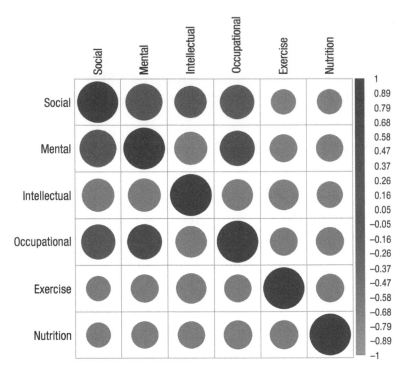

Figure 4.13. Correlation Heat Map With Circles.

You can also use heatmaps in a variety of scenarios. Figure 4.14 has a heat map of 12 participants from a large study with several constructs of wellness. Darker red indicates higher values on that domain for that participant.

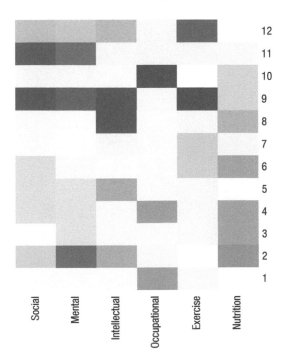

Figure 4.14. Heat Map of Participants and Wellness Scores.

Geographic heat maps, like the one in **Figure 4.11**, are very common now. **Figure 4.15** displays a Centers for Disease Control and Prevention map of adults with obesity from 2020. With geographic based maps, the minuteness of the data affects the level of detail in the visualization. There are 15 states with rates of 35% to less than 40%.

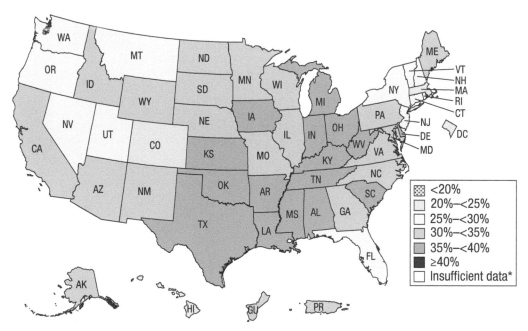

Figure 4.15. Rates of Obesity Among Adults, 2020.

Two Continuous Variables

Scatterplots, aka scattergrams, consist of two *continuous* normally distributed variables that are linearly related, thus the graphic version of the **Pearson Correlation Coefficient** (Chapter 8). The basic scatterplot displays the individual data pairs of two variables. **Figure 4.16** is a scatterplot of two variables, ambiguity and stress. The two variables look positively related because as one increases the other appears to increase. In actuality, the correct interpretation is the lower the ability to tolerate ambiguity the higher the stress. This is a reminder to make sure the coding of the data is understood when reading the scatterplot and explain it to the reader. There are also a few data points that may be multivariate outliers. On the right side of the scatterplot, one data pair at (38:ambiguity,41:stress) is located at several points (distance) from the rest and may be a multivariate outlier that could create a residual problem in later analyses (Chapter 8).

The assumptions for a Pearson correlation are both variables are normally distributed (looks like a bell curve), interval or ratio, no outliers, and the underlying relationship between the two is linear (straight line). If these assumptions are not tenable, you can still create the scatterplot and it will highlight any problems.

In addition to the basic scatterplot, including the histograms of each variable can be informative and sometimes eye opening. **Figure 4.17** displays the two variables from **Figure 4.16**, Stress and Ambiguity, with the densities included. Both are relatively normally distributed, see the distributions at top and right side. This is a reminder that perfect normality is not seen in applied research (see Geary, 1947 in Chapter 3).

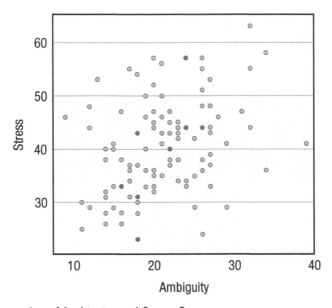

Figure 4.16. Scatterplot of Ambiguity and Stress Scores.

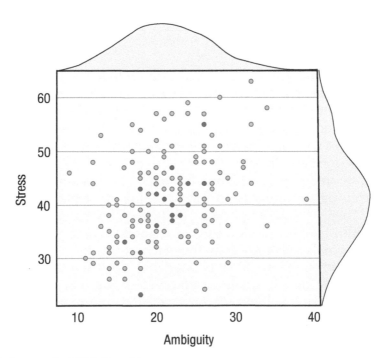

Figure 4.17. Scatterplot With Densities.

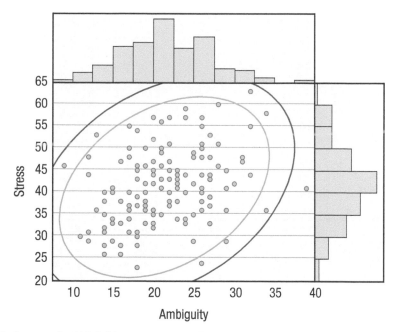

Figure 4.18. Scatterplot With Histograms and Confidence Interval Ellipses.

Next, ellipses around the data points to look for multivariate outliers is possible in some software programs. Figure 4.18 displays the data points with ellipses and histograms. The ellipses around the data points are set at 95% and 99% compatibility levels, but the ellipses can be set at any desired level. The red 99% ellipse (outer) excludes only the one point in the far right of the image that was discussed previously. The green (inner) ellipse is the 95% confidence and displays eight potential multivariate outliers. Notice that the same value from Figure 4.17 is outside the 99% compatibility interval. Software packages have different functions, some do not automatically draw an ellipse, thus this can easily be accomplished by drawing an ellipse on printout.

There are other options for scatterplots with histograms, regression lines, and different calculations of the correlation value. In Figure 4.19, the Ambiguity and Stress data points with histograms are displayed. The histograms also include smoothed distribution lines. The scatterplot has a bivariate regression line (Chapter 8) to show the magnitude of the correlation. Finally, there are two correlation calculations, Pearson's r and Spearman's rho (ρ). Spearman's rho is used when the assumptions of Pearson's are violated. This is discussed in further detail in Chapter 8. Finally, the regression line displayed in the top right corner has a slope equal to the Pearson correlation value, 0.349.

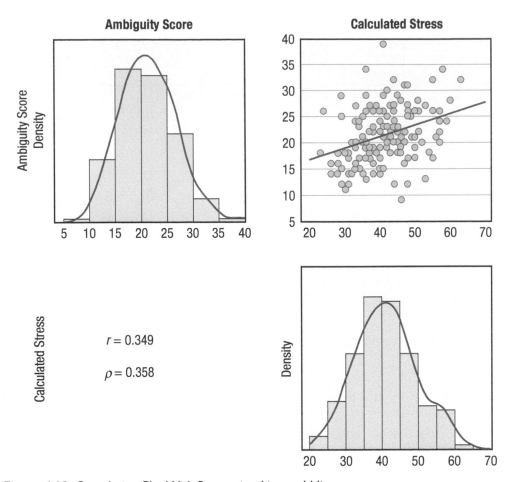

Figure 4.19. Correlation Plot With Regression Line and Histograms.

When there are more than two continuous variables that need to be examined, scatterplot matrices can be created. Figure 4.20 displays a scatterplot matrix with six wellness variables, with histograms down the diagonal, scatterplots to the left and correlations on the right. The histograms also include a frequency polygon. The correlation font size is relative to the correlation size, and the red stars indicate the traditional "statistical significance."

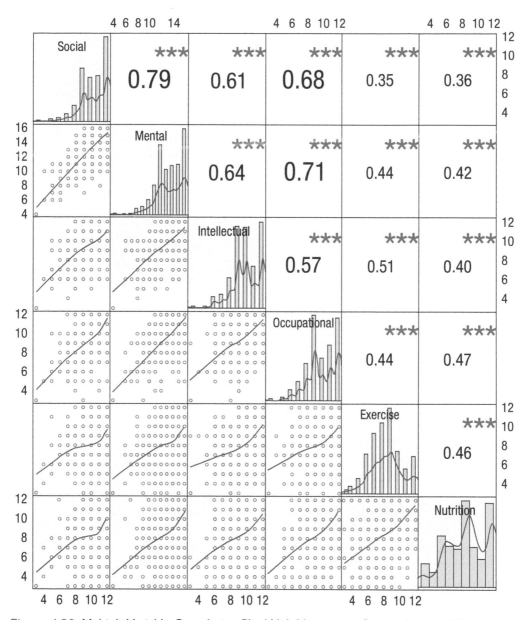

Figure 4.20. Multiple Variable Correlation Plot With Histograms, Scatterplots, and Regression Lines.

Two Continuous With One Categorical Variable

There are also data situations when a scatterplot needs to be separated by groups. Figure 4.21 provides an example of the wellness data for Social and Mental wellness along with three different groups as the categorical variable. There is some overlap of the datapoints, making the Small group look dominant. Another way to discuss this is there is not much separation among the groups.

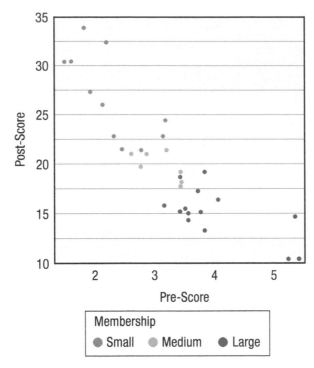

Figure 4.21. Scatter Plot With Separate Groups by Color.

Data Wrangling-Visualization

Visualization can be used for data wrangling, thus it holds two jobs at the same time. Data visualization helps clean the data, and it can also assist in telling the data story. For telling the story, getting the data into proper format is always important, but for visualization it can take more work. Missing data is a key issue for visualization. Some programs will use a pairwise delete for the correlation heatmap, for example. This means that each correlation may have different sample sizes depending on how the missing data is distributed in the data set. A second issue is making sure the data is coded properly for type, such as continuous, ordinal, and so on. Finally, the normal wrangling discussed previously in Chapter 3 should be completed, such as looking for incorrectly coded data.

NONTRADITIONAL REPRESENTATION

The visualizations previously presented are traditional in data analysis. The visualizations you decide to create can be as creative as desired. Thus, visualization provides an opportunity to explore the data in a variety of unique ways or to simply preplan and design visualizations that you want. We recommend taking time to learn to visualize data by looking at things that happen in daily life.

Data of Daily Life

A great process for learning to visualize data is to focus on what happens in your daily life. Jim has his students use a book by Lupi and Posavec (2018). The book

Sit down and recall all the trips (vacations/holidays) you've taken for leisure in your life up until now; note the year, the place, who you were with, and how you traveled there, and draw this data on the abstract map on the right-hand page!

How does the grid work?

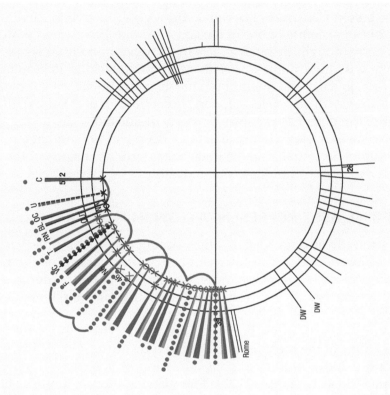

When you were born

It's a circular timeline, from when you were born up until now

3. Other continent
2. My continent
1. My country

The 3 circles indiate where you traveled in your own country, on your continent, or on other continents

(If you are 25 years old, your circle will be divided into 25 parts)

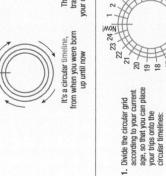

1. Divide the circular grid according to your current age, so that you can place your trips onto the circular timelines:

Now! 1 2 3 4 5 6 7 8 9 10 11 12 13 14 15 16 17 18 19 20 21 22 23 24

2. Mark each vacation with a cross, add a colored line toward the edges of the page to indicate who you were with, and a black line indicating how you got there. Decide your colors, and follow the examples for the types of lines:

Line color
Who were you with?
● Family
 Friends
 Classmates
○ Girlfriend/boyfriend
○ Fiance
○ Alone
● Spouse

Line type
How did you get there?
—— Car
– – – Train/bus
...... Plane
∿∿∿ Boat
〰〰〰 Other

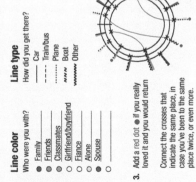

3. Add a red dot ● if you really loved it and you would return

Connect the crosses that indicate the same place, in case you've been to the same place twice, or even more.

Data collected on _____

Figure 4.22. Data Visualization of Travel.

provides a guide for engaging in data of daily life that has a scaffolded approach to creating better visualizations overall through an active journaling process. Figure 4.22 is an example of one of the activities that Jim created with his class.

The process through the book assists in the development of shape and color choice along with improving your data interpretation skills. Researchers should take their own journey and attempt unique visualizations for their data. There is no need to start with statistical software, sometimes a piece of paper and some crayons or colored pencils can answer many of questions. By taking time to visualize the data as a researcher or analyst, a deep and rich understanding of the data is possible. By visualizing the data, the interrelationships of the variables, researchers can create a unique visual narrative.

BEST OF THE BEST REPRESENTATION IN HISTORY

The real strength of data visualization occurs when multiple variables are included which provides rich interconnected information for the reader in a small space. An added bonus with visualizations is the reader gains a computational advantage for memory of the elements of the picture (Kulhavy & Stock, 1996; Schreiber et al., 2002; Schreiber & Verdi, 2003). Researchers do not use this technique very often, but the technique is extremely useful for investigating data. One of the most famous, and maybe the best statistical graph ever created (Tufte, 2001), is Minard's visualization of Napoleon's march to (and retreat from) Moscow (Figure 4.23). The visualization combines six different variables: time, temperature change, military size changes, and location and directionality, along with contrasting colors and easy to read numbers all contained in two dimensions.

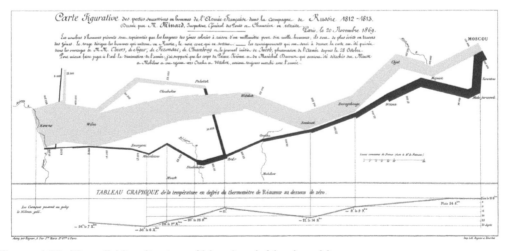

Figure 4.23. Minard's Visualization of Napoleon's March to Moscow.

William Playfair (1759–1823) was also noted for his data visualizations, specifically the book *Commercial and Political Atlas* of 1786, which includes 43 time series plots and a bar chart. This book was the first to contain statistical based graphs. *Statistical Breviary* (1801) contained the very first pie chart. **Figure 4.24** shows a time series analysis of revenues, expenditures, debt, price, and imports of stocks and bread spanning over 50 years.

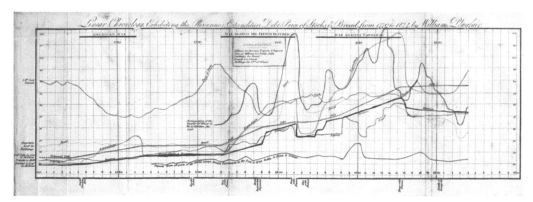

Figure 4.24. Playfair's Time Financial Time Series Graph.

Stocks are in blue, Revenue is in dark red, Expenditures are in Green, Debt is in pink with dashes, Bread is in yellow with very small dashes, Exports are in Violet, and Imports are in a blue/green at the bottom. The graph is easy to read and interpret and includes contextual information such as "American War," and "Death of George III."

There are many rich resources for learning about data visualization, and their references are at the end of chapter denoted with an asterisk (e.g., D'Ignazio & Klein, 2020; Friendly & Wainer, 2021). There is also a massive amount of data available through your local, state, and federal governments along with data housing websites that can be obtained to practice on and improve visualization skills. Data visualization is a process, art, and science that is worthy of learning. Researchers will be better analysts by taking the time to visualize the data.

SUMMARY

Visualizing data is important to complete because it aids in understanding each variable and their interrelationships. There are times where the visualization makes it much easier to see what is going on because basic descriptive statistics can mask issues, since they are aggregating the data. Each basic visualization, for example, histogram and box plot, has assumptions about the data and needs to be used carefully and aligned to your goals. Our recommendation is taking the time to visually display the data using multiple techniques. Those visualizations will help make analytic decisions, such as transforming, and will point the way to conclusions based on the inferential statistical analyses, for example, *t*-tests and regression, that will be completed after the visualizations are done.

END-OF-CHAPTER RESOURCES

REVIEW QUESTIONS

Answers and rationales for the review questions are located in the Appendix at the end of the book.

1. Discuss why visualization of the collected data is a critical element of data analysis.

2. Describe the general goal(s) associated with the following data visualizations:

   histograms: see the shape of the distribution

   bar charts: visually compare groups

   line charts or box plots: trend analysis

   scatterplots or heat maps: see a relationship or connection

   pie charts or stacked bars: investigate part of something

3. TRUE or FALSE?

   Heat maps are a univariate visualization useful for determining the density of the data distribution.

4. TRUE or FALSE?

   A desirable shape of the univariate histogram visualization is a bell shape, but it almost never occurs in dealing with real data in applied research.

5. TRUE or FALSE?

   Box plots are useful for identifying univariate outlying values beyond either "arm" of the plot representing Quartile 1 and Quartile 4.

6. TRUE or FALSE?

   When using a pie chart where the segments represent proportions or percentages of the sample, it is not necessary to note the total sample size.

7. Each data point on a scatterplot represents the values of two variables for one participant, and the overall plot visually depicts which type of statistical analysis?

   a. analysis of variance

   b. *t*-test

   c. Pearson correlation coefficient

   d. standard deviation

8. When examining the data point distribution pattern of a bivariate scatterplot, what is a desirable pattern that represents a strong positive relationship between the variables?

9. A potential issue that can arise in planning your data visualizations using a statistical analysis software package is:

   a. the data story cannot be told

   b. the software may delete cases with missing data

   c. the sample size will never be the same

   d. the variables' levels of measurement are not relevant

10. Which of the following is an important reason for visually displaying your data using several different strategies? Select *all* that apply

    a. Visualizing the data prevents the investigator from making analysis errors.

    b. Visualizing the data shows where missing data is occurring in the data set.

    b. Visualizing the data can help reveal information about the data set not seen in descriptive analyses.

    c. Visualizing the data helps the investigator decide whether to consider transforming the data prior to analysis.

    d. Visualizing the data assists the investigator in knowing if the underlying assumptions of the planned data analyses are met.

 SPRINGER PUBLISHING **CONNECT™** A robust set of instructor resources designed to supplement this text is located at http://connect.springerpub.com/content/book/978-0-8261-6582-4. Qualifying instructors may request access by emailing textbook@springerpub.com.

REFERENCES

*Battle-Baptiste, W., & Rusert, B. (Eds.). (2018). *WEB Du Bois's data portraits: Visualizing black America*. Princeton Architectural Press.

Cronin, M. A., Gonzalez, C., & Sterman, J. D. (2009). Why don't well-educated adults understand accumulation? A challenge to researchers, educators, and citizens. *Organizational behavior and human decision processes*, 108(1), 116–130.

*D'ignazio, C., & Klein, L. F. (2020). *Data feminism*. MIT press.

*Friendly, M. (2008). A brief history of data visualization. In *Handbook of data visualization* (pp. 15–56). Springer Publishing Company.

Friendly, M., & Denis, D. J. (2001). Milestones in the history of thematic cartography, statistical graphics, and data visualization. *32*, 13. http://www.datavis.ca/milestones

*Friendly, M., & Wainer, H. (2021). *A history of data visualization and graphic communication*. Harvard University Press.

Ivanjek, L., Planinic, M., Hopf, M., & Susac, A. (2017). Student difficulties with graphs in different contexts. In *Cognitive and affective aspects in science education research* (Hahl, Kaisa, Kalle Juuti, Jarkko Lampiselkä, Anna Uitto, and Jari Lavonen, eds) (pp. 167-178). Springer, Cham.

Kulhavy, R. W., & Stock, W. A. (1996). How cognitive maps are learned and remembered. *Annals of the Association of American Geographers, 86*(1), 123–145. https://doi.org/10.1111/j.1467-8306.1996.tb01748.x

Lupi, G., & Posavec, S. (2018). *Observe, collect, draw!: A visual journal*. Princeton Architectural Press.

*Mulbrandon, C. (2013). *Visualizing economics*. https://www.visualizingeconomics.com/viewincomeguide

Schreiber, J. B., Verdi, M. P., Patock-Peckham, J., Johnson, J. T., & Kealy, W. A. (2002). Differing map construction and text organization and their effects on retention. *The Journal of Experimental Education, 70*(2), 114–130. https://doi.org/10.1080/00220970209599502

Schreiber, J. B., & Verdi, M. (2003). Dual coding and conjoint retention: Past, present, and future. *Alternation, 10*(1), 250–270.

Shah, P., & Hoeffner, J. (2002). Review of graph comprehension research: Implications for instruction. *Educational psychology review*, 14(1), 47-69.

*Tufte, E. R. (1983). *The visual display of quantitative information graphics press*. Cheshire, Connecticut.

Tufte, E. R. (2001). *The visual display of quantitative information* (Vol. 2). Graphics press.

*Tukey, J. W. (1970). Exploratory data analysis. Addison-Wesley.

*Tukey, J. W. (1988). *The collected works of John W. Tukey: Graphics: 1965–1985* (Vol. 5). Chapman & Hall.

*Yau, N. (2011). *Visualize this: The Flowing Data guide to design, visualization, and statistics*. John Wiley & Sons.

FURTHER READING

Tabachnick, B. G., Fidell, L. S., & Ullman, J. B. (2007). *Using multivariate statistics* (Vol. 5). Pearson.

*Tufte, E. R. (1990). *Envisioning information*. Graphics press.

Tufte, E. R. (2006). *Beautiful evidence*. Graphics press.

*Tufte, E. R., & Robins, D. (1997). *Visual explanations* (p. 52). Graphics.

CHAPTER 5

Traditional Study Design

CORE OBJECTIVES

- Explain differences between different designs (e.g., experimental and nonexperimental) and randomization
- Use ROX system to display different study designs
- Explain and identify different types of limitations to study designs
- Explain the different models and designs of quality improvement studies

INTRODUCTION: THE KEY TO GOOD DESIGN

The research design has to be durable. By durable, we mean that is must support the whole study and be able to withstand critics. Critics looks for weaknesses in the design. We like to discuss this with the concept of a fort. Fort Murud-Janjira is an island fortification off the coast of Murud, India (**Figure 5.1**). Its strength lies in the fact that one can see attacks coming, it has enormous stone walls, and three massive cannons. The fort was attacked multiple times and never failed.

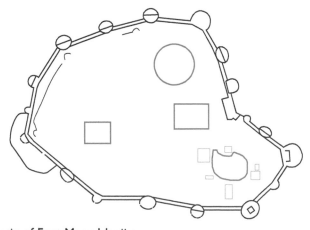

Figure 5.1. Schematic of Fort Murud-Janjira.

The designs researchers use in their studies are critiqued (attacked) when being reviewed. This attack is a normal and important part of science. The design should be able to withstand that critique. Thus, researchers need to think about the strengths and weaknesses of the design, measurement (Chapter 2), and statistical analysis during the development stage. Finally, it is important to understand how the research questions, design, sampling, data collection, and data analysis interact with and are affected by each other.

VARIABLES: INDEPENDENT AND DEPENDENT

In general, the independent variable (IV) is the variable that is argued to cause or be associated with some outcome—the dependent variable (DV) (Kirk, 2013). For example, the number of hours you study (IV) may increase your performance on an essay exam (DV or outcome) in your research methods course. Within each design below, these two variables will have more explicit attributes that separate them, but it is important to begin to separate IVs and DVs early in the design stage. Naturally, they should easily flow from the literature review and your research question(s). The example above could be rewritten as a research question: Are the number of hours studying (IV) predictive of the essay exam score (DV) in a research methods course?

Number of hours studying is typically not manipulated by the researcher. The researcher might assign participants to studying different organizations of material. For example, some participants are told to read a story; read a story and take notes; and read a story, take notes, and predict what happens next. The story reading has three versions and levels, where each level is a different manipulated version of the IV.

EXPERIMENTAL AND NONEXPERIMENTAL DESIGNS

Experimental designs have one thing in common, an IV (or variables) that is manipulated by the researcher (Kirk, 2013; Schreiber & Asner-Self, 2010). Nonexperimental designs do not have a variable that is manipulated. Variable manipulation is the core distinction between the two. But this can be confusing because participants being randomly assigned to experimental conditions is normal in research. These are two different topics, design and assignment. There are also quasi-experimental designs where there are experimental groups or experimental and control, but participants are not randomly assigned (Cook et al., 2002). Pre-experimental designs are a weaker version of quasi-studies and are probably best used as pilot tests of the design and data collection. These designs are also commonly termed nonexperimental (Schreiber & Asner-Self, 2010). We will begin with a discussion of random assignment and selection.

Random Assignment/Selection

Random assignment occurs when each participant from a sample is randomly assigned to one of the experimental or control conditions. For example, 100 participants were randomly assigned to four dosage conditions: 25 mg, 15 mg, 10 mg, and a placebo. This would typically produce 25 participants in each group. **Random selection** occurs when participants are randomly selected from the population of potential participants. Random assignment of participants is common, but random selection and then random assignment is rare in social science research but a staple in randomized controlled trials (RCTs). The random selection from the population and the random assignment to the control is an important assumption for many experimental studies but is not commonly pursued because it is not very feasible to accomplish during recruitment. There is an abundance of sampling processes that are out of the scope of this book, but they are important for what the researcher gets to say later (Henry, 1990; Hess, 1985; Schreiber & Asner-Self, 2010).

Experiments

As stated, **experimental** designs have one thing in common, an IV (or variables) that is manipulated by the researcher. A **"true"** experiment is where at least one IV is manipulated by the researcher and participants are randomly assigned to experimental groups. Each design can be described symbolically/ graphically using a group of letters based on Campbell and Stanley (1963) where R = random assignment, O_i = observations and the subscript tells which time period; first, second third, X_i indicates which group the participants are in or the treatment group, that is, activity in which the participants engage. We use X_c, others use X_o, to indicate no treatment, which is a control group. R indicates *random assignment* only of participants to one of the groups and G indicates a group without random assignment. The designs are also commonly drawn with squares and rectangles that show the design by individual participants, where R means random assignment, X_{ijk} indicates an observation for participant X and i is the participant number, j is for the grouping, and k is the group number. For example, RX_{112G3} is randomly assigned participant number 112 in group 3. The subscripts vary quite a bit depending on preferences, but the general pattern is the same. We use a few different versions to highlight the variability. Table 5.6 displays several more designs along with other information.

Independent Groups

Independent groups are those designs where the participants in each group are not linked in any way to each other. Thus, a participant cannot be in two groups, and there cannot be a relationship between participants within or between the groups, for example, twins, spouses, and so on. The focal question for independent groups design is "How much of a difference exists between the groups?" The design for two groups, experimental and control group with random assignment (Post-Test Only Control Group) is in Figure 5.2.

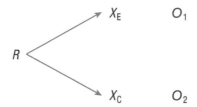

Figure 5.2. Independent Group Design With Randomization.

Table 5.1. Independent Group Design With Randomization.

Group 1	Group 2
RX_{1E}	RX_{1C}
RX_{2E}	RX_{2C}
RX_{3E}	RX_{3C}
.	.
.	.
.	.
RX_{iE}	RX_{iC}

In Figure 5.2, the participants are randomly assigned to X_E or X_C, such as dosage amounts. The observation (O) is the collection of the **dependent variable** of interest, for example, blood pressure. In **Table 5.1**, RX_{1E} indicates randomly assigned participant number one to experimental group. The IV in this design is the group assignment. The analysis most commonly used with this design is the **independent t-test** (Chapter 6), but others such as ANOVA and regression can be implemented (Tabachnick & Fidel, 2007). Caution is needed because "independent" is used several times in design and analysis, that is, IV, independent groups, and independent t-test.

This design can easily be expanded to more groups, that is, greater than two. **Figure 5.3** displays a three-group design, two experimental groups and one control (often called a One-way ANOVA). As an example, groups one and two could be different dosages and group three gets a placebo. The DV and IV are the same as the independent groups. The focal question is, "How large are the differences between the groups?" The common analysis is a One-Way ANOVA (Chapter 6). **Table 5.2** displays the design in block form with the individual participants indicated.

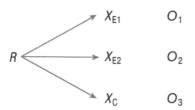

Figure 5.3. Three Independent Groups (One-Way ANOVA).

Table 5.2. Three Independent Groups.

Group 1	Group 2	Group 3
RO_{1E1}	RO_{1E2}	RO_{1C}
RO_{2E1}	RO_{2E2}	RO_{2C}
RO_{3E1}	RO_{3E2}	RO_{3C}
.	.	.
.	.	.
.	.	.
RO_{iE1}	RO_{iE2}	RO_{iC}

Factorial Designs

Factorial designs also have independent groups, but the distinguishing characteristic is more than one IV is manipulated. There are now two focal points for the research questions. The first is the same as before, "How large are the differences in the outcome variable between the groups?" The second focal question is, "Do the two IVs interact (interaction)?" Interaction types are discussed in detail in Chapter 7. The traditional analysis for this design is a Factorial ANOVA. **Figure 5.4** has an example of a factorial design where exercise and sleep are the two IVs and myocardial function is the outcome variable. Exercise and sleep have two groups, 15 minutes and 30 minutes a day for exercise and a minimum of 7 or 8 hours of sleep. If there are two levels to each IV, such as the current example, this design is also called a 2x2 (Exercise by Sleep).

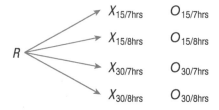

$$R \begin{cases} X_{15/7hrs} & O_{15/7hrs} \\ X_{15/8hrs} & O_{15/8hrs} \\ X_{30/7hrs} & O_{30/7hrs} \\ X_{30/8hrs} & O_{30/8hrs} \end{cases}$$

Figure 5.4. Factorial Design.

Table 5.3. Factorial Design

		Hours	
Exercise Amount		7	8
	15	$RO_{1\text{-}15/7hrs}$ $RO_{2\text{-}15/7hrs}$ . . . $RO_{i\text{-}15/7hrs}$	$RO_{1\text{-}15/8hrs}$ $RO_{2\text{-}15/8hrs}$ . . . $RO_{i\text{-}15/8hrs}$
	30	$RO_{1\text{-}30/7hrs}$ $RO_{2\text{-}30/7hrs}$ . . . $RO_{i\text{-}30/7hrs}$	$RO_{1\text{-}30/8hrs}$ $RO_{2\text{-}30/8hrs}$ . . . $RO_{i\text{-}30/8hrs}$

Factorial design can be easily extended out. For example, if a third exercise group is added, 1 hour, the design becomes a 3x2 ANOVA (3 exercise groups by 2 sleep groups).

Each of the previous designs have been displayed with random assignment to groups. Random assignment is not always the case and there are times where intact "groups," participants that are linked in some way, are used for each experimental group. For example, an experiment is developed by clinical faculty concerning the effect of the type of patient unit (orthopedic, cardiac telemetry, post-stroke) where a student has their adult med-surg clinical on students' clinical judgment skills at the end of the term. Because the students cannot be randomly assigned to different experimental groups (they cannot run different groups in the same clinical rotation), the whole clinical rotation group is assigned to each experimental group. Thus, the groups are considered "in-tact." The problem with this is the unit of assignment is the clinical group, yet the unit of analysis is based on the individual participants. This difference is a common problem in research and there are ways to address this.

Repeated Measures/Dependency

The **repeated measures** key feature is at least one variable has been collected multiple times on each individual participant (Ferguson & Takane, 1989; Tabachnick & Fidel, 2007). For example, blood pressure, pulse, and oxygen rate are continually collected on patients in the hospital. Dependency occurs when there is a link or relationship between participants. A research study interested in couples and their health behaviors would collect the same data on both people. Because both people are a couple, they are not independent; there is a dependency between them.

Paired Designs

Paired designs (one-group, pre-test, post-test) are possibly the most common repeated measure. Simply, the same data are collected twice for individuals or groups of individuals. The focal question for paired designs is "How much of a change has occurred between data collection?" If a researcher was interested in resting heart rate after changes in exercise, resting heart rate would be collected before the program started and then after the program ended. In this example, the IV (exercise, but manipulated) is the intervention and the DV is the resting heart rate. The paired t-test is the traditional analysis for this design. **Figure 5.5** displays the design.

$$G \quad O_1 \quad X_{\text{Intervention}} \quad O_2$$

Figure 5.5. Paired Design.

The G indicates that this is a group design and leaving the G out would indicate a single participant design. Overall, The first observation is made (O_1), then the intervention occurs ($X_{\text{Intervention}}$), and then the second observation is made (O_2).

Repeated Designs

When there are more than two repeated observations, the designs are commonly referred to as *repeated measures*. The focal question is "How much change over time is exhibited by the participants?" This can also be phrased as "trajectory" or "patterns" depending on how much data is collected (Tabachnick & Fidel, 2001). The designs can be based on a group or individual. **Figure 5.6** shows a repeated measure for a group, where multiple baseline observations were taken, then the intervention was implemented, and then multiple postintervention observations were made. Again, the IV (exercise, but manipulated) is the intervention and the DV is the resting heart rate. There are a few analyses that can be conducted, but it is common to see a paired *t*-test based on the average of the baseline values and the average of the post-intervention values.

Designs such as the one in **Figure 5.6** are most common with individuals related to behavioral changes (Schreiber & Asner-Self, 2010). The design can have multiple interventions or switch or counter-balance different interventions, thus changing which participants see which intervention first (Schreiber-Asner-Self, 2010). Tracking large numbers of participants over time can be resource intensive. One example is the anxiety research in the Pittsburgh Youth Study (Jolliffe et al., 2019).

$$G \quad O_1\, O_2\, O_3\, O_4\, O_5\, X_{Intervention}\, O_6\, O_7\, O_8\, O_9\, O_{10}$$

Figure 5.6. Repeated Measures Design With Intervention.

Paired/Repeated With Independent/Experimental Groups

A very strong design is a **one-within and one-between group** design. In this design there is a paired or repeated component and two independent groups. This design is popular with randomized assignment and in-tact group studies. The focal questions for this design are "How large are the group differences?", "How large are the changes over time points?", and "How large is the interaction between time points and the groups?" The Repeated-Measure ANOVA is the most common approach, but there are examples of ANCOVA being used, though that can be fraught with problems (Chapter 7). **Figure 5.7** displays the letter version of the design using the exercise part of the previous sleep and exercise design. The participants are randomly assigned, and for interpretation $O_{15,1}$ indicates 15 minutes of exercise group and time point 1.

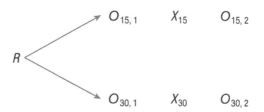

Figure 5.7. One-Within One-Between.

Table 5.4 displays this design in the block format where $RO_{1,15,2}$ is the second observation for participant one in the 15-minute exercise group.

Table 5.4. One Within One Between Block Display.

Exercise Amount	Group	Repeated Measures	
		Time 1	Time 2
	15	$RO_{1,15,1}$ $RO_{2,15,1}$ . . $RO_{i,15,1}$	$RO_{1,15,2}$ $RO_{2,15,2}$ . . $RO_{i,15,1}$
	30	$RO_{1,30,1}$ $RO_{2,30,1}$ . . $RO_{i,30,1}$	$RO_{1,30,2}$ $RO_{2,30,2}$ . . $RO_{i,30,2}$

And as with many of these designs, they can be extended to having more groups and more repeated time points.

Longitudinal

Longitudinal designs are extended versions of repeated measures that may or may not have an intervention, that is, IV (**Figure 5.8**). The focal question tends to be:

$$G \quad O_1\,O_2\,O_3\,O_4\,O_5\,O_6\,O_7\,O_8\,O_9\,O_{10}$$

$$G \quad O_1\,O_2\,O_3\,O_4\,O_5 \text{ Intervention } O_6\,O_7\,O_8\,O_9\,O_{10}$$

Figure 5.8. Longitudinal Design With and Without Intervention.

"What does the pattern/trajectory look like over time?" For example, "What is the pattern of calories expended by age over the lifetime?" or, "How much does our caloric need change from birth to age 65?" (Herman et al., 2021). With an intervention, the question would change to "How much does the trajectory change after intervention?" Researchers will look at the trajectory by groups as a way to understand the pattern, such as grouping by geographical location. In this instance, the geographical region becomes an IV, but it was not part of the core design. Finally, there is no formal indicator for the number of observations needed to call a study longitudinal, though we think a minimum of four observations over an extended time period (e.g., weeks) is a good rule of thumb.

COMMON EPIDEMIOLOGICAL DESIGNS

There are three epidemiological designs we think are important to discuss here, RCTs, **cohort studies**, and **case-control** (Gordis, 2004). Each has a slightly different goal and reason for being used. Some of this will be a repetition of the basic designs above, but it is important to see these three independently.

Randomized Controlled Trials

The RCT is considered the ideal design for evaluating both the effectiveness and the side effects of new forms of intervention in clinical trials, such as evaluating new drugs and other treatment modalities, assessing new programs for screening or early detection, and assessing new ways of organizing and delivering health services (Table 5.5). The focal questions are similar to "How much of a difference does the treatment make?" or "Does the treatment reduce the progression of the disease?" The most general design is an independent groups design where participants are randomly assigned to an intervention or a placebo group. Then the individuals are examined later to determine if they improved or did not get the disease. The Sars-COV-2 vaccine studies followed this basic pattern. The traditional analyses are driven by the design, but t-test ANOVAs are common when the outcome is continuous. When the outcome is categorical, logistic and multinomial regression are common. RCTs can also include switch overs that are planned or based on if the person gets the disease or does not improve. In Figure 5.9, each participant is randomly assigned to a treatment or placebo group. As the study progresses, some participants are moved from their original randomly assigned group to another group, a cross-over design.

Table 5.5. RCT Two Group Example.

Intervention	Placebo
$RX_{1\,Int}$ $RX_{2\,Int}$ $RX_{3\,Int}$	$RX_{1\,P}$ $RX_{2\,P}$ $RX_{3\,P}$
. . . $RX_{i\,Int}$	. . . $RX_{i\,P}$

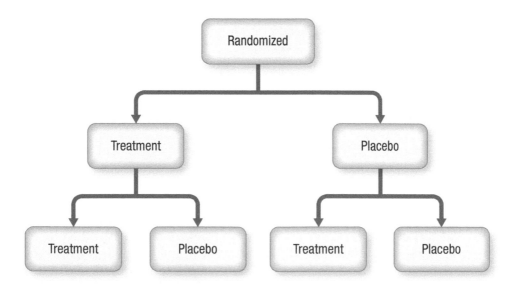

Figure 5.9. RCT Design With Cross-Over.

For example, a participant could begin in the placebo group and then be randomly assigned to the treatment group after a specified period of time. In other designs, a placebo participant might be moved to the treatment group if the participant becomes ill and needs the experimental treatment. Finally, factorial designs are common in RCTs because of the ability to manipulate multiple variables, examine interactions, and make specific claims with the results.

In addition to the randomization, there is masking. A single-masked (blinded) study means the participant does not know which group they are assigned to. In a double masked study, the participant and the researchers do not know. Double-blinded RCTs are a very powerful way to understand the effects of treatments and interventions. Masking is included in research design to decrease the potential for bias on the part of the participant and the researcher.

Cohort Studies

Cohort studies are based on cohorts of individuals and are an attempt to understand what lead to a disease state. Thus, they tend to follow an exposure → disease argument. The researcher starts with the outcome variable, and then examines multiple variables to determine which ones might be the IVs associated with the outcome. There are two types of cohort studies, existing (retrospective) and prospective. Retrospective cohort studies are examined after individuals have developed the disease, or the DV of interest. For example, heart disease and diet are common topics in retrospective cohort studies (Figure 5.10). The researchers essentially look back in time to try to understand which variables are associated with the outcome variable. They are looking to figure out the exposure status prior to the outcome variable. Thus, the focal questions are similar to "Which variables are associated with Y variable?", such as, "How much red meat consumption is associated with myocardial infarction?"

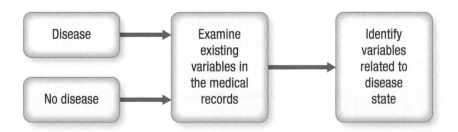

Figure 5.10. Retrospective Cohort.

Prospective cohort studies start with a group of individuals and track them over time. The Nurses' Health Study (Belanger, et al., 1978) is an example of a prospective study where more than 120,000 female nurses were enrolled who were free of cancer and heart disease and then tracked. During the development phase, researchers must carefully decide which variables to collect at the beginning and during the study. Once participants begin to be diagnosed with the disease or outcome variable of interest, then researchers can begin to examine which variables are associated with the disease (Figure 5.11).

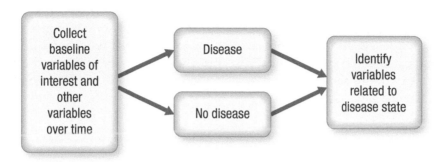

Figure 5.11. Prospective Cohort.

For example, weight change over time could be a variable of interest and then examined to see if it is associated with heart disease. Comparatively, prospective studies are much stronger than retrospective cohort designs. Cohort studies can have a range of analyses associated with them, such as multivariate regression to deal with confounding variables, and using propensity score matching to match participants in the disease and no disease groups.

Case Control

Case-control studies begin with identifying participants with the outcome variable of interest, then identifying control participants, those without the outcome of interest. It is also an exposure -> disease argument model (Figure 5.12). The control participants should be matched. Matching is the process of identifying those without the outcome of interest who are similar on a set of variables, such as age, geographic, location, education, and so on. Matching is not easy and has problems (King & Neilsen, 2019; Mervis & Klein-Tasman, 2004), and therefore is an area where a great deal of reading is needed before implementing it. The control group participants should also be at a similar level of developing the outcome variable of interest, that is, same risk of disease. There can be concerns with overmatching, which can reduce the potential number of participants and make recruitment difficult.

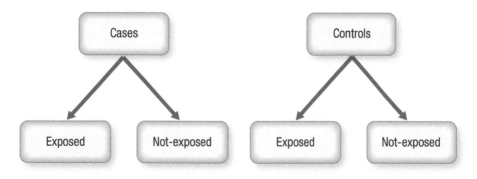

Figure 5.12. Case-Control.

Figure 5.12 displays the cases, those with the outcome variable, controls who were exposed and not exposed to the variable of interest and the controls where were also exposed and not exposed. For example, those who have been diagnosed with a specific cancer and those not diagnosed are compared based on exposure to chemicals in ground water. Odds ratios are used to analyze the data. Incidence rates cannot be used unless it is a full population study with all cases included.

NONEXPERIMENTAL

Nonexperimental designs look the same as experimental, but there is simply no random assignments, that is, in-tact groups. Nonexperimental are also commonly called observational studies. Paired, repeated measures and longitudinal are commonly nonexperimental, which was evident with the lack of randomization previously discussed. By far the most common nonexperimental designs come from surveys. Surveys are used to collect a large amount of data typically at a single point in time. The IV(s) from surveys are a wide range from demographic values (e.g., education level) to psychological constructs. The same for the DVs. The focal questions generally are phrased as "How much of an association is there between variable X and variable Y?" Other questions related to differences (e.g., independent group) are also possible. Thus, survey data is quite flexible. The data collected generally include many variables across multiple surveys. The presentation of the surveys should be counterbalanced (Figure 5.13) as part of the design. Counterbalancing helps to alleviate concerns of items from one survey affecting the responses of later surveys. In Figure 5.13, there are three surveys, thus there are six patterns. The pattern a participant receives can be randomized, but it is not as common, and this randomization is not the same as an experiment where a variable is manipulated. Research organizations, such as Pew, do conduct experiments with counterbalancing of items and wording on a survey, but these are explicitly completed as experiments. Many studies still fail to counterbalance, and this should not be the case. With the advent of easy-to-use online survey systems, counterbalancing is very easy to complete. The analyses commonly associated with surveys are correlation and regression, though depending on the data, independent t-tests, and other analyses are possible.

G1 O Survey 1   O Survey 2   O Survey 3

G2 O Survey 1   O Survey 3   O Survey 2

G3 O Survey 2   O Survey 1   O Survey 3

G4 O Survey 2   O Survey 3   O Survey 1

G5 O Survey 3   O Survey 1   O Survey 2

G6 O Survey 3   O Survey 2   O Survey 1

Figure 5.13. Counterbalancing Design Example.

DESIGN LIMITATIONS

There is not enough discussion of design limitations. We believe they should be integrated into the discussion and not separate sections. For example, the differences between the two experimental groups were 300 calories burned, but this is limited by potential external validity effects because this was a convenience sample. We provide the types of limitations along with discussion of each below. Table 5.6 provides a design by limitation reference sheet. These limitations create problems in determining, and arguing for, why the results occurred.

Table 5.6. Designs, Analysis, and Limitations.

Name	ROX Setup	Typical Analysis	Threats	Potential Threat	Controlled
One Group Post-test-Only	*X O*	*Measures of Central Tendency and Variability*	HI, SEL, MAT,SX	SR, INST, ATT, EE TR, SE	
One Group Pre-test-Post-test	*G O X O*	*Paired (Dependent) t-test*	HI, PRE, MAT, TX, SX	ST, INST, EE,TR,SE, SC, RA	
Nonequiv. Group Post-test Only	*G1 X O* *G2 O*	*Independent t-test*	SEL	EVERY-THING BUT PRE-TEST-ING	
Nonequiv Groups Alternate Treatment Post-test Only	*G1 X_1 O* *G2 X_2 O*	*Independent t-test*	WITHIN GROUP HI, ATT,	SR, INST, MAT, DOT, EE, SE, TR	
Post-test Only Control Group	*R X_E O* *R X_C O*	**ANOVA/ Independent t-test**		HIS, INST, ATT, DOT, EE, TR, SE, SC	SEL, MAT
Pre-test-Post-test Control Group Design	*R O X_E O* *R O X_C O*	**ANCOVA or one-within/one between (repeated measure)**		ATT, DOT, EE, TR, SE, SC	HI, INST, SEL, SR, PRE, MAT
Pre-test-Post-test Control/ Comparison Group	*R O X_{E1} O* *R O X_{E2} O* *R O X_{E3} O* *R O X_C O*	**ANCOVA or ANOVA with one-between (repeated measure)**		HI, INST, ATT, DOT, EE, TR, SE, SC	SEL, SR, PRE, MAT
Solomon Four Group	*R G1 O X O* *R G2 O* *R G3 X O* *R G3 O*	ANOVA or ANCOVA		HI, MAT ATT, DOT	Protects against the remaining threats
Nonequivalent Groups Pre-test Post-test Design	G1 O X_E O G2 O X_C O	ANCOVA Or One-Within/ One Between (Repeated Measure)	SEL, MAT	HI, SR, INST, ATT, DOT, EE TR, SE, SC	

(continued)

Table 5.6. Designs, Analysis, and Limitations *(continued)*.

Name	ROX Setup	Typical Analysis	Threats	Potential Threat	Controlled
Nonequivalent Groups Pre-test-Post-test Comparison	G1 O X_{E1} O G2 O X_{E2} O G3 O X_{E3} O	ANCOVA Or ANOVA With One-Between (Repeated Measure) Three Levels	SEL, MAT	HI, SR, INST, ATT, DOT, EE TR, SE, SC	
Single Group Time Series Also ABA or ABAB	G OOO-XOOOO	Averaged Dependent t-Test	H,	SEL, PRE, INST, ATT, TR, SE, SC	SR, MAT, EE
Single Group Time With Control	G1 OOO-X_EOOO G2 OOO-X_COOO	Averaged Dependent t-Test		SEL, INST, ATT, TR, SE, SC, EE, SC	HI, SR, PRE, MAT

ATT = attrition; DOT = diffusion of treatment; EE = experimenter effect; HI = history; INST = instrumentation; MAT = maturation; MT = Multiple Treatments; PRE = pre-testing; RE = reactive; SC = statistical conclusion; SE = subject effects; SEL = selection; SR = statistical regression; SX = selection interaction; TR = treatment replication; TX = testing interaction.

Source: Adapted from Schreiber, J. B., & Asner-Self, K. K. (2010). *Educational research.* John Wiley and Sons.

Internal Validity

Internal validity threats are concerns within the study, such as participants leaving, which can lead to a problem with the quality of the arguments being made based on the data collected. These threats fall into seven major categories. The names of the threats are based on these concerns. Campbell and Stanley (1963) sometimes merged these with more common phrasing (Schreiber & Asner-Self, 2010).

Historical Effects: These are unplanned events that happen while the study is ongoing. For example, during an online experiment conducted recently by colleagues the server hosting the experiment for one of the groups crashed and then started back up and the participants continued. But this is now a historical effect that can affect the results and the interpretation of those results.

Maturation: Maturation concerns are based on the natural developmental changes that occurs over time. The longer the study, the higher the probability of a maturation effect. Studies with very young children and longitudinal are most susceptible to this validity problem. It is important for the researcher to demonstrate that maturation is not the main cause of the change.

Testing Effects: Testing effects occur when the participant has experience with the instrument or activity. Students who have previous clinical experience not associated with the program appear to perform much better than students who are in clinical rotations for the first time.

Instrumentation Threats: Instrumentation threats occur because of mistakes or other inconsistencies with the data collection method. This can occur with the instrument (e.g., survey) being used such as typographical errors, interviewer, observer, or evaluator change. If raters are not using the instrument in the same way, scores will vary due to rater differences and not actual participant differences.

Regression to the Mean: The regression to the mean phenomenon demonstrates that individuals who score on the outer extremes (either very high or very low) of the score continuum will naturally score closer to the mean when retested.

Mortality: For some studies, mortality does indicate the death of participants. For the vast majority of social science research, mortality happens when participants leave the study formally or simply never return. Participant departure or drop-out can affect the results and lead to incorrect inferences.

Selection Threats: The previous internal validity threats are considered single-group threats because the focus is on the sample group of interest. Multiple-group designs (e.g., experimental and control group) have the same threats as single groups. Selection threats occur when problems occur with the comparison group due to problems with the sampling process. The problem becomes a rival hypothesis. There are five selection threats:

Selection-history occurs when one group experiences a related event that the other group or groups do not. For example, one group of nurses in a new procedure experiment experience a large number of patients and use the new procedure and the remaining groups in the study do not have that experience. This is a common occurrence in in-situ research.

Selection-maturation occurs when one group matures faster than the other. This is most common in studies with children but can occur in any study.

Selection-testing occurs when one group has previously taken the instrument or completed the activity. Control groups, by definition, should not be exposed to the intervention or treatment, but often are or are told by people in the experimental group about it. Subsequently, the control groups can be observed to outperform the experimental groups.

Selection-mortality occurs when one group of participants leaves the study at a higher rate compared to other groups. This is a more specific version of mortality. For example, appropriate inferences can be compromised when specific sub-groups leave the study (e.g., transfemale participants). This concern also arises during the data examination or cleaning phase. Thus, the researcher must examine the demographics and response patterns of participants who stay, leave, and are removed from the data set during cleaning.

Selection-regression occurs when one group has a larger proportion of very high or very low scorers. One group of nursing students began with lower clinical skills scores than a second group. When examining a postintervention skill, the first group had much higher gains in clinical skills compared to the first because they started off lower and had more room to improve.

Internal Social Effects

We are social creatures who want to interact with each other. As social creatures, there are sometimes interactions during the actual experiment or study. Social creatures interact during experiments. How the researchers interact with the participants can make a difference in behaviors. A correct inference problem occurs because of this. And inferences to the larger population are no longer possible because of the social effects.

Diffusion or Imitation of Treatment: If participants (and sometimes those running the study) have knowledge of the study's purpose, or the expected difference in treatment, it can lead to a diffusion or imitation of treatment. Take two groups of participants who are receiving two different treatments. The first group is getting a medication for lower leg pain, and the second is getting the medication and a leg massage once a week. Participants in the first group hear about what the second group is getting and decide to get leg massages on their own. This is a diffusion of treatment. This can also be considered a historical event in the study.

Compensatory Rivalry or the John Henry Effect: This effect occurs when the control group attempts to outperform the experimental group. It is based on the story of John Henry attempting to lay railroad track faster than a machine. This is one of the reasons placebos are used so that everyone knows they are in the study, just not which group.

Resentful Demoralization: This is the reverse of the compensatory rivalry. It happens when the control group tries to perform even worse. The later differences between the groups are exacerbated and inferences are made that the intervention worked. This is incorrect because the large difference is due to the changes in behavior of the control group.

Compensatory Equalization of Treatment: This problem occurs when those running the study have outside individuals ask for the same treatment that the experimental group is getting or some other bonus. They are trying to equalize the groups. This occurs a great deal in applied educational settings when parents get involved.

Novelty: Simply, people behave differently when they are in a study. Therefore, the treatment may look effective because it is a novelty and not because it is better than other treatments or no treatment. To deal with this situation, one should conduct the study over a longer period of time, so this effect can wear off.

External Validity

External validity (aka generalizability) relates to the inferences made to the larger population of interest based on the sample in the study. A major goal of a quantitative study is to make inferences from the sample to the population.

Selection Treatment: Random assignment does not always lead to external validity. Biases in the sampling process can interact with the experimental variables. Convenient random sampling occurs quite commonly where a convenience sample, those the researcher has easy access to, are randomly assigned to experimental groups. This is how most studies that use undergraduate research study pools work. The convenience sample may or may not represent the whole population of interest and may interact with the experimental variable differently than the rest of the population. Thus, it reduces the quality of the inferences made from the results.

Pre-test Treatment Interaction: Pre-test treatment interaction happens when the pre-test activities essentially tell the participants what the study is looking for. This then affects their behavior, which, in turn, affects the post-test behaviors. If the activities of the study are very unique, it is more likely this effect will be seen.

Multiple Treatment: When multiple treatments or interventions are used, one treatment can interfere, positively or negatively, with the other treatments. This is solved by counterbalancing the treatments and testing for this problem.

Reactive or Participant Effects: This is similar to novelty but is more general and is termed the Hawthorne Effect. A study at the Hawthorne Works plant of the Western Electric was being conducted related to productivity and light intensity. The higher the light intensity, the better the production and vice versa. The researchers came to understand that it was not the light, but the observation of the workers that was affecting productivity. We simply behave differently when we are being watched. This is also why reality TV is not reality.

Specificity of Your Variables: Chapter 2 discusses measurement issues, and this is a measurement issue. The variables of interest have to be clearly specified otherwise the inferences made from the results are useless. Additionally, the researcher needs to clearly detail data collection procedures for replication purposes.

Experimenter Effects (Rosenthal): Researchers are their own limitation because they can consciously, or unconsciously, affect the results through how they engage with the participants. Relatedly, the researcher's gender, age, race, or outgoingness, and so on can change the behavior of the participants. This why some studies are double-blinded or a third party does the scoring or coding of the data.

Ecological Validity

Ecological validity is simply how real the material or context is in the experiment. The specificity of variables, multiple treatments, pre-test effect, and any Hawthorne effect can also be considered an ecological validity problem. Jim was involved in a long history of experiments on graphical displays and related text studies in order to understand cognitive processes. After many years of these studies, the group ran a series of studies that were more life-like, which was similar to what students see in textbooks. The final results supported the previous basic research work and were needed because the original experiments suffered from an ecological validity problem.

Statistical Validity

Statistical validity is simply using the most appropriate statistical analysis in relation to the research question, design, and data (and type of data). The non-alignment of these in studies remains a constant problem. This requirement seems obvious when one reads it, but it is a common mistake.

QUALITY IMPROVEMENT

Quality improvement projects (QI) are not a traditional research design, though some of the methods and analyses are sometimes the same. There are a range of methods for QI (Boaden et al., 2008; Health Foundation, 2013). There is the Model for Improvement, which is planning, doing, studying, and acting (**PDSA cycles**) and **lean** (aka, Toyota Production System). Two other methods are the Clinical Microsystems and Experience-Based Co-Design. A great deal of the quality improvement's use and growth can be attributed to individuals such as Shewhart (1950) or Deming (1982). We provide very brief descriptions of the methods below.

The PDSA cycles are centered around three core questions (Institute for Health Science, 2021; Langley et al., 2009):

- What are we trying to accomplish? (What are our goals and objectives?)

- How will we decide if the change is an improvement? (What do we mean by improvement?)

- What changes can we make that would lead to this improvement?

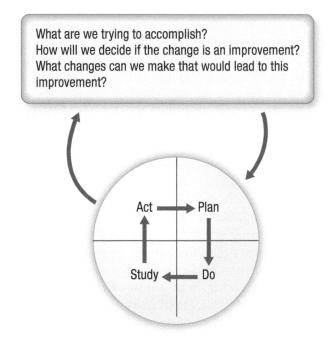

Figure 5.14. PDSA Cycle With Core Questions.

These questions feed into the PDSA cycle (Figure 5.14). Every PDSA cycle will include an abductive reasoning process where hunches and ideas are provided by team members that will build a knowledge base or schema for the situation. This knowledge base then can be used for informing action. The PDSA cycle is an ongoing process.

Lean in healthcare settings focuses on the patient and that the patient is central to all activities (Smith et al., 2020). Lean uses a five-part process:

1. Define what is value-added to the patient.
2. Map the pathways that deliver care.
3. Make the value streams more efficient through the removal of waste, duplication, and delay.
4. Let patients pull resources (e.g., staff) toward them so their care is central and needs are met.
5. Pursuing perfection as a continual goal.

Clinical microsystems are based on small groups of people who focus on specific groups of patients regularly (Godfrey et al., 2010). The quality of care along with safety is determined by what is occurring in each microsystem for this method. The model focuses on the 5 Ps: patients, people, patterns, processes, and purpose. Through assessing the 5 Ps, improvement areas can be identified.

Experience-based co-design was developed for the National Health System in the United Kingdom. The focus is on data from interviews with patients where emotional important touch points are identified. Videos and other information from the patient experience interviews are then shown to staff. Once that information is shared, staff and patients come together in small groups to work on improvements.

Regardless of method, there are issues with implementing QI, we discuss a few (Dixon-Woods et al., 2012). The first and foremost is convincing peers there is actually a problem. There will be peers that do not see the issue being raised as a problem. Intertwined with that is the issue that what is being identified is a problem versus a symptom. One way to view this is as an area of concern (Schreiber et al., 2007). An **area of concern** is not yet the potential problem, for example, central-line-associated blood stream infection (CLABSi) rates in a hospital. The rate is not the problem, it is an area of concern, and a **symptom** of a potential problem, such as not following protocol or lack of training. Other areas to examine are the data and the monitoring system. These need to be considered together. The data are what has been decided to be measured. We think it can all be measured in some way, but some data are easier than others to capture. And someone or some team has to be monitoring the data as it comes in and making sure that it does come in. Relatedly, there needs to be multiple measures captured in a reasonable time frame. The data should also be plotted over time in a traditional run chart. **Figure 5.15** is a run chart of simulated data for CLABSi rates over time with different events occurring. You will notice that this is essentially a longitudinal design.

Focusing the project on the correct amount of time needed is another area of concern. Too short, and no improvement will be seen, which is common in one-off training sessions. Too long, and the change will never become practice. The leadership team must also be supportive of the project and side effects, or downside risks should be discussed along the way. A **downside risk** is an unexpected result of the change. Jim once worked for a company that used pure

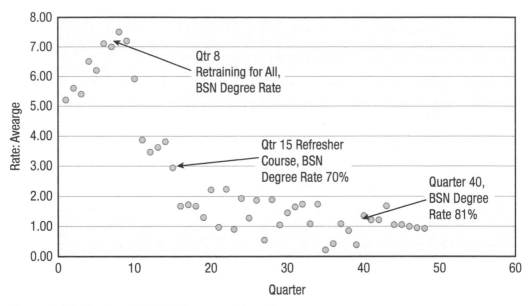

Figure 5.15. Simulated CLABSi Rates in a Run Chart.

virgin aluminum. Purchasing was charged with being more efficient and reducing costs, which they did. When the aluminum from a new supplier arrived at the plants it jammed all the fabricating machines and caused a massive backlog of product orders, which then affected sales, and quarterly bonuses for sales representatives. Finally, QIs are complex systems with many individuals and parts and it can take time to put it all together and make a sustained change in an organization.

SAMPLING AND ERROR

This is a good moment to discuss, again, sampling and error. Error is simply not discussed enough. This is important because during the design phase, researchers need to deal with these issues and not wait until the data are collected. First, there is sampling error. These occur when the sample from a study does not fully represent the population of interest. The values obtained from the sample are estimates, and when the sample is not fully representative of the population the estimates are incorrect—maybe too high or too low.

Sampling error leads into the second error, standard error. Standard error, which we detail in later chapters, is the estimate of how far a calculated value, for example, sample mean value, is from the population mean. Due to the calculation, the larger the sample size, the smaller the standard error estimate. The standard error is only an estimate because if the researcher has a large sample, but the sample is predominantly from the lower end of the distribution (Chapter 3), the standard error value may not be large enough to estimate the difference between the sample mean and the population mean.

Sampling and standard error are also related to power versus accuracy. Power is based on trying to get to $p < 0.05$. The ultimate goal is to make sure the researcher has enough power (sample size) to show "statistical significance." This again, is not the best way to think about science. Accuracy, that is precision, with sample size is focused on how close the researcher wants to be to the population value and at what confidence level (Trafimow & McDonald, 2017). For example, if the researcher wants to be 95% confident that they are within 0.1 standard deviation (precision) of the mean for a two-group independent design (two means) 500 participants are needed (Trafimow & McDonald, 2017). If the researcher is willing to be less confident, 85%, the sample size need drops to 300, and at 75% it is 225. Changing the precision to 0.3 standard deviations, a two-group design with 95% confidence of the means, the sample size is less than 100. But 0.3 standard deviations is not very precise.

Accuracy also applies to the actual measures, a third source of error, as discussed in Chapter 2. Lower reliability adds error into the analysis and inferences. Now, couple that with lack of precision based on sample size, and the amount of error in the results can become quite large. Risk is also related to this. As the risk level of the study increases, accuracy across all aspects of the design becomes important. This is why clinical trials have to have very large sample sizes that represent the population. We believe researchers need to spend more time focusing on error and accuracy and less time on power to reach 0.05.

CAUSALITY (AND BACK TO ARGUMENTATION)

Researchers want to be able to make causal claims that generalize to the larger population based on their study results, and thus their study designs. These claims are arguments (Abelson, 2012) and the ability to do that is affected by the quality of the design and the reducing the limitations of designs. Based on the number of potential and actual design limitations previously discussed, this can be difficult. Replications with representative samples help increase the causality argumentation, along with larger sample sizes. If the researcher wants to make causal claims, very accurate measures, precision on sample size, and a strong design that allow for the claims are needed. We will end this with one caveat. There are areas we have worked in, for example, apraxia, where large sample sizes are not possible. But the sample sizes we use are large in comparison with the actual population size.

SUMMARY

This chapter discussed experimental and nonexperimental designs. Core examples were provided, but design is a creative area where the possibilities are quite open. For example, a researcher may want 4 raters, with a 2x2 factorial design with three repeated measures. This becomes a 4x2x2x3, technically. It is also quite a complicated design. The analysis possibilities are also open a bit, because the researcher could use the four raters as a factor or a covariate or simply use an average of their scores. Each design has strengths and limitations and those need to be carefully considered during the development stage of the study. Quality improvement is a subsection of design with different goals and its own models, yet the methods sometimes overlap with traditional research design and statistical analysis. Finally, we rediscussed error and causality because the topics do not get enough attention in research design and statistical analysis.

END-OF-CHAPTER RESOURCES

REVIEW QUESTIONS

Answers and rationales for the review questions are located in the Appendix at the end of the book.

1. You are deciding between designing an experimental study and a quasi-experimental study. What are the features of these two designs that overlap? What feature distinguishes an experimental design from a quasi-experimental design?

2. Discuss the difference between random assignment (i.e., randomization to groups) and random selection.

3. TRUE or FALSE?

   A quasi-experimental design is stronger than an experimental design.

4. TRUE or FALSE?

   In factorial designs, there is more than one IV being manipulated, and one of the research questions is interested in whether there is an interaction between the IVs.

5. TRUE or FALSE?

   In a cross-over design, all participants eventually receive all the treatment conditions.

6. TRUE or FALSE?

   In a double-blinded randomized controlled trial, only the participants do not know to which study group they have been assigned.

7. The Nurses' Health Study, which follows a group of individuals over time to investigate the factors associated with developing heart disease, is an example of which of the following designs?

   a. case control

   b. randomized controlled trial

   c. prospective cohort

   d. retrospective cohort

8. A researcher is conducting a study to examine the effect of an educational intervention among school age children on fruit and vegetable intake in a local school district. If one of the elementary schools launches its own "healthy eating campaign" at the same time the intervention is being delivered to several schools, this is an example of which type of threat to internal validity?

9. A nonexperimental design is used in the form of a survey to determine the number of recruitment strategies that are associated with the highest enrollment in the Medicare Diabetes Prevention Program by eligible older adults. The researcher also collects information about the number of older adults enrolled. Which of the following is an appropriate statistical analysis for this study?

   a. correlation

   b. Chi-square

   c. factor analysis

   d. t-test

10. Which of the following is an example of the internal threat to validity known as compensatory rivalry?

    a. Participants in the intervention group share the new treatment they are receiving for osteoporosis with the comparison group taking an NSAID.

    b. Participants in the group receiving the standard of care for heart failure treatment try to do better on their exercise tolerance test than the group receiving the new cardiac rehab therapy protocol.

    c. Participants in a 24-month trial of a new therapy for Parkinson's disease drop out of the study because they think the treatment is not working.

    d. Participant scores on cognitive function that are very high at baseline will naturally move closer to the average score when retested 6 months later.

11. Trained observers for a study on adherence to handwashing protocols note that most healthcare workers they observe are closely following the steps of the procedures described in the handwashing protocol. This is an example of which threat to external validity?

    a. experimental effects

    b. reactive (Hawthorne) effect

    c. multiple treatment

    d. novelty

12. Select all that apply: Which of the following is an example of a contributing source of error in a study on functional mobility among adults aged 65 and older?

    a. the tool used to measure mobility has questionable reliability

    b. the sample of participants was drawn only from nursing home residents

    c. the standard error of the mean is representative of the population standard error

    d. the sample size of participants is determined by a power analysis focused on precision

---

A robust set of instructor resources designed to supplement this text is located at http://connect.springerpub.com/content/book/978-0-8261-6582-4. Qualifying instructors may request access by emailing **textbook@springerpub.com.**

REFERENCES

Abelson, R. P. (2012). *Statistics as principled argument*. Psychology Press.

Belanger, C. F., Hennekens, C. H., Rosner, B., & Speizer, F. E. (1978). The nurses' health study. *American Journal of Nursing, 78*(6), 1039-1040.

Boaden, R., Harvey, G., Moxham, C., & Proudlove, N. (2008). *Quality improvement: Theory and practice in healthcare*. NHS Institute for Innovation and Improvement. https://www.england.nhs.uk/improvement-hub/publication/quality-improvement-theory-practice-in-healthcare/

Campbell, D. T., & Stanley, J. C. (1963). *Experimental and quasi-experimental designs for research*. Houghton-Mifflin.

Cook, T. D., Campbell, D. T., & Shadish, W. (2002). *Experimental and quasi-experimental designs for generalized causal inference*. Houghton Mifflin.

Deming, W. E. (1982). *Quality, productivity, and competitive position*. Massachusetts Institute of Technology.

Dixon-Woods, M., McNicol, S., & Martin, G. (2012). *Overcoming challenges to improving quality*. Health Foundation.

Ferguson, G. A., & Takane, Y. (1989). *Statistical analysis in psychology and education* (6th ed.). McGraw-Hill.

Godfrey, M., Nelson, D., & Batalden, P. (2010). *Supporting microsystems. Assessing, diagnosing and treating your microsystem.* http://clinicalmicrosystem.org/knowledge-center/workbooks

Gordis, L. (2004). *Epidemiology* (5th ed.). Elsevier.

The Health Foundation. (2013). *Quality Improvement made simple: What everyone should know about quality improvement.* The Health Foundation. https://www.health.org.uk/publication/quality-improvement-made-simple

Henry, G. T. (1990). *Practical sampling.* SAGE Publications.

Herman, P., Yosuke, Y., Hiroyuki, S., Philip, A., Lene, A., Anderson, L., Arab, L., Baddou, I., Bedu-Addo, K., Blaak, E., Blanc, S., Bonomi, A. G., Bouten, C. V. C., Bovet, P., Buchowski, M. S., Butte, N. F., Camps, S., Close, G., Cooper, J. A., … Speakman, J. (2021). Daily energy expenditure through the human life course. *Science, American Association for the Advancement of Science, 373*(6556), 808–812. https://doi.org/10.1126/science.abe5017

Hess, I. (1985). *Sampling for the social research surveys 1947–1980.* University of Michigan.

Institute for Health Science. (2021). *How to improve.* http://www.ihi.org/resources/Pages/HowtoImprove/default.aspx

Jolliffe, D., Farrington, D. P., Brunton-Smith, I., Loeber, R., Ahonen, L., & Palacios, A. P. (2019). Depression, anxiety and delinquency: Results from the Pittsburgh Youth Study. *Journal of Criminal Justice, 62,* 42–49. https://doi.org/10.1016/j.jcrimjus.2018.08.004

King, G., & Nielsen, R. (2019). Why propensity scores should not be used for matching. *Political Analysis, 27*(4), 435–454. https://doi.org/10.1017/pan.2019.11

Kirk, R. E. (2013). *Experimental design: procedures for the behavioral sciences* (4th ed.). SAGE Publications.

Langley, G. L., Moen, R., Nolan, K. M., Nolan, T. W., Norman, C. L., & Provost, L. P. (2009). *The improvement guide: A practical approach to enhancing organizational performance* (2nd ed.). Jossey-Bass Publishers.

Mervis, C. B., & Klein-Tasman, B. P. (2004). Methodological issues in group-matching designs: α levels for control variable comparisons and measurement characteristics of control and target variables. *Journal of Autism and Developmental Disorders, 34*(1), 7–17. https://doi.org/10.1023/B:JADD.0000018069.69562.b8

Schreiber, J. B., & Asner-Self, K. K. (2010). *Educational research.* John Wiley and Sons.

Schreiber, J. B., Moss, C. M., & Staab, J. M. (2007). A preliminary examination of a theoretical model for researching educator beliefs. *Semiotica, 164,* 153–172. https://doi.org/10.1515/SEM.2007.023

Shewhart, W. A. (1950, December). *Statistical control* [Paper presented]. American Statistical Association and Institute of Mathematical Sciences, Chicago.

Smith, I., Hicks. C., & McGovern, T. (2020). Adapting Lean methods to facilitate stakeholder engagement and co-design in healthcare. *BMJ, 368,* m35. https://doi.org/10.1136/bmj.m35

Tabachnick, B. G., & Fidel, L. S. (2001). *Using multivariate statistics.* Allyn & Bacon.

Tabachnick, B. G., & Fidell, L. S. (2007). *Experimental designs using ANOVA.* Thomson/Brooks/Cole.

Trafimow, D., & MacDonald, J. A. (2017). Performing inferential statistics prior to data collection. *Educational and Psychological Measurement, 77*(2), 204–219. https://doi.org/10.1177/0013164416659745

CHAPTER 6

Variability Between and Within Groups

CORE OBJECTIVES

- Define and describe variability between and within groups
- Create research questions for independent and dependent *t*-tests, and One-Way ANOVA analyses
- Explain results from independent and dependent *t*-tests, and One-Way ANOVA analyses
- Explain sums of squares, degrees of freedom, mean square error, and effect sizes
- Explain a priori and post hoc analyses for One-Way ANOVA
- Explain options for nonparametric analysis
- Explain assumptions for each analysis

INTRODUCTION: UNDERSTANDING VARIABILITY

Variability, as stated in Chapter 3, is the difference in values a variable can take. If a variable can only have one value, there is nothing to examine or understand (Kirk, 2013). A test score that can range from 0 to 100 and has observed scores from 10 to 96 has a good deal of variability. If the observed scores range from 80 to 90, it has much smaller variability. Researchers want to understand this variability. One path to understanding variability is to examine the observed scores of two different groups on a variable of interest, such as academic motivation. Researchers might also want to examine differences in academic motivation over time for a group of people to see how much change occurs. In Figure 6.1, there are two distributions of two normally distributed variables. Variable one, in green, has a lower mean value (about 40) and smaller variability, the values are much closer to the mean, a smaller range. This distribution, therefore, has less variability within the group. Variable two, in orange, has a higher mean (about 50) and a much larger variability, the values spread out away from the mean. Therefore, it has a larger range and more variability within the group. The distributions overlap—not much distance between the means—and therefore have little *between group variability* (Tukey, 1986).

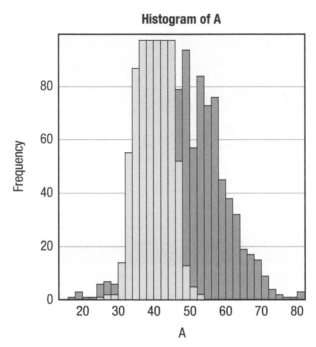

Figure 6.1. Two Distributions With Different Means and Variability.

How Much Focus

Focusing "how much" variability centers understanding on the distributions of the observed variable and the mean values of each distribution. **Figure 6.2**, like **Figure 6.1**, depicts two groups, with the distribution of scores for each group and an indicator of how far apart the mean scores are between the two groups. This difference is the separation of the mean values for each distribution. Then, we have the *within variability* for each group (green and orange) and *between variability* (red). The within variability, the variance, is commonly described with the standard deviation: the "how much" of the spread of scores. Focusing on how much allows one to spend more time examining the distribution—the within and between variances—and location of the means. This also helps one to better understand the data and explain it to others.

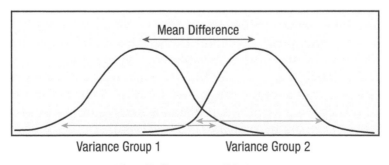

Figure 6.2. Two Distribution by Mean Difference and Variance.

PURPOSE AND QUESTION FOCUS

The purpose of between and within two group analyses is to examine how much variation, or difference, groups have on an observed variable (between group) and how much variation the observed scores have within each group. The first three analyses associated with between and within differences are independent t-test, dependent t-test, and One-Way ANOVA. **Independent t-tests** examine differences *between groups*, and **dependent t-tests** examine change *within one group*. **One-Way ANOVA** extends the independent groups when there are more than two groups (Ferguson & Takane, 1989; Kirk, 2013). The questions, as discussed in Chapter 5, focus on how much, such as:

■ Independent t-test: How much difference is there between nursing students and physician assistant (PA) students on academic related stress?
  ● The independent variable is healthcare group-nursing and PA students. The dependent variable is academic related stress.
■ Paired/Dependent t-test: How much does academic stress lower after mental health intervention for nursing students?
  ● The independent variable is time (pre-post intervention). The dependent is academic stress.
■ One-Way ANOVA: How much difference is there between traditional Bachelor of Science in Nursing (BSN), second degree BSN, and PA students on academic related stress?
  ● The independent variable is study degree type. The dependent variable is academic related stress.

A reminder, the questions should focus on how much of a difference and not just that a difference exists. Too many research articles have only focused on *if* there is a difference and not *how much* and if it is meaningful or actionable (Greenland, 2019; Greenland et al., 2016; Meehl, 1954; Schreiber, 2019; Ziliak & McCloskey, 2008).

Designs Associated With Two Group Analyses

The design of studies for the independent t-test can be experimental or nonexperimental. Experimental designs may have an experimental and control group or two different experimental groups (e.g., different dosages of medicine). Nonexperimental designs might have two in-tact or existing groups (e.g., students in two sections of a simulation course) or naturally occurring groups such as children and adults. This is common in large data surveys which have naturally occurring groups that often employ independent t-tests for analyses. Paired t-tests are non-experimental (sometimes quasi-experimental) because there is one set of participants of cases and, therefore, cannot be randomly assigned to different groups.

GRAPHICAL AND CONCEPTUAL REPRESENTATIONS

This next section provides a foundation of each analysis in this chapter. Conceptual and graphical representations are provided by analysis. We feel it is important to have a solid conceptual grasp of what is actually occurring in these analyses before seeing technical information. Additionally, we believe if you truly understand a topic, you can draw it.

Independent *t*-Test

The **independent *t*-tests** in **Figure 6.3** show three different examples of "how much" difference and are focused on ***between group*** differences, but a major component in the calculation is the error (Student, 1908). Each figure displays the histogram of the data along with a smoothed curved line to highlight the shape of the distribution. **Figure 6.3A** highlights two groups that are not very different, the means are close together (peak of the distribution) and the distributions overlap a great deal. Now, looking at this, one might say, "there is not much difference here." This observation would be correct, yet one of the historical problems in statistical analysis is, if the sample size was large enough, this small difference would have been considered "statistically significant" with $p < 0.05$. It must be noted that for some fields of research, a small difference such as this, would be considered very important and meaningful. **Figure 6.3B**, has a difference that most researchers would be quite happy with, but there is still a great deal of overlap between the distributions.

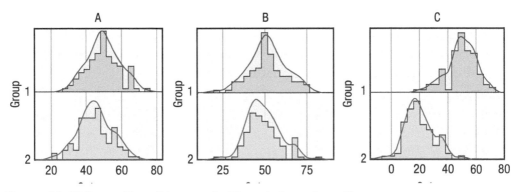

Figure 6.3. Different Mean Distances for Three Independent *t*-Tests.

Figure 6.3C shows a very large difference between the means of two groups. Additionally, the amount of within group variability can affect the results. If the amount of variability is reduced, not much overlap but the means stay the same in **Figure 6.3C**, the "how much" would be larger because there is little overlap of the distributions.

For researchers, **Figure 6.3C** would be quite exciting because it shows a large difference between groups, and there is not much overlap of the two distributions. For example, if this was a drug trial where one group received a placebo and one group received the actual drug and the outcome was number of days until feeling better, the lack of overlap indicates the drug works very well compared to the placebo because there is not much overlap. For *t*-tests, the best-case scenario for a result is two groups whose distributions are far apart; no overlap of the distributions and means far apart. Therefore, it is very important to examine, graphically, the distributions of the groups at the same time (i.e., on the same graph).

Paired *t*-Test

The **paired *t*-test**, also known as **dependent *t*-test**, is used for studies that are interested in how much change over time of a single set of participants or cases. This can also be termed a **within-group difference analysis** or a **repeated measure analysis**. This analysis is very common for pre-test and post-test studies, though that is not necessary; the key attribute is the scores are dependent or connected in some manner. For example, scores on a survey completed by a couple would be dependent because there is a relationship between the people and thus the scores. For **Figure 6.3A**, instead of being two groups, *change* the focus to time one and time two. Therefore, in **Figure 6.3A**, the change over time is small and **Figure 6.3B** shows a larger change. Finally, **Figure 6.3C** shows a very large change from time one to time to time two. Paired and independent *t*-tests both focus on the overlap and difference of two distribution of values, but independent have two groups that are not related, and paired *t*-tests have one set of participants, two times.

One-Way ANOVA

The **One-Way ANOVA** in Figures 6.4A and 6.4B show two different examples of "how much" difference and is focused on *between group* differences. **Figure 6.4A** highlights three groups of students, different programs, that are not very different, the means are close together and the distributions overlap a great deal. As with the independent t-test example one might say,

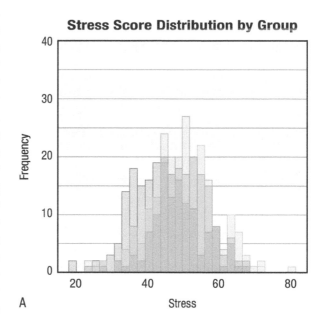

A

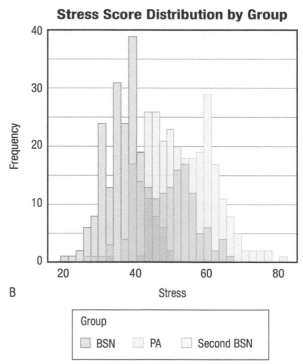

B

Figure 6.4. Two Different Amounts of Distribution Overlap.

"there is not much difference here." Again, this observation would be correct, and again with this sample size (600 total) and the *p*-value would be less than 0.05. And to repeat, for some fields of research, a small difference such as this, would be considered very important and meaningful. **Figure 6.4B**, has a difference that most researchers would be quite happy with, but there is still a great deal of overlap between the distributions.

TECHNICAL SECTION

There are several assumptions that should be tested and other technical pieces of information that should be included in addition to the core information just discussed. Independent and paired *t*-tests are considered **parametric** tests because the data are assumed to be continuous and normally distributed. As a reminder, a variable that is normally distributed will look symmetrical on both sides of the mean (i.e., bell-shaped curve, see Chapter 3). For the paired *t*-test, a histogram of the difference of the two scores is needed. Data should always be graphically displayed so that one can see what is occurring. There are statistical tests that can be used to examine normality. The testing of normality of the distribution is commonly completed with the **Shapiro-Wilk** or **Kolmogorov-Smirnov**. There is one main caveat about both of these tests. The first is, as sample sizes increase and there is even a small deviation from normality (e.g., mean > median), the result will indicate nonnormality. If the sample size is small, under 50, the Shapiro-Wilk (SW) is better than the Komogorov-Smirnov (KS), because it has better power to detect nonnormality. In the previous independent *t*-test example, the KS value was 0.05, *p* = 0.864. When testing for normality, the general rule is to have a *p*-value over 0.05. But, values close and still greater than 0.05 indicate a need to examine the data more closely. With these values, we can assume normality. We can also look at a Q-Q (Quantiles) plot and see if the data fall along a 45 degree line. In our example, the Q-Q plot looks quite good (**Figure 6.5**) with just one value (bottom left) that appears to be a little bit away from the 45 degree line. In reality, as the sample size increases past 50 for these analyses, nonnormality becomes less of an issue with *t*-tests. In statistical terms, this is called "robustness of the test." If the distribution is determined to be nonnormal, the data can be transformed (Chapter 3) or a different technique can be used, such as Mann-Whitney U (MW)

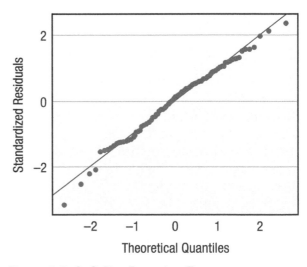

Figure 6.5. Q-Q Plot Example *t*-Test.

(see the nonparametric section later). Finally, the normality of the outcome variable within each group should also be tested.

A second assumption, only for the independent t-test, is the variance is assumed to be equal between the two groups, termed **homogeneity of variance** (Satterthwaite, 1946; Sawilowsky, 2002; Welch, 1938). A quick examination of the standard deviations can provide initial insight into this. If the standard deviations for the two are relatively close, there is typically no problem, and the two variances can be assumed to be equal. In the independent t-test example, the standard deviations are 9.55 and 10.66, which are relatively close. As the standard deviations become farther apart, one is much larger than the other, then the assumption fails. **Homogeneity of variance** is examined with the Levene's test (Levene, 1960). If the test fails, the variances cannot be assumed to be equal. When failure occurs, an adjustment is made to the degrees of freedom, which then adjusts the t-value that is obtained. Most statistical software offers the option of a Welch's test to adjust or automatically provide that information. In our example, Levene's test value was 0.543, $p = 0.50$, indicating that we can assume homogeneity of variance.

The last assumption for independent t-tests is the observations are independent of each other and randomly sampled from the population. This means than each individual score for an individual participant or case is not related to any other participant or case.

For the paired t-test, as stated previously, the main assumption is the difference between the two sets of paired values is normally distributed. By this, we mean that each matched paired score (i.e., pre-test and post-test) is subtracted from each other, and the new values, the difference scores, from the subtraction should be normally distributed. These new scores can be graphed and tested for normality just like the independent t-test.

The t-Value

The **t-value** for an independent t-test, if the variances are equal, is based on this equation:

$$t = \frac{(\bar{x}_1 - \bar{x}_2) - 0}{\sqrt{\dfrac{s_1^2(n_1 - 1) + s_2^2(n_2 - 1)}{n_1 + n_2 - 2}} \times \sqrt{\dfrac{1}{n_1} + \dfrac{1}{n_2}}} \qquad \text{eq. (6.1)}$$

where

t is the t-ratio, a value we will use to compare to critical values on a t-distribution table,

$\bar{x}$ is the sample mean, one for each group

s^2 is the sample variance, one for each group, and

n is the sample size, one for each group.

If the variances are unequal (aka Behrens-Fisher problem, see Sawilowsky, 2002) we use:

$$t = \frac{(\bar{x}_1 - \bar{x}_2) - 0}{\sqrt{\dfrac{s_1^2}{n_1} + \dfrac{s_2^2}{n_2}}}$$

eq. (6.2)

In both equations, the researcher is essentially examining

$$\frac{(observed\ values) - (expected\ value)}{standard\ error}$$

Using our previous drug dosage study example and (Table 6.1) assuming variances are equal, we substitute the values in the variances equal equation (eq. 5.2) and obtain,

Table 6.1. Means, Standard Deviation, and Group Size From Independent t-Test.

	Mean	sd	n
Group A	33.9	9.55	57
Group B	63.0	10.6	57

$$
\begin{aligned}
t - value &= \frac{(33.90 - 63.00) - 0}{\sqrt{\dfrac{9.55^2(57-1) + 10.6^2(57-1)}{57+57-2}} \times \sqrt{\dfrac{1}{57} + \dfrac{1}{57}}} \\[2ex]
&= \frac{-29.1}{\sqrt{\dfrac{5107.34 + 6292.16}{112}} \times \sqrt{\dfrac{2}{57}}} = \frac{-29.1}{\sqrt{10.09} \times \sqrt{0.35}} = -15.39
\end{aligned}
$$

Notice it is a negative t-value. That is simply an artifact of subtracting the larger mean from the smaller mean. Also notice, that the t-value is a bit smaller than before. The smaller value is due to some rounding error. The t-value is simply a value. But what does it mean? The t-value is a standardized value that describes where a value is on t-distribution (Chapter 3). Thus, we are comparing our value to something we know, the t-distribution. A t-value of 15 is very far away from the mean of the t-distribution, or "far out on the curve." A t-value of 3 would be three standard deviations away from the mean on a t-distribution and would look like the tip of the curve (Chapter 3). Fifteen is 15 standard deviations away. This is our first comparison, but we also need to the degrees of freedom to complete this comparison.

In our example, the **degrees of freedom** is 112. But where did this come from? Well, it came from the sample size. In all, the sample size in each group is 114, but the degree of freedom is 112. This is because we adjust by 2—one for each group—$n_1 + n_2 - 2$ is the calculation. A degree of freedom, in essence, allows space to move. Imagine having friends over for lunch. There are 12 seats and

12 guests. This looks great, one seat for each guest. But, as the host starts to set the name plates down, they realize they cannot sit Auntie Meg next to cousin Marvin. So, the host begin to switch around and is struggling to get this right. They have no degrees of freedom. If the host has 12 chairs and 11 guests, they would have a degree of freedom and could make it work. We use the degrees of freedom and the t-value to calculate the p-value.

We can look at the t-distribution table to see if it would be greater than a critical value cut off that we chose while designing the study. This has historically been 0.05 (Chapter 1). Generally, any t-ratio over 2, with a moderate sample size greater than 60 will surpass the traditional critical value. At this point, most individual researchers will look to see if the p-value related to this t-ratio and degrees of freedom is less than 0.05. This behavior is fine, we do not expect that to stop and, descriptively, this should be done. But the p-value is not the end of the story. Now, examine the table in Appendix 6.1. The first thing to notice is it looks like just a bunch of numbers. Yet, these numbers follow a pattern. The first is degrees of freedom, which are needed. If the researcher has an older table, it might say v_1. The degrees of freedom for our example is 112, but it is not on the chart. Thus, we can interpolate because we have 30 and then jumps to 120. At 112, it is close to the 120 and we can use the 120 for estimation. The two-tailed test with the alpha at 0.05, gives us a value of critical t-value of 1.99. Our t-value is over 15. Since 15 is greater than 1.99, our p-value is less than 0.05. The exact p-value is actually quite small, less than 0.001, thus we normally write $p < 0.001$. We will use this critical t-value again for the compatibility values.

The standard error is not always reported or discussed but should be. The **standard error** provides an estimate of the amount of variability there is in a statistic, like a t-value, across samples from the population. For the t-value, the standard error is simply the denominator of the t-value equation. The standard error is a statistical error from sampling, not a measurement error, which is a different issue (Chapter 2). Sampling error is just the estimated difference between the values a researcher obtains from the sample of participants and the true population value. The standard error values are 1.27 for Group A and 1.40 for Group B indicating some sampling error. For the difference value (29.2), the sampling error example is 1.88, which also indicates a little error. The larger the number the more the error. Focusing on the denominator of equations 6.1 and 6.2, notice that if the sample size doubled, the standard error would decrease. And, most importantly, the t-value would increase! Specifically, if using 114 for each group, the t-value increases to −21.77 and the standard error reduces to 1.33. This is why people often say a larger sample size is better. What is meant is a large sample size will decrease the sampling error, increase the t-value and reduce the standard error. The standard error is also used to calculate confidence intervals.

Compatibility Intervals: t-Test

This phrase is normally read as "Confidence Interval" and not "Compatibility Interval." Confidence is a bad name for this, but is the most common phrasing. Confidence implies one should have confidence, but one should not, unless the sample size is very large and is representative of the population of interest. Why? These intervals assumes that the study is run over and over and over again. Therefore, we will be using **Compatibility intervals (CIs)**, more commonly known as confidence intervals (Gelman & Greenland, 2019) because it highlights that these are all estimates of a possible range of values that could be very wrong and not exact values.

CIs examine how wide the potential range of values could be if the study continued to be replicated. For the independent *t*-test, the confidence interval equation is,

$$CI95 = (\bar{x}_1 - \bar{x}_2) + t_{\alpha/2} \times standard\ error \qquad \text{eq. (6.3)}$$

which provides two values because of the addition and subtraction (±) aspect of the equation.

The α/2 of the $t_{\alpha/2}$ is the size of the compatibility bandwidth in question. The α/2 indicates the alpha level associated with the band and it is divided by 2 (two-tailed test). Most researchers choose 95%, or alpha of 0.05 (α/2 = 0.025) width but any value can be used. Common ones are 68, 95, and 99, which correspond to specific spots on the normal curve. For example, 68% corresponds to one standard deviation above and below the mean. The $t_{\alpha/2}$ value used in the equation is based on the degrees of freedom and the α/2. For 95% (α/2 = 0.025) with our degrees of freedom (112) the value would be 1.99. Notice this is also our critical *t*-value from earlier when determining if our observed *t*-value is greater than our critical *t*-value. In our example, the substituted values would be:

$$CI_{95} = 29.10 + 1.99 \times 1.89 = 32.80 \quad \text{This is the upper bound.}$$

$$CI_{95} = 29.10 - 1.99 \times 1.89 = 25.40 \quad \text{This is the lower bound.}$$

Thus, if one were to conduct this study again and again and again . . . with a new sample of 114 participants randomly assigned to two groups, 95% of the mean differences of the group values would potentially be between 25.4 and 32.8. There is also the possibility the value will be outside of this. And there is no guarantee that someone else replicating the study will find their difference to be in the CI (Greenland et al., 2016). CIs are very sample specific and thus affected by the sampling process (Schreiber & Asner-Self, 2010).

Effect Sizes

Regardless of the sample size of a study, the calculation of effect sizes, especially for meta-analytic studies, has been important for the past 40 years (Glass, 1976). More recently, with the larger data sets available for analyses, the role of effect size, to us, has become more important. For the example data, we can use Cohen's *d* which is the difference between the groups and the standard deviation for both groups (i.e., the pooled sd) (Cohen, 1977).

$$\text{Cohen's } d = \frac{\bar{x}_1 - \bar{x}_2}{\sqrt{\dfrac{sd_1^2 + sd_2^2}{2}}} \qquad \text{eq. (6.4)}$$

For example, if the first group has mean equal to 33.90 and standard deviation (sd) equal to 9.55, and the second group has mean equal to 63 and a sd equal to 10.6, Cohen's d would equal,

$$\text{Cohen's } d = \frac{33.90 - 63.00}{\sqrt{\dfrac{9.55_1^2 + 10.6_2^2}{2}}} = \frac{-29.10}{\sqrt{\dfrac{91.20 + 112.36}{2}}} = \frac{-29.10}{10.09} = -2.89.$$

The negative value, gain, is just an artifact of which mean was first. We want the absolute value of the effect size. This value would be considered a very large effect size. The traditional values for interpretation are small effect ~ 0.30, medium effect ~0.50, and large effect ~0.80 and above. The value is interpreted as the mean difference between the groups is *2.89 standard deviation units* apart. Cohen's d works well if the standard deviations are about the same size and the sample sizes are the same or close. Hedges' g is used when group sizes are unequal and Glass' delta (Δ) is calculated when there is a control group in an experiment. Glass' delta and Hedges' g use the same cut off values as Cohen's d (Glass, 1977; Hedges, 1982; Smith & Glass, 1977).

Paired t-Tests

Paired t-tests are used when the data are matched (e.g., time one, time two) or some dependency makes the responses related (e.g., spouses) and one would expect an association.

Paired t-tests are also known as nonrandomized one group pre- and post-test design. For paired t-tests, much of the technical information will look the same. Normality examination is completed the same way as the independent t-test, but it is completed on the difference of the two related scores. From the example earlier, with a pre-test and a post-test, one would test the normality of their difference,   post-test-pre-test.

In the paired t-test example, the normality of the pre- and post-test is problematic, there are only two values, 2 and 3 (**Figure 6.6**), because our sample size is very small and we do not have a wide range of scores between the pre- and post-tests.

The reason we look at the normality of the difference score is due to the fact the actual test in on the difference score and not on the pre- and post-tests. This can be seen in the equation used.

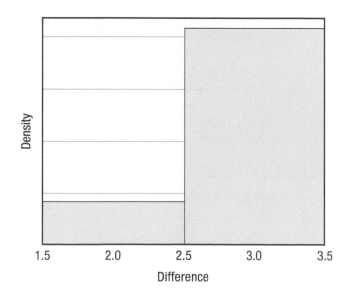

Figure 6.6. Difference Score Histogram.

$$t\text{-dependent} = \frac{\overline{D}}{s_{\overline{D}}} \qquad\qquad \text{eq. (6.5)}$$

where $\overline{D}$ is the mean of the difference scores and the square root of $s_{\overline{D}}$ is standard error.

To calculate by hand, start with the standard error calculation,

$$s_{\overline{D}} = \frac{s_D}{\sqrt{(N)}} \qquad\qquad \text{eq. (6.6)}$$

where

N is the sample size,

S_D is standard deviation of the difference score.

If the mean difference because the pre-test and post-test is 2.84, and the standard deviation of that difference is 0.408, with a sample size of 6, the t-value can be calculated from the equations above starting with,

$$s_{\overline{D}} = \frac{s_D}{\sqrt{(N)}} = \frac{0.408}{\sqrt{6}} = \frac{0.408}{2.44} = 0.167$$

Then take equation 6.6, with the mean of the difference (2.84) and the $s_{\overline{D}}$ value (0.167) and substitute them in,

$$t\text{-dependent} = \frac{\overline{D}}{s_{\overline{D}}} = \frac{2.84}{0.167} = 17.0.$$

The t-value of 17.0 is just a number and needs to be compared to the t-distribution with the degrees of freedom to understand it. To determine the descriptive p-value, we can take our t-value from above of 17.6 and degrees of freedom and compare it to the critical value on the t-distribution table (Appendix 6.1). The degrees of freedom is calculated as $N - 1$. For a sample size of 6, this leaves us with 5 degrees of freedom. Using the traditional two-tailed cut-off value for 0.05, the critical value is 2.57. Thus, observed t-value of 17.0 exceeds the critical value.

The standard errors for the means for the pre- and post-test and the standard error for the paired t-test should also be included. The standard error is simply the standard deviation divided by the square root of the sample size. For the pre-test that is $1.47/\sqrt{6} = 0.601$, for the post-test it is $1.63/\sqrt{6} = 0.667$, and for the difference, it is 0.16, which was calculated for the t-value (equation 6.6).

Compatibility Intervals Paired t-Test and Effect Size

CIs should also be calculated on the results. The confidence interval equation is

$$CI95 = (\overline{D}) \pm {}^{s_{\overline{D}}} \times t_{cutoff}$$

Substituting in values gives,

$$\text{Lower CI95} = (2.84) - 0.167 \times 2.57 = 2.41$$

$$\text{Upper CI95} = (2.84) + 0.167 \times 2.57 = 3.24.$$

Thus, the CI95 is [2.41, 3.24]. This indicates a small distance between what was observed and what the mean overall difference value could be if the study was replicated multiple times. The last piece of information that should be included in the narrative is the correlation between the pre- and post-test scores. In this case, the Pearson correlation is −0.028. As stated earlier, this is a small correlation between the pre- and post-test indicates that each person decreased at different rates. The Cohen's d effect size can be calculated using the t-value and the

$$\text{sample size, ES} = d = \frac{(t)}{\sqrt{N}}, \qquad \text{eq. (6.7)}$$

$$\text{For these results that is } d = \frac{17.00}{\sqrt{6}} = 6.94.$$

One-Way ANOVA

The major assumptions for the One-Way ANOVA analysis are the same as the independent t-test. The outcome variable is assumed to be normally distributed, and preferably normally distributed within each group. Homogeneity of variance between the groups. Finally, the cases/participants are independent. Homogeneity of variance is an assumption again, but now it is for more than two groups and should be tested.

Source Table and Compatibility Intervals

The major technical component of a One-Way ANOVA is the calculation of the source table (Table 6.2). The source tables provide the values for how the variance is accounted for across the groups, within the groups (error) and total. Additionally, the degrees of freedom, mean square for between and within, along with the F-ratio are calculated. For this analysis, there three sums of squares: between-group some of squares (SS_B), within-group or error sum of squares (SS_E) and total sum of squares (SS_T). The SS_T is just the composite of the SS_B and SS_E,

$$SS_T = SS_B + SS_E.$$

The between group sums of squares calculates the differences, the *deviances*, among the group means by calculating the variation of each mean ($\overline{Y}_{.j}$) around the grand mean ($\overline{Y}_{..}$). Within each group, each participant has a value, those within a group have a mean value. If there are three groups, there are three mean values. There is also a grand mean, that is the mean for all of the participants on the outcome variable. Thus, the equation below shows the between sums of square calculation, where,

$$SS_B = n\Sigma(\overline{Y}_{.j} - \overline{Y}_{..})^2,$$

n is the number of observations in each group. If you have three groups, you will take the mean of each group, subtract the grand mean, square that value, add them together and multiply by the sample size. This calculation works when the sample sizes are all the same. In a three group study such as BSN, second BSN (BSN after a different bachelor degree), and PA, the n size would have to be the same across groups, such as 50 in each group. If sample sizes are different, a slightly different calculation is used. The SS_E calculates the error variation or *deviances* of individual scores around each group mean. Since it is not associated with the grand mean, this is the variation not due to the independent variable.

$$SS_E = \Sigma\Sigma(Y_{ij} - \overline{Y}_{.j})^2$$

The SS_T is computed by adding the SS_B and the SS_E.

Table 6.2. ANOVA Source Table.

	Sums of Squares	Degrees of Freedom	Mean Square	F ratio
Between	$SS_B = n\Sigma\,(\overline{Y}_{.j} - \overline{Y}_{..})^2$	$df_B = k - 1$	$MS_B = \dfrac{SS_B}{df_B}$	$F = \dfrac{MS_B}{MS_E}$
Within (error)	$SS_E = \Sigma\Sigma(Y_{ij} - \overline{Y}_{.j})^2$	$df_E = N - k$	$MS_w = \dfrac{SS_E}{df_E}$	
Total	$SS_T = SS_B + SS_E$	$df_T = N - 1$		

The degrees of freedom (df) for each sums of squares has a different calculation as described previously (Table 6.2). For the between sums of squares $df_B = k - 1$, where k is the number of groups (Table 6.1). Note that the letter k is also used. For the error sums of squares the $df_E = N - k$ or $(N - 1) - (k - 1)$ where k equals the number of groups, and N is the total sample size. For the total sums of squares is a $df_T = N - 1$. For explanation of mean square and F-ratio, see ANOVA Core Results.

CIs are calculated for the means for each group is the same way they were calculated for the means in the independent t-test analysis, there are just more means to work with in One-Way ANOVA.

Effect Sizes

Effect sizes for the One-Way ANOVA are easily calculated by based on sums of squares. The most common effect sizes for a one-way ANOVA are eta-squared, omega squared, partial eta-squared, and Cohen's f. Eta-squared is calculated by taking the between sums of squares of the and dividing it by the total sums of squares, $\eta^2 = \dfrac{SS_B}{SS_T}$. For One-Way ANOVA partial eta-squared will be the same value. For more complicated ANOVAs it is different. Omega-squared $(\omega^2) = \dfrac{SS_B - (k - 1)(SS_E)}{SS_T + MS_E}$ adjusts the eta-squared numerator by the number of df of between and error sums of squares along with an adjustment to the denominator with the mean square error. Thus, both adjustments are about error.

$$\eta^2_{parital} = \frac{SS_{Between}}{SS_{Between} + SS_{Error}}$$

Cohen's f is easily calculated by using the eta-squared results. Cohen's $f =$

$$f = \sqrt{\frac{\eta^2}{(1 - \eta^2)}}$$

Using an eta/partial eta-squared value of 0.09, and substituting that value Cohen's f is

$$f = \sqrt{\frac{0.097}{(1 - 0.097)}} = 0.32$$

The value of $f = 0.32$ would also be considered a moderate effect size. Table 6.3 has the general and historical cut-offs for these three effect sizes. The calculated effect size should also be discussed in relation previous research to provide a better context to the results and their implication.

Table 6.3. Effect Sizes One-Way ANOVA.

Effect Size	Small	Moderate	Large
η^2/partial η^2	0.01	0.06	0.14
omega-squared	0.01	0.06	0.14
Cohen's f	0.10	0.25	0.40

It is also common for researchers to calculate a Cohen's d between pairs of groups in a One-Way ANOVA.

Multiple Comparisons

With three or more groups, researchers want to know how much are the differences between each of the groupings, for example BSN vs. second, BSN vs. PA, and so on. The researcher cannot just calculate multiple t-tests, that is problematic. What should be done is either a priori planned comparisons, or appropriate post-hoc comparisons. A priori planned comparisons are designed to compare specific groups before the analysis is run. For example, the researcher might be interested in differences between BSN and PA and second degree and PA, but not in BSN and second degree. If that were the case, two a priori comparisons would be completed. In this scenario, the ANOVA does not always need to be run, it is just common to do so.

The researcher could also plan before the analysis to test all the combinations post-hoc analyses. These are called post-hoc because they are run after the ANOVA is run. There are several and this is where being a scholar becomes important—and this is a rich area of research.

Why do we need to do this? Post hoc tests are a way to examine group differences without inflating the Type 1 error—saying there is a difference when there is not. This is about null hypothesis statistical testing (Chapters 1 and 2). Running several t-tests on the groups will inflate the possibility of making that type of inference error in the 0.05 framework. Thus, post-hoc tests that control for Type 1 error were developed to examine the differences. The researcher is adjusting for multiple statistical tests being completed at one time.

There are many post-hoc tests and we discuss a few. Each post-hoc test has a different mathematic focus. Table 6.4 provides a summary of multiple tests. Scheffé (1953) is a suitable test regardless of whether the sample sizes are equal or the variances (standard deviations across groups) are equal. It was very popular because it was easy to calculate by hand. The **Bonferroni** is even more popular because it is even easier to calculate. If the researcher has 6 comparisons to make, the researcher takes 0.05 and divides it by 6, which is 0.0083 for the new cut off value. The **Dunn-Bonferroni** (D-B) is similar to Bonferroni and uses a *t-value* cut off. To calculate the value, you need the number of tests, your p-value limit such as 0.05, and degrees of freedom. For example, if you had 5 contrast tests, a 0.05 cut-off, adjusted cut-off (0.05/5 = 0.01), and there are 20 degrees of freedom for the error, the cut-off value is 2.845 (0.01 at 20 df) as your threshold on a "two-tailed test." CIs can also be calculated because it is based on the *t*-distribution. The **Dunn-Sidak** (D-S) is very similar to the D-B. D-B and D-S are simultaneous because they run all possible contrasts. Both will allow for

Table 6.4. Types of Post-Hoc Analyses.

Contrast	Confidence Interval	Group Size (*n*) Not Total Size N	Variances in the Population	What Should You Do?
Planned	Y	Does not matter	Equal	DB or DS
	Y	Does not matter	Not	DB or DS
	N	Does not matter	Equal	Hochberg
	N	Does not matter	Not	Hochberg
Control Group	Y	Equal	Equal	Dunnett
	Y	Not equal	Equal	DB or DS
	Y	Does not matter	Not equal	DB or DS
All Pairwise Comparisons	Y	Equal	Equal	Tukey
	Y	Not Equal	Equal	Tukey-Kramer
	Y	Does not matter	Not equal	G-H or Dunnett's T3
	N	Does not matter	Equal	F-H
General post hoc	Y	Does not matter	Equal	Scheffé
	Y	Does not matter	Unequal	Scheffé

CIs to be calculated. Sequential methods help sustain power in the 0.05 framework, such as Hochberg's. **Hochberg's** will take the group comparisons and rank their *p*-values. Hochberg's controls well for 0.05 cut-off and is more powerful at detecting differences than D-B. There is no way to calculate CIs. Finally, **Games-Howell (G-H) or Dunnett's T3** are used with unequal variances. Dunnett's T3 is more powerful. G-H has a problem controlling for type one error when sample sizes are small.

The number of tests can be overwhelming. The key is to see which are available based on the software being used. Then from that group, decide which matches what needs to be done for the study and the research questions. We have only shown a few popular ones; more can be seen in Seaman et al. (1991).

Bootstrapping

Still not as common as it should be, **bootstrapping** is a statistical technique where the original data is resampled thousands of times, and the analysis is completed again thousands of times. Each resampled dataset is a subset of the original data (Efron, 1979). For example, with 100 participants, the bootstrap can take a random sample of 90 participants and rerun the analysis but do that 1,000 or 10,000 or however many times chosen. Once the bootstrap is complete the distribution of results can be examined. For example, a researcher may bootstrap the *t*-value 1,000 times for an independent *t*-test and then examine the full range of *t*-values, along with the mean and median *t*-values along with the standard deviation of the bootstrapped *t*-values. If the mean *t*-value from the bootstrap is the same or close to the one observed, and the standard deviation is very small, the research can be a little more confident about the *t*-value for the analysis.

Traditional Power and Alpha

We have not discussed traditional power analysis and alpha (Cohen, 1977; Faul et al., 2009) to this point for these analyses. The reason for this is the goal of power analyses is not for accuracy but for reaching 05. Thus, if reaching the magical 05 is not the goal, traditional power analyses are not helpful. We think the goal should be accuracy or stability of results. This is a growing area of research. Trafimow and MacDonald (2017) make this argument that accuracy is a better way to think about power. Trafimow and MacDonald (2017) argue that the focus should be on accuracy of the estimate and how much error one is willing to accept. For two groups, such as our independent *t*-test, of we want to be 95% confident that we are within 1 standard deviation of the population means, we need a sample size close to 500. If we are willing to sacrifice that confidence down to 65%, we only need about 160. Or we could sacrifice a bit of accuracy, and with 95% confidence and within 0.2 standard deviations, we would need about 150 participants (Trafimow & McDonald, 2017). Therefore, we think researchers should be focusing more on accuracy and confidence and less on power and reaching 0.05.

CORE RESULTS

The core results for these three analyses are similar and can look the same, but each has unique components to it. For the new researcher, it is important to understand the differences in order to evaluate an article or to run the analysis. Below, we present the core results by analysis.

Independent t-Test

The narrative for the core results for an independent t-test analysis are 1) t-value, 2) the degrees of freedom, 3) the p-value, 4) the means and standard deviations of the two groups, and 5) effect size. This is the information most individuals reading an article with a t-test analysis want to know. There are other pieces of information that are important, but these have been the core historically. A typical result section with this information would read as such, "the independent t-test had a $t(112) = 8.21$, $p = 0.001$. Group A had a mean of 35.27 (9.87) and Group B had a 63.48 (11.65). Group B outperformed Group A on the task. The effect size, Cohen's d, was 2.90, a very large effect size."

There are tables that are also used to summarize the results. Table 6.5 shows the same information from the narrative along with a mean difference value between the groups, and the sample sizes for each group (n).

Table 6.5. Example of Independent t-Test Table.

Test	df	t-value	p-value	Mean Difference
Independent t	112	15.46	0.001	29.10

	Mean	sd	n
Group A	33.9	9.55	57
Group B	63.0	10.6	57

In the technical section of this chapter, there is a discussion of degrees of freedom, calculation of degrees of freedom and calculation of the t-value, along with other key components of this test.

Graphically, the two distributions are displayed in Figure 6.7. The separation of the distribution can be noted quite clearly, and they are separated enough—little overlap—that statistical analyses will simply confirm what is visible. The distance between the means of the distributions and the small amount of overlap can be seen in the effect size value, 2.90.

Effect sizes provide a standardized estimate of the size of the difference that is not affected by the scale of the variable (Glass, 1976). Scale of a variable can be thought of as the possible range. A variable that has values that from 1 to 5 is a different scale than a variable that ranges from 1 to 20. Effect sizes for independent t-tests are calculated by using the mean difference of the groups and the standard deviations. There are three common effect sizes for the independent

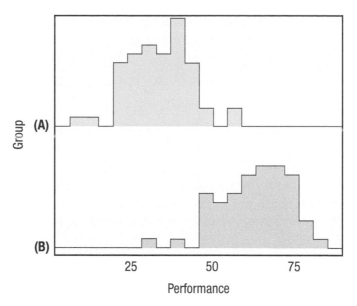

Figure 6.7. Display of Group A and B Distributions.

t-test, Cohen's *d*, Hedge's *g*, and Glass' delta. Cohen's *d*, the effect size in this example, is interpreted as, the scores are 2.90 standard deviations apart and would be considered a very large effect size (0.3 is small, 0.5 medium, and 0.80 large). Additionally, effect sizes and how "large" they are is partially driven by the research domain. These are general cutoffs, but it is very important to understand the effect sizes in one's research domain and the best way to interpret them. Finally, note that the large effect size in this example is just an artifact of the simulated data.

Paired *t*-Test Core Results

The core narrative for the results of a paired *t*-test will look similar to those from the independent *t*-test. For example, "A dependent *t*-test indicated an average drop of 2.84 problem behaviors after intervention, with $t(5) = 17.00$, $p < 0.001$. Cohen's *d* was 6.94, a very large effect for the difference between the two sets of scores from pre-test to post-test." Table 6.6 shows the sample size for each test, mean, median, standard deviation, and correlation between the scores. The pre-test scores are higher than the post-test scores, and in this case shows improvement, lower scores indicate fewer problems. The standard deviations are similar in size and indicate the two distributions have a similar spread of scores. The correlation between the two sets of scores is an indicator of similarity in change of scores for the participants. At −0.028, there is not much similarity; in this case individuals scores dropped at different rates, though the overall average drop is 2.84. As a reminder, correlation values closer to 1 indicate the scores are strongly related, and the positive or negative component just signals the direction.

Table 6.6. Descriptive Statistics Paired *t*-Test.

	N	Mean	Median	sd	se
Pre	6	7.17	7.50	1.47	0.601
Post	6	4.33	4.50	1.63	0.667

Correlation Pearson's r −.028

Table 6.7 provides the paired *t*-test results. The *t*-value is −17.00 with 5 degrees of freedom and a *p*-value <0.001. These results would be desirable from the *t*-value/*p*-value perspectives. The large mean difference and large effect size would indicate excellent results. In detail, the mean difference is 2.84 (i.e., 7.17 − 4.33 with a little rounding), the standard deviations are about 1.5 points, which is a good sign in general if the difference is larger than the standard deviations of the groups. Cohen's *d* here is interpreted as, the scores are 6.94 standard deviations apart and would be considered an extremely large effect size. Effect sizes for paired *t*-tests are expected though not always provided but are finally becoming more common in published research.

Table 6.7. Paired Samples *t*-Test.

			t-value	df	*p*	Effect Size
Post	Pre	Student's *t*	−17.0	5.00	<0.001	6.94

One-Way ANOVA: Core Results

The narrative for the core results for One-Way ANOVA analysis are the source table and the means and standard deviations by group. The source table is designed to demonstrate how the variability is split up between the groups and within the groups. The within component in a One-Way ANOVA is considered error because this is variability not explained by being in a group. Table 6.8 has the source table for the three student groups and stress from Figure 6.4.

Table 6.8. Source Table for One-Way ANOVA Results Example.

	Sums of Squares	df	Mean Square	F-Ratio
Between (Groups)	3980	2	1990.00	32.39
Error (Within)	36679	597	61.44	
Total	40659	599		

The sums of squares explains the total variation in the outcome variable based on independent variables and error. In this example, the Group is the independent variable with three categories (BSN, second degree, PA). The group and error sums of squares add up to the total. The degrees of freedom for the between component is based on the number of groups minus 1 ($k − 1$). There are three groups, so that leaves two as the degrees of freedom. The error degrees of freedom are the total sample size minus one and then minus the degrees of freedom for the between component $(N - 1) - (k - 1)$. In this example that is $(600 - 1) - (3 - 1)$, which equals 597. The total degrees of freedom is the sample size minus 1, or 599 in this example.

The mean squares are the sums of squares divided by the degrees of freedom. For the between component, the mean square represents the variation between the sample means. For the error component, the mean square represents the samples (within groups). The F-ratio is calculated by dividing the mean square between by the mean square error. In this case that is, $1990/61.44 = 32.39$. Similar to the t-value, the F-ratio has to be compared to a table using degrees of freedom for the between and the error. But note that at 32.39, the F-value is quite large. In general, if you have F-ratio over 5, even with just 3 groups and 12 participants, the p-value will be less than 0.05.

A typical result section with this information would read as such, "A One-way ANOVA was performed to examine the effect of group membership on stress level, $F(2, 597) = 32.39$, MSError $= 61.44$, $p < 0.05$. BSN students had a mean score of Group 39.50 (8.18) and second degree BSN students had a mean of 44.50 (7.09), while PA students had a mean stress score of 45.4 (8.2). The effect size, partial eta squared was 0.097, (3,980 / (3,980 + 36,679), and is considered a moderate effect size."

There are tables that are also used to summarize the basic results. Table 6.9 displays the same information from the narrative with a mean, standard deviation (sd) and the sample sizes for each group (n).

Table 6.9. Descriptives From One-Way ANOVA Example.

	Mean	sd	n
BSN	39.50	8.18	200
Second BSN	44.50	8.20	200
PA	45.40	7.09	200

FULL INDEPENDENT t-TEST EXAMPLE

Now that we have covered the basics, the core results, and read about the technical information, it is time to see a detailed example of an independent t-test. Table 6.10 presents a subset of data from two groups of participants and their scores on a risk assessment instrument. The research question is:

■ How large is the difference between BSN trained nurses and second degree BSN on their self-perception of stress during their first six months?

The traditional null hypothesis is there is no difference, $H_0: \mu_1 - \mu_2 = 0$. Alternative and directional hypotheses can be applied. The traditional alternative or research hypothesis is the means are not equal: $H_0: \mu_1 - \mu_2 \neq 0$. A directional test is informed by the previous research and may indicate the BSN trained nurses have less stress than second degree BSN trained nurses, $H_0: \mu_1 < \mu_2 = 0$. This is part of the null hypothesis statistical testing, and it has its own problems (Szucs & Ioannidis, 2017) but is a good way to start thinking about what is expected. We personally prefer theoretically informed directional tests, but those are not common in the literature.

Table 6.10. Group Descriptive Statistics.

	Group	N	Mean	Median	sd	se
Stress Level	BSN (second)	62	42.1	42.5	8.74	1.11
	BSN	48	38.0	37.5	8.44	1.22

The mean perceived stress score for the second degree BSN nurses is higher than for traditionally trained BSN students (Table 6.11). The scores have a potential range from 13 to 52, where 13 would indicate very low stress. The two distributions substantially overlap as can be seen in Figure 6.8. The stress score is assumed to be normally distributed, both visually (Figure 6.9) and with SW (0.985, $p = 0.241$) and Kolmogorov-Smirnov tests (0.06, $p = 0.864$). Each group also had normally distributed data. Skewness was 0.25 and slightly platykurtic (−0.43). No outliers were observed based on visual examination and examination of the standardization of the variable. Therefore, no transformation of the outcome variable is warranted.

Homogeneity of variance was examined by Levene's test ($F(1,108) = 1.06$, $p = 0.746$) and based on those results, homogeneity will be assumed ($F(1,108) = 1.06$, $p = 0.746$. The analysis results show a mean difference of 4.06 with a standard error of the difference of 1.66 ($t(108) = 2.45$, $p = 0.016$) (Table 6.11). The second degree BSN students have a higher stress level score on average. The effect size is 0.47 and indicates the groups are almost 1/2 of a standard deviation apart, a moderate effect, along with an indication that the distributions of the two groups still overlap substantially. Note, a bootstrap (1,000 times) on the mean difference provided a mean difference of 4.06 with a range from 1 to almost 8.

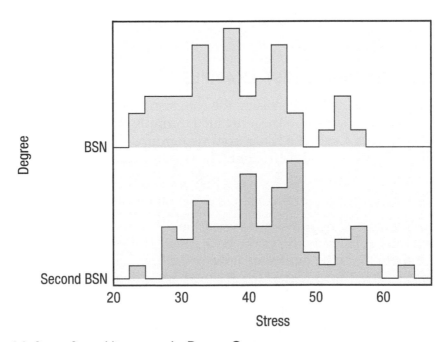

Figure 6.8. Stress Score Histograms by Degree Group.

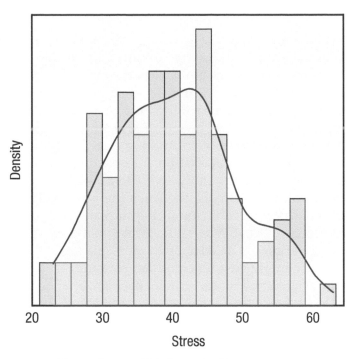

Figure 6.9. Histogram of Stress Scores With Smoothed Line.

Table 6.11. Independent Group Results for Stress.

| | t-value | df | p | Mean Difference | se Difference | 95% Confidence Interval | | Cohen's d |
						Lower	Upper	
Stress	−2.45	108	0.016	−4.06	1.66	−7.34	−0.777	−0.471

NONPARAMETRIC ANALYSES

When the normality assumption fails, or data are not normally distributed, non-parametric analyses are utilized. **Nonparametric** simply means the restrictive assumptions of parametric tests (e.g., *t*-test assumptions) are not implemented. The results between a parametric test and nonparametric test may not vary depending on the sample size and amount of nonnormality, but understanding how much of a difference exists will be greatly improved. Examples of dependent variables that are nonnormal are those ordinal in nature (ordered categorical) such as Likert items (e.g., a 5-point scale from "strongly agree" through to "strongly disagree") or continuous, but nonnormal, such as income. Income, for example, is heavily positively skewed (Mulbrandon, 2013). The independent variable in question has two categorical, independent groups, just like the independent *t*-test. Examples of independent variables that meet this criterion include, smoker (2 groups: yes or no), or education (college degree or high school diploma).

Mann-Whitney U

The MW is the analog for independent t-test and is implemented when comparing differences between two independent groups and the dependent variable is either ordinal or nonnormally distributed. There is a process for the MW analysis where the first step is to order the data for each group lowest to highest. The next step is to rank the data. When ranking the data, any data that are tied must be given the same rank across both groups. For example, if there are two scores of 10 in group 1 and two scores of 10 in the group 2, all four of those scores would end up with the same rank. The third step is to add up the rankings for each group. A quick examination of the average rank for each will provide an initial clue if there will be differences between the groups. The last step is the actual calculation of the MW value for each group and take the lower of those two values and compare it to a MW table. With small data sets, this process is easy, as data sets get larger $n > 20$, it becomes more and more tedious and almost all MW analyses are completed with computer software.

The statistic U is calculated twice, once for each group. Then, the lower of the two numbers is used. Once the U value is determined, it is compared to a MW table-similar to the process in the t-test example. Instead of using degrees of freedom the sample sizes of each group are used.

Assumptions

Just as with independent t-tests, paired t-test, and ANOVA, the observations should be independent of each other, with no participant being in more than one group. Second, there must not be a linking relationship between participants. Homogeneity of variance is not an assumption because with nonnormal data, the expectation of variances being equal is suspended. Using the nursing example from the independent t-test, the research questions would be the same.

Research Questions, Hypotheses, Designs

As with the independent t-test, the focus is on how much of a difference there is between the two groups related to the outcome variable. For example,

- How large is the difference between BSN trained nurses and second degree BSN on their self-perception of stress during their first 6 months?

The traditional null and alternative hypotheses for the MW two group nonparametric are written as:

$$H_0 : Z_i = Z_j$$
$$H_A : Z_i \neq Z_j$$

Note that these hypotheses look very much like the ones for the independent group hypotheses with just different letters to indicate the different distribution test.

As with independent t-tests, there are a variety of study designs from survey, to nonexperimental, quasi-, and true experimental which will use a MW analysis. We see many manuscripts where the dependent variable is nonnormal and nonnormal within each group, and the authors decide to just use the MW option. A researcher may also purposefully implement both the *t*-test and MW analyses with a discussion of the implications of both.

Mann-Whitney Results

The results for the MW are in Table 6.12. The U statistic is 1,097, which is difficult to understand because it is just a number until compared to a MW table. The two-tailed *p*-value is 0.018. The mean difference between the groups is 4. The negative, again, is just related to how the subtraction was completed, higher from lower. The CI is next. The effect size calculated used a Rank Biserial Correlation (Chapter 8). This is the appropriate correlation for nonnormal continuous data being associated with a binary value (two groups). A value of 0.26 would be considered a small to moderate effect size.

Table 6.12. Mann-Whitney Results.

		Statistic	p	Difference	95% Compatibility Interval Lower	Upper	Effect Size	
Stress	Mann-Whitney U	1097	0.018	−4	−8	−1	Rank biserial correlation	0.26

Wilcoxon Signed Rank Test

In many statistical packages, Wilcoxon Signed Ranks test is implemented for paired or matched data. With the Wilcoxon test, the paired differences will be examined using a Z distribution or S. The S distribution is very useful, but that is more mathematical in nature and not a focus of this book (Kendall, 1948). Researchers might also use a Friedman test in this scenario. The results of a Wilcoxon and Friedman traditionally provide the same result, though a difference may be observed on a rare occasion, depending on the data.

Research Questions, Hypotheses, Designs

Research questions are similar to paired and repeated measures and typically concern amount of change or differences over the repeated measures. For example,

> How much of a difference over time is there on satisfaction rating?

> Which product of the three had the highest rank?

The traditional null and alternative hypotheses for the Wilcoxon Signed Ranks Tests paired nonparametric analyses are written as:

$$H_0 : Z_i = Z_j$$
$$H_A : Z_i \neq Z_j$$

These look like the previous ones with the interpretation for paired t-test equal for the null, and the medians are not equal for the alternative, with a different letter that indicates a different distribution. "Me" may also be used for median instead of Z to indicate the medians are the same or different. The Wilcoxon Signed Rank Test can be analyzed through a sum of ranks procedure and the sum of ranks compared to a critical value table. As such, a sum or ranks value or a $\underline{Z}$-value or both may be produced in the results. The designs are the same from paired-tests, nonexperimental group with two repeated measures. Pre- and post-test designs with an intervention between the two times points is the most common.

Wilcoxon Results

Table 6.13 provides results as an example from two semester tests of undergraduate students in a core course for their major. Test 2 scores are slightly higher than Test 1 scores. Highest possible score was 45.

Table 6.13. Descriptive Statistics for Wilcoxon Signed Rank Test.

	N	Mean	Median	sd	se
Test 2	35	38.80	38.60	3.36	0.567
Test 1	35	38.20	38.00	4.41	0.745

			Statistic	p	Mean Difference	se Difference	Rank Biserial Effect Size
Test 2	Test 1	Wilcoxon W	362	0.45	0.64	0.58	0.15

The Wilcoxon results (Table 6.11) indicate a small difference between the groups with a test statistic of 362 and a p-value of 0.45. The test statistic (W) of 362 is the sum of the largest of the ranks. The standardized test statistic (Z) is 0.77, not shown. Both of these test statistics are compared to examine their critical value tables to determine the p-value. This is the same as traditional independent and paired t-test. The effect size is 0.15 and would be considered small.

Kruskal-Wallis

Researchers with more than two groups in their analyses cannot use the MW, and need to move to another analysis, just like moving form t-tests to ANOVA. The **Kruskal-Wallis H (K-W)** nonparametric test is used when there are three or more independent conditions, for example, that cannot be in more than one group and the dependent variable is nonnormally distributed. Though ANOVA is more powerful, sometimes the switch must be made or was planned in the design phase. Now, ANOVA is robust against nonnormality and as you read earlier there are adjustments when there is unequal variance. Thus, we generally recommend staying with ANOVA and transforming the outcome variable.

The Kruskal-Wallis H test is an *omnibus* test. The result will tell you overall something is occurring, but it will not tell you which group has more or less.

Research Questions

The basic research question for Kruskal-Wallis is the same as the One-Way ANOVA, such as:

■ How much of a difference exists in blood pressure reduction among diet change, diet change plus increase is walking, and diet change and yoga for high school students who have been classified as overweight using the body mass index (BMI)?

The questions can be written more directionally, such as,

■ Is the difference between diet change plus increase is walking and diet change and yoga 50% as much?

Most research questions researchers write are based on just seeing if a difference exists based on the 0.05 cutoff (two-tailed). These questions, because of how they are written, fail to look at how much, the costs, the risks, and so on. An example is, "Are there differences between three diet and exercise techniques?" The focus of the question is if there are differences, which is a 05 statement, and not how much or what could that mean from multiple perspectives.

Traditional Hypotheses

The traditional hypotheses for a three-group Kruskal-Wallis study are:

$$H_0 : Z_a = Z_b = Z_c$$
$$H_a : Z_a \neq Z_b \neq Z_c$$

You will notice, just as with Mann-Whitney, similarity to independent groups, these hypotheses look very much like the ones for the One-Way ANOVA hypotheses, with just different letters. This is due to the fact both Mann-Whitney and Kruskal-Wallis are the nonparametric versions of those parametric analyses.

Assumptions

As with all of these analyses, there are assumptions. And, again, when analyzing data, one or more of these assumptions will likely be violated. This is common. As stated earlier, the dependent variable is ordinal or continuous but nonnormal such as Likert-type scales, which are ordinal in nature (strongly agree to strongly disagree). Though, many researchers treat them as continuous, they are not. K-W analysis is used when you have three or more categorical, independent groups as your independent variable and a nonnormally distributed dependent variable. Examples of categories or created categories are high-medium-low income levels, year in high school, degree granted, and many more.

The participants or cases in your study should be independent with no relationship between them. Thus, you cannot be in two groups at the same time or a statistical dependency between group members, for example, spouses. Now, that being said, there are studies where you design for some pairing between people and then randomly assign to groups, but this is a study design planned component. If you have a dependence issue, you will need to switch to the Friedman test, for example.

As the Kruskal-Wallis *H*-test does not assume normality in the data and is much less sensitive to outliers, it can be used when these assumptions have been violated and the use of a one-way ANOVA is inappropriate. In addition, if your data are ordinal, a one-way ANOVA is inappropriate, but the Kruskal-Wallis *H*-test is appropriate. The *H* statistic follows a Chi-Square distribution and the test compares the ranks of the values for the groups. Special note: If you wish to take into account the ordinal nature of an *independent variable* (e.g., the number of minutes exercising, increases for each group, 10, 15, 20) and have an ordered alternative hypothesis, you could run a Jonckheere-Terpstra test instead of the Kruskal-Wallis *H*-test.

Kruskal-Wallis Results

The results for most nonparametric tests in statistical software packages are quite limited. As we stated earlier, ANOVA is a stronger analysis. Tables 6.14 and 6.15 provide the results of a Kruskal-Wallis with four independent groups (meditation type) by relaxation score as the dependent variable. The omnibus test is Chi-Square = 3.74, df = 3, p = 0.28 with a small effect size 0.03. The pairwise comparisons agree with the overall test. Note there are times when the individual comparisons will indicate some difference between groups when the omnibus tests do not.

Table 6.14. Kruskal-Wallis Results.

	χ^2	df	p	ε^2
Relaxation	3.7393	3	0.291	0.0343

Table 6.15. Dwass-Steel-Critchlow-Fligner Pairwise Comparisons.

		W	p
1	2	0.4715	0.987
1	3	2.1988	0.405
1	4	0.2889	0.997
2	3	2.2671	0.377
2	4	−0.3360	0.995
3	4	−2.5844	0.261

MOST DEFINING ATTRIBUTES

When reading or writing analytic results, there are multiple topics that should be included. This information should be available in the articles being read and should also be provided in any articles or reports published.

Independent t-Test Attributes

For the independent t-test, the overall checklist for running the analysis, writing the analysis, or reviewing an analysis is below.

1. Dependent variable for normality
2. Dependent variable by group for normality for each group
3. Outliers/missing data
   a. Discussion of removal of outliers, removal of missing data, or imputation of missing data
4. Levene's test for equal variances
5. Core Information to discuss in narrative
   a. Means, sd, and n-size for both groups
   b. Standard errors for both groups
   c. Levene's results
   d. t-value, adjusted t if Levene's is a problem
      i. e.g., $t(\text{df}) = X. XX$
   e. Degrees of freedom,
   f. Descriptive p-value,
      i. e.g., $p = 0.17$
   g. Mean difference
   h. Standard error of difference
   i. Compatibility intervals
   j. Effect size, Cohen's d, for example

Paired (Dependent) t-Test

1. Check both dependent variables (e.g., time 1 time 2) for normality
2. Identify any potential outliers (if outliers are suspected, run analysis twice, one with and one without outliers)
3. Make sure the difference between the two measures is normally distributed
4. Check normality of the difference between the two groups
   a. A new variable needs to be created to do this
5. Information to include in narrative.
   a. Means, sd, and n-size for both groups
   b. Standard errors for both groups
   c. Correlation between the two time periods
   d. Mean difference, sd or difference, se or difference

    e. *t*-value

        i. e.g., t(df) = X. XX

    f. Degrees of freedom

    g. Descriptive *p*-value

        i. e.g., $p = 0.17$

    h. Compatibility intervals

    i. Effect size

ANOVA

1. Check dependent variable for normality
2. Check dependent variable by group for normality
3. Outliers/missing data and how they were handled
4. Levene's test for equal variances
5. Core Information to discuss in narrative/tables
   a. Means, sd, and *n*-size for all groups/categories
   b. Standard errors for all groups/categories
   c. Levene's (homogeneity of variance test) results and any adjustments if needed
      i. MSe at a minimum (full source table is best)
   d. degrees of freedom, *F*, omnibus
   e. descriptive *p*-value
      i. e.g., $p = 0.17$
   f. Contrasts/post hoc
      i. Full details on contrasts
      ii. Full details on post-hoc chosen and why
   g. Mean differences
   h. Standard error of differences
   i. Compatibility intervals
   j. Effect size, partial eta-squared for example

Nonparametric

1. Total *N* and *n* by group/missing data
2. Means and median by group
3. Test statistic *U, W, or Z*

4. Descriptive p

5. Degrees of freedom

6. Acknowledge how any tied values were handled and the number of ties

7. Calculate effect size

8. Mean rank for each group (not always produced by statistical software)

9. Sum of ranks for each group (not always produced by statistical software)

10. Pairwise comparisons for K-W

SUMMARY

Variability between and within groups is a foundational topic in understanding research. Independent t-tests focus on the difference between the groups while examining the variability within each group. Dependent *t*-tests are focused on the changes within a group over two time periods. There are several assumptions for each of these analyses, such as normality of the data. When the assumptions are not tenable, adjustments or changes in analyses must occurs. For example, when the normality of the data assumptions fails, there are nonparametric options, such as Mann Whitney U and Wilcoxon Signed Rank test, to use to answer the research questions.

END-OF-CHAPTER RESOURCES

REVIEW QUESTIONS

Answers and rationales for the review questions are located in the Appendix at the end of the book.

1. TRUE or FALSE?

   The scores for a variable measuring caring behaviors among new nurses are narrow in range around the mean score, indicating a large amount of variability.

2. TRUE or FALSE?

   The range of the distribution of scores for a group, or the variance around the mean, is known as within group variability.

3. TRUE or FALSE?

   A statistical test that investigates how much of a difference there is in the mean of two groups is known as the dependent *t*-test.

4. TRUE or FALSE?

   To calculate the degrees of freedom for an independent t-test, use df $= n - 2$ where n is the total number of participants.

5. Which of the following is an example of a research question that would lend itself to statistical analysis using ANOVA?

   a. What is the effect of a mindfulness-based intervention on weight loss among second semester freshman students?

   b. How much difference is there in test anxiety between first-generation college students and college students who are not first generation?

   c. How much difference is there in intention to leave the profession between new nurses participating in a 3-month, 6-month and 12-month residency program?

   d. How much of a difference is there in perceived level of exertion from baseline to 6 months among participants in a cardiac rehab program?

6. Which of the following is an example of a research question that would lend itself to statistical analysis using an independent t-test?

   a. What is the effect of a mindfulness-based intervention on weight loss among second semester freshman students?

   b. How much difference is there in critical thinking skills between nursing students who graduate from a diploma program and nursing students who receive a BSN?

   c. How much difference is there in burnout between nurses, physicians, nurse practitioners, and physician's assistants during the COVID-19 pandemic?

   d. How much of a difference is there in perceived level of exertion from baseline to 6 months among participants in a cardiac rehab program?

7. Discuss the components of the narrative description for the results of a paired (dependent) t-test?

8. What is an effect size, why is it relevant, and what are some common tests of effect size?

9. Which of the following is <u>not</u> a method of assessing the assumption of normality?

   a. Levene's test

   b. histogram

   c. SW test

   d. Q-Q plot

10. Which of the following are parametric tests that can be utilized if the data are normally distributed? Select <u>all</u> that apply.

    a. independent t-test

    b. dependent (paired) t-test

    c. Wilcoxon signed rank

    d. one-way ANOVA

    e. Mann Whitney U

11. An investigator has completed a project to examine if there are differences in an outcome between three groups and uses an ANOVA to examine this. Because the ANOVA only tells us if there is an overall difference between the groups, post-hoc analyses such as the Bonferroni are used to determine what?

    a. whether you have committed a Type 1 error

    b. exactly which of the groups had a difference in means

    c. the size of the effect of the difference between groups

    d. the accuracy of the parameter being estimated

12. An investigator is trying to determine how much of a difference there is in medication adherence between a group that received usual care and a group that received a medication bottle with a reminder function. In examining the data, she sees that the outcome variable is not normally distributed for the usual care group. Which statistical analysis could she choose to use with the data as it is now?

    a. dependent t-test

    b. independent t-test

    c. Wilcoxon signed rank

    d. Mann Whitney U

REFERENCES

Cohen, J. (1977). *Statistical power analysis for the behavioral sciences* (Rev ed.). Academic Press.

Efron, B. (1979). Bootstrap methods: Another look at the Jackknife. *Annals of Statistics, 7*(1), 1–26. https://doi.org/10.1214/aos/1176344552

Faul, F., Erdfelder, E., Buchner, A., & Lang, A.-G. (2009). Statistical power analyses using G*Power 3.1: Tests for correlation and regression analyses. *Behavior Research Methods, 41,* 1149–1160. https://doi.org/10.3758/BRM.41.4.1149

Ferguson, G. A., & Takane, Y. (1989). *Statistical analysis in psychology and education* (6th ed.). McGraw-Hill.

Gelman, A., & Greenland, S. (2019). Are confidence intervals better termed "uncertainty intervals"? *BMJ, 366,* l5381. https://doi.org/10.1136/bmj.l5381

Glass, G. V (1976). Primary, secondary, and meta-analysis of research. *Educational Researcher, 5,* 3–8. https://doi.org/10.3102/0013189X005010003

Greenland, S. (2019). Valid p-values behave exactly as they should: Some misleading criticisms of p-values and their resolution with s-values. *The American Statistician, 73*(sup1), 106–114. https://doi.org/10.1080/00031305.2018.1529625

Greenland, S., Senn, S. J., Rothman, K. J., Carlin, J. B., Poole, C., Goodman, S. N., & Altman, D. G. (2016). Statistical tests, P values, confidence intervals, and power: A guide to misinterpretations. *European Journal of Epidemiology, 31*(4), 337–350.

Hedges, L. V. (1982). Estimation of effect size from a series of independent experiments. *Psychological Bulletin, 92*(2), 490–499. https://doi.org/10.1007/s10654-016-0149-3

Kendall, M. G. (1948). *Rank correlation methods.* Charles Griffin and Co.

Kirk, R. E. (2013). *Experimental design: procedures for the behavioral sciences* (4th ed.). SAGE Publications.

Levene, H. (1960). Robust tests for equality of variances. In I. Olkin, H. Hotelling, et al. (Eds.). *Contributions to Probability and Statistics: Essays in Honor of Harold Hotelling* (pp. 278–292). Stanford University Press.

Meehl, P. E. (1954). *Clinical versus statistical prediction: A theoretical analysis and a review of the evidence.* University of Minnesota Press.

Mulbrandon, C. (2013). *An illustrated guide to income in the United States.* Worthy Shorts.

Satterthwaite, F. E. (1946). An approximate distribution of estimates of variance components. *Biometrics Bulletin, 2*(6), 110–114. https://doi.org/10.2307/3002019

Sawilowsky, S. S. (2002). Fermat, Schubert, Einstein, and Behrens-Fisher: The probable difference between two means with different variances. *Journal of Modern Applied Statistical Methods, 1,* 461–472.

Scheffe, H. (1953). A method for judging all contrasts in analysis of variance. *Biomctrika, 40,* 87–104.

Schreiber, J. B. (2019). New paradigms for considering statistical significance: A way forward for health services research journals, their authors, and their readership. *Research in Social and Administrative Pharmacy, 16*(4), 591–594.

Schreiber, J. B., & Asner-Self, K. (2010). *Educational Research.* Wiley and Sons.

Seaman, M. A., Levin, J. R., & Serlin, R. C. (1991). New developments in pairwise multiple comparisons: some powerful and practicable procedures. *Psychological Bulletin, 110*(3), 577.

Smith, M. L., & Glass, G. V. (1977). Meta-analysis of psychotherapy outcome studies. *American Psychologist, 32*(9), 752–760.

Student. (1908). The probable error of a mean. *Biometrika,* 1–25.

Szucs, D., & Ioannidis, J. P. (2017). When null hypothesis significance testing is unsuitable for research: A reassessment. *Frontiers in Human Neuroscience, 11,* 1–21.

Trafimow. D, & MacDonald J. A. (2017). Performing inferential statistics prior to data collection. *Educational and Psychological Measurement, 77,* 204–219. https://doi.org/10.1177/0013164416659745

Tukey, J. (1986). The collected works of John H. Tukey. In L. V. Jones (Ed.), Philosophy and Principles of Data Analysis: 1965–1986 (Vol. 4). Wadsworth & Brooks/Cole.

Welch, B. L. (1938). The significance of the difference between two means when the population variances are unequal. *Biometrika, 29*(3/4), 350–362. https://doi.org/10.1093/biomet/29.3-4.350

Ziliak, S. T., & McCloskey, D. N. (2008). *The cult of statistical significance: How the standard error cost us jobs, justice, and lives.* University of Michigan Press.

FURTHER READING

Wasserstein, R. L., Schirm, A. L., Lazar, N. A. (2019). Moving to a world "p<.05". The American Statistician, 73:1–19. https://doi.org/10.1080/00031305.2019.1583913

APPENDIX 6.1

	t-distribution			
One Tailed	0.005	0.025	0.05	0.1
Two Tailed	0.01	**0.05**	0.1	0.2
df				
1	63.66	**12.71**	6.31	3.08
2	9.92	**4.30**	2.92	1.89
3	5.84	**3.18**	2.35	1.64
4	4.60	**2.78**	2.13	1.53
5	4.03	**2.57**	2.02	1.48
6	3.71	**2.45**	1.94	1.44
7	3.50	**2.36**	1.89	1.41
8	3.36	**2.31**	1.86	1.40
9	3.25	**2.26**	1.83	1.38
10	3.17	**2.23**	1.81	1.37
11	3.11	**2.20**	1.80	1.36
12	3.05	**2.18**	1.78	1.36
13	3.01	**2.16**	1.77	1.35
14	2.98	**2.14**	1.76	1.35
15	2.95	**2.13**	1.75	1.34
16	2.92	**2.12**	1.75	1.34
17	2.90	**2.11**	1.74	1.33
18	2.88	**2.10**	1.73	1.33
19	2.86	**2.09**	1.73	1.33
20	2.85	**2.09**	1.72	1.33
21	2.83	**2.08**	1.72	1.32
22	2.82	**2.07**	1.72	1.32
23	2.81	**2.07**	1.71	1.32
24	2.80	**2.06**	1.71	1.32
25	2.79	**2.06**	1.71	1.32
26	2.78	**2.06**	1.71	1.31
27	2.77	**2.05**	1.70	1.31
28	2.76	**2.05**	1.70	1.31
29	2.76	**2.05**	1.70	1.31
30	2.75	**2.04**	1.70	1.31
120	2.62	**1.98**	1.66	1.29

CHAPTER 7

Variability Between and Within Groups Expanded

CORE OBJECTIVES

■ Describe conceptual and technical differences between factorial, repeated measures, and ANCOVA analyses

■ Describe three types of interactions

■ Describe effect sizes for each analysis and their inferences

■ Understand which pieces of evidence need to be included in results sections

■ Describe the assumptions associated with each analysis

INTRODUCTION: EXPANDING GROUPS

What happens when a researcher wants to manipulate more than one variable, or add in multiple time points? Maybe the researcher wants to have a pre-test or baseline information included in the analysis. Well, independent groups and One-Way ANOVAs provide limited options for these types of issues, and as was described in Chapter 5, the design of a study can be quite creative and complex. Luckily, the underlying analytic framework is quite flexible and allows for the addition of other variables. The caveat is there are more technical issues to deal with. In this chapter, we discuss four designs than can be integrated with each other, but we look at them relatively independently. The four designs are factorial, repeated measures, repeated measures with independent groups, and ANCOVA (analysis of covariance).

QUESTION FOCUS AND PURPOSE

Each of the analyses in this chapter have specific questions and purposes. As such, we have separated each by their focus and the types of research questions. The actual design can be mixed across these and even combined. There are studies that are factorial ANCOVAs with repeated measures.

Factorial

Each design and subsequent analysis is aligned with a different purpose and set of research questions. The first analysis, **factorial**, is utilized when the researcher wants to manipulate more than one variable (Kirk, 2013). In Chapter 5, the example was a 2x2 design. In this design, there would be four groups. **Figure 7.1** redisplays the example from Chapter 5. The analysis for the design is commonly named, factorial ANOVA or Two-Way ANOVA. There are three core research questions:

■ What is the main effect for Factor A? For example, how much of a difference is there between 15 minutes and 30 minutes of exercise and myocardial function?

■ What is the main effect for Factor B? For example, how much of a difference is there between 7 and 8 hours of sleep and myocardial function?

■ Is there an interaction between Factors A and B? For example, how much does myocardial function vary by hours slept and amount of exercise?

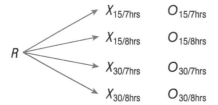

Figure 7.1. Factorial Design.

Why are the terms main effect and interaction used? These are used to demonstrate to the reader what the different groups are, which variables are manipulated, and that an interaction is involved. They are termed **main effects** because they are what the researcher is interested in examining, the main differences between these groups (Kirk, 2013; Maxwell & Delaney, 2017). Main effects may also be discussed as factors (e.g., Factor A and B) with different levels in a factor (e.g., different dosage rates: 10 mcg vs 25 mcg). **Interactions** occur when the main effects do not vary in the same manner. Interactions, historically, have been discussed three ways, ordinal, disordinal, and parallel (Kirk, 2013).

In **Figure 7.2**, **Ordinal Interactions** occur when changes between the groups have different rates of change across the levels of a factor. **Disordinal** interactions occur when the rates are different and those rates cross each other, for example, one groups improves and one group declines in health status. In essence, the outcome variable scores across levels invert. Interestingly, as one level changes, for example, no medication (NM) to medication (M), the other levels change differentially. **Parallel**, or no interaction, occurs when the changes across main effect levels stays the same—they look parallel.

Ordinal and disordinal interactions create an interesting dilemma for the researcher. When there is an interaction, ordinal or disordinal, should the focus of the results stay on the main effects and add in the interaction discussion? This makes sense on the surface, because the focus of the study was examining differences between those groups. Or should the focus be on the interaction? This argument makes sense, because you cannot talk about A or B alone because

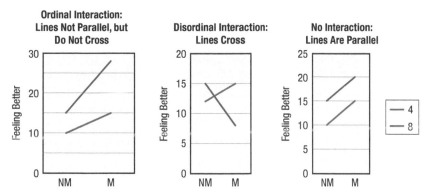

Figure 7.2. Ordinal, Disordinal, Parallel.

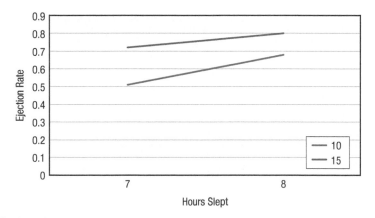

Figure 7.3. Ordinal Interaction.

they interact with each other! Another is you have to talk about all three effects equally. Historically, the debate about what to talk about just hinged on which of the three reached the $p < 0.05$ station. We feel, because the focus should be on "how much," the discussion should be all three equally. If there is a considerable interaction (i.e., large proportion of the sums of squares discussed later), the focus should be on the interaction and what that means theoretically, empirically, and in practice. In **Figure 7.3**, we have displayed a ordinal interaction (slopes are not parallel) with amount of sleep and exercise and myocardial function using ejection fraction.

The ejection fraction rates between groups (hours slept) are not the same for 10 and 15 minutes of exercise each day. Because they are not parallel, there is an interaction.

Repeated Measures

The purpose of repeated measures with one group design is to examine changes (or sometimes lack of change) on a variable of interest over time (Glass & Hopkins, 1995; Schreiber & Asner-Self, 2010) (**Figure 7.4**). These studies usually do not manipulate a variable because the interest is in natural changes. The core research question is,

■ How much of a change over time is observed?

$G\ O_1\ O_2\ O_3\ O_4$ Figure 7.4. Repeated Measures with Four Observation Points.

They may not appear to be exciting, but these studies provide an important source of information. The current "All of Us" Study (https://allofus.nih.gov/about) is hoping to enroll over one million participants in a longitudinal study designed to examine the development or lack of development of disease. There are not variable manipulations, just the collection of data over time. Some data will be collected repeatedly, others will only be collected once. Other repeated measures studies (see Chapter 5) do add in an intervention.

Repeated Measures With Groups

Some researchers want to manipulate at least one variable and track participants over time (**Figure 7.5**).

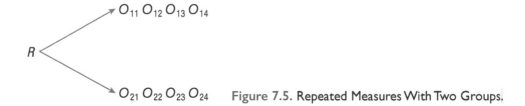

Figure 7.5. Repeated Measures With Two Groups.

The core research question is,

■ How different are these groups over time on the outcome variable (i.e., variable of interest).

For example, a researcher might assign participants to one of two groups (once a month check-in with doctor/nurse practitioner or weekly 5-minute telehealth meetings) in reference to weight management and track their weight over six months. In addition to the differences between the groups over time, there is also an interaction between groups and time. For example, Does one group change much faster over time than the other group? Though this is an important research question, it is not always the primary focus of a repeated measure design with groups. There can be a wide variety of repeated measures, such as an intervention between specific observations (See Chapter 5).

ANCOVA

The purpose of ANCOVA is to add in a covariate (a variable that is not of particular interest in the study but may affect the outcome) or covariates that the researcher is concerned about before analyzing how much the groups are different on an outcome variable (Ferguson & Takane, 1989; Glass & Hopkins, 1995). The covariate is collected typically after random assignment (**Figure 7.6**).

■ The core research question for ANCOVA is, how large are the differences between the groups after accounting for variable X?

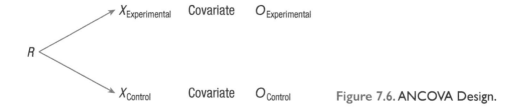

Figure 7.6. ANCOVA Design.

For example, how large are the differences between weight maintenance programs after accounting for starting weight? There are many technical issues with ANCOVA, which we will discuss later, but we want to write this caveat now: ANCOVA will not save a bad design or bad data and in general fancy statistics will not do that either.

Hypotheses

The hypotheses that are normally written in research articles will focus on expected research observations and not the null. In factorial ANOVAs, for example, the research hypotheses could be written such as, "The high dosage group will outperform the low dosage group on the sleep quality indicator. The longer exercise group will outperform the shorter exercise group on the sleep indicator, and the longer exercise and high dosage group, will perform the best." This provides the research hypotheses for both main effects and the interaction.

Repeated measures has one main research hypothesis, such as "Over time, there will be an increase (or decrease) in health knowledge as participants age." Because there is just one group that is watched over time, the options are limited in what the research hypotheses can be. The values of the outcome variable can go up, down, or vary (up and down) over time.

Repeated measures with groups has the same core research hypothesis as repeated measures. Where it differs, is between the groups and the potential interaction. For example, "The experimental group will increase their healthy behaviors over time at a faster rate than the control group." This research hypothesis statement is covering each group and their interaction all at once. The change within each group is important because both are increasing, but the experimental group has a faster change of the two. So, the interaction is between the group variable and the time variable.

ANCOVA analyses will have a caveat at the beginning or end of the research hypothesis. For example, "After controlling for baseline diabetes self-care knowledge scores and age, the experimental group that receives the educational intervention will score higher on diabetes self-care knowledge post-test than the control group."

GRAPHICAL REPRESENTATIONS

For all four of these analyses, conceptually, the differences between the group means and the differences within each of the groups is being analyzed, the between and within. But this is truly about distributions and their overlap.

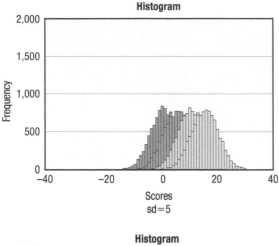

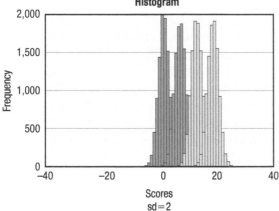

Figure 7.7. Factorial ANOVA Using Distributions.

Figure 7.7 provides distributions from two different factorial ANOVAs. The first shows the four groups overlapping a great deal. The first group (orange) with a mean about 0 is relatively far away from the last group (yellow) with a mean of 15. But overall, the groups overlap. In the upper display, the means are 5 points apart with a standard deviation of 5 for each distribution.

In the lower figure, the distributions are farther apart (standard deviation is smaller) and you can see a gap between them. To deeply understand factorial results, the researcher should graph the distribution of scores of each group to examine the differences between the groups (between analysis) and how spread out each group is (within analysis).

For repeated measures, the graph in Figure 7.7 can be used again to discuss changes over time because what is important is the distribution shape and the overlap with the other distributions. In the top figure, the changes over time are closer together and the group is making progress, but at each time interval, there is still a great overlap with scores from the previous time. In Figure 7.8, there is a display of distributions over time that are more separated with small standard deviations. The mean scores are clearly separated for each group and there is much less overlap in the distribution of scores. The first (farthest left) and the last (farthest right) do not actually overlap at all.

Repeated measures with groups simply adds a second set of distributions to examine. Figure 7.9 shows two groups, control on top and experimental on the bottom. Both groups start at about the same mean, around six. But by the second time point, the first group has only moved up a small amount, but the by the fourth time period the experimental group has quite a bit of an increase. The difference between time points and between groups would most likely indicate an interaction is occurring.

ANCOVA is where just looking at the distributions becomes problematic. The reason is due to technical components of the analysis (See technical section below). Overall, ANCOVA is ANOVA and regression (Chapter 8) combined

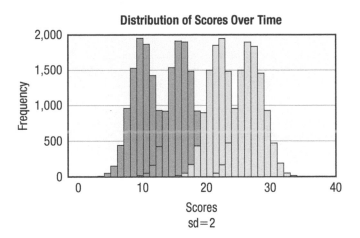

Figure 7.8. Repeated Measures Using Distributions.

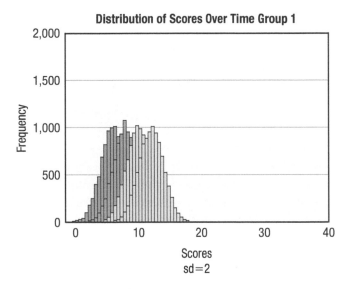

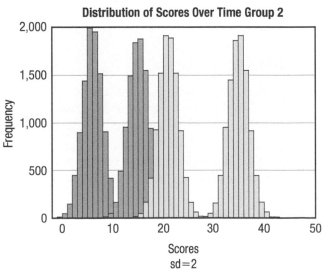

Figure 7.9. Repeated Measures With Two Groups Using Distributions.

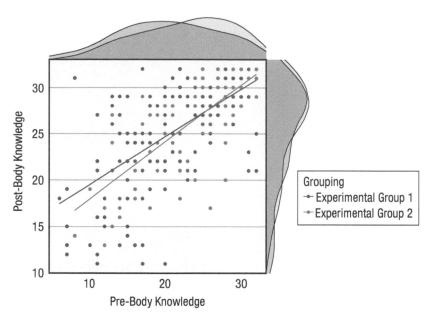

Figure 7.10. ANCOVA Using Distributions, Scatterplot, and Regression Lines.

because of the covariate (Glass & Hopkins, 1995). The best way to look at what is going on is to graph the outcome, the covariate, and the between group variable. Figure 7.10 shows two groups of children randomly assigned to two experimental groups and their knowledge about their body parts for a pre-test and a post-test. The different experimental groups are color coded, and the distributions of the data by group are provided. The distributions for both groups and both tests are not perfectly normally distributed. The post-test knowledge is higher than the pre-test knowledge on average. Notice that the distribution on the post-test overlaps a great deal along with the individual data pairs in the scatter plot, thus the groups are not separated–not different. Finally, the two regression lines' slopes are almost parallel, which is an important assumption in ANCOVA.

TECHNICAL SECTION

Though there are overlapping assumptions across these four designs, we have separated the technical section by analysis because it makes it a bit easier to learn the first time. Additionally, many of these assumptions will be familiar from Chapter 6. All four of these tests are considered parametric tests because the outcome data are assumed to be normally distributed. If the covariate in the ANCOVA is continuous, it is also assumed to be normally distributed.

Factorial ANOVA

Factorial ANOVA assumptions include that the independent variables are categorical and that participants cannot be in multiple categories at the same time (Stevens, 2002; Tabachnick & Fidell, 2007). For example, if the researcher is interested in manipulating treatment plans, participants can only be in one treatment plan at a time. Factorial ANOVA is relatively robust to nonnormality of the dependent variable. By **robust**, we meant that the results will not be drastically affected by nonnormality. In general, though the researcher wants the outcome variable to be close to normally distributed. The variances are also expected to be equal, or at least close to equal, thus **homogeneity of variance**. Participants are assumed to be randomly sampled as is uncommon in these analyses. Finally, the errors are independent (not correlated) between participants and groups.

Source Table

The main information for the factorial ANOVA comes from the source table. This is the same source table as the ANOVA with an expansion for the second independent variable and the interaction. Table 7.1 displays a fictitious source table for a 2x2 factorial design with 12 participants. In the source table, the "source" again comes from the independent variables, the interaction and the error. The sums of squares are the calculation of where the variability is split up across the source. Each source value added up will equal the total at the bottom. In this example, the main effect A has the largest sums of squares values indicating it is quite important in explaining the total variability in the outcome. Most importantly, error is not taking up much of the total sums of squares. In general, researchers want the Error source value to be very small because that indicates that the variables are explaining the outcome. This is commonly missed or forgotten when researchers only focus on the p-value. Next, are the degrees of freedom (df), which are based on the sample size of the study and the number of groups. In this 2x2 example, the first factor A has two levels so the degrees of freedom are $k - 1$, $2 - 1$, or 1—same for the next factor B. A × B is the interaction, and is calculated by multiplying the degrees of freedom of the two factors together, in this example $1 \times 1 = 1$. The error df is the sample size of the study minus one and then subtract the degrees of freedom for the two factors and the interaction. Finally, the degrees of freedom for the total is the sample size minus one. And yes, the factors, interaction, and error degrees of freedom have to equal the total degrees of freedom.

Table 7.1. Source Table One-Way ANOVA.

Source	Sums of Squares	df	Mean Square	F-ratio
Main Effect A	34.26	2 – 1 =1	34.26/1	34.26/2.87 = 11.94
Main Effect B	15.39	2 – 1 =1	15.39/1	15.39/2.87 = 5.36
A × B	21.78	(2 – 1) × (2 – 1) = 1	21.78/1	21.78/2.87 = 7.59
Error	22.95	(12 – 1) – (1 + 1 + 1) = 8	22.95/8 = 2.87	
Total	94.38	12 – 1 = 11		

Mean square is the source sums of squares divided by the degrees of freedom for that source. For example, the between sums of squares for main effect A is 34.26 and the degrees of freedom is one, so the mean square between value is 34.26/1 = 34.26. For the error, the mean square is *15.39/1= 15.39* and for the interaction it is *21.78/1 = 21.78*. Now the *F*-value is calculated for each component, main effect A, B, and the interaction. Each mean square value is divided by the error mean square. Those three values are then compared to an *F*-distribution table with df of each component and the error df of 8. Thus, main effect B, would have a cut-off value on the *F*-distribution table ($F(1,8) = 5.32$). Since main effect B of 5.36 >5.32, the researcher would state that the observed *p*-value is less than 0.05 ($p < 0.05$). Most statistical packages will produce an exact p-value. In this example, the value would be 0.0485.

Compatibility Intervals and Effect Sizes

Compatibility intervals (CI) and effect sizes are calculated similarly to independent *t*-tests for the means and One-Way ANOVA for the source table. In research studies, there are Cohen's *d* commonly used for looking at effect sizes for mean, CIs for means of each group. The effect sizes for the source table are generally eta, partial eta-squared and omega-squared, one for each main effect and one for the interaction–three in total. Some statistical packages also produce effect sizes (Cohen's *d*) for post-hoc analyses, such as Scheffe or Tukey. Those effect sizes for the post-hoc tests provide the researcher a good deal of information about "how much" difference there is between groups.

Sample Size

Sample sizes for factorial analysis are currently based on number of cells, for example, a 2x2 has four cells, the expected effect size, 0.05 cut off, and the desired power. But again, this is still focusing on the *p*-value. The old rule of thumb was 30 participants per cell. A traditional power analysis with 0.05 cutoff, 0.80 as power, and a moderate effect size (eta squared of 0.06), indicates 32 per cell would be needed or 128. As a reminder, it is important to think about accuracy from Chapter 4 in relation to sample size. Additionally, the importance or risk level is an essential consideration. As the importance or risk of being wrong increases, sample size with a focus on representation should take precedence over traditional power analysis.

Repeated Measures

In a repeated measures analysis, there is an assumption that the participants were randomly selected from the population, just like the independent *t*-test, ANOVA, and factorial ANOVA. Additionally, and with all of the previous parametric analyses, repeated outcome variables are assumed to be normally distributed. Next, homogeneity of variance is also assumed. A unique assumption in repeated measures is termed **sphericity**, also called **compound symmetry**. Sphericity is the assumption that the variance of difference scores in the population is equal. For example, a researcher collects data three times on the same measure. To meet this assumption, the variances scores between the first score and the second, the first score and the third, and the second and the third should be equal:

$$\text{Variance}_{A-B} = \text{Variance}_{A-C} = \text{Variance}_{B-C}$$

Table 7.2 provides a small example of three time points of a fictitious study where nurses were asked their stress level right before their shift started as the hospital was filling up with patients. The variances for the three differences are pretty close, 2.50 to 2.68. There most likely is not a sphericity issue with this data.

Table 7.2. Sphericity Variance Example.

A	B	C	A–B	A–C	B–C
2	7	6	−5	−4	1
4	3	7	1	−3	−4
4	6	7	−2	−3	−1
1	3	5	−2	−4	−2
2	5	9	−3	−7	−4
5	7	9	−2	−4	−2
1	4	5	−3	−4	−1
3	7	8	−4	−5	−1
5	6	7	−1	−2	−1
1	3	3	−2	−2	0
		sd	1.64	1.48	1.58
		variance	2.68	2.18	2.50

The test for sphericity is completed with the Mauchly test. There are some issues with this test because it has been shown to have accuracy problems when the normality assumption is violated and with small sample sizes. If the sphericity assumption is not tenable, there are adjustments built into most statistical software programs, such as Huynh-Feldt Epsilon, (Huynh & Feldt, 1976) and Greenhouse-Geisser Epsilon (Greenhouse & Geiser, 1959).

Finally, linearity of the trajectory of the data is assumed. Thus, the change in scores is assumed to move in a linear fashion, up or down. As time points increase, the possibility of this assumption being violated increases, and therefore tests of nonlinear patterns (e.g., curvilinear) need to be completed.

Source Table and Sums of Squares—Repeated Measures

There are multiple tables in a repeated measure design. The data from the stress at start of work sphericity example is used here. The first is the sphericity test table with Mauchly's test (Table 7.3), then the Within Subjects table (Table 7.4). Notice the Mauchly's W test p-value is quite large indicating there is not

Table 7.3. Mauchly's Test.

Tests of Sphericity				
	Mauchly's W	p	Greenhouse-Geisser ε	Huynh-Feldt ε
Stress	0.986	0.944	0.986	1.000

Table 7.4. Within-Subjects Test Repeated Measures.

Within Subjects Effects								
	Sphericity Correction	Sum of Squares	df	Mean Square	F	p	η^2	η^2_p
Stress	None	73.267	2	36.633	29.882	<0.001	0.469	0.769
	Greenhouse-Geisser (G-G)	73.267	1.972	37.155	29.882	<0.001	0.469	0.769
	Huynh-Feldt	73.267	2.000	36.633	29.882	<0.001	0.469	0.769
Residual	None	22.067	18	1.226				
	Greenhouse-Geisser (G-G)	22.067	17.747	1.243				
	Huynh-Feldt	22.067	18.000	1.226				

a problem, so no correction needed. The within subjects effects table looks like a traditional source table. The only difference is there is no between groups component because there is only one group in this example. The repeated measure stress is first, and error is next (Table 7.4). Error is commonly referred to as residual. Next in the table is the type of correction, then sum of squares and so on.

In the Within-Subjects results, the sums of squares is the same, but the difference occurs with the degrees of freedom for G-G. This adjustment is based on the adjustment value from Table 7.3 (.986). The adjusted degrees of freedom is calculated by using the no correction degrees of freedom (2) and multiplying it by the G-G correction (2 × 0.986) which equals 1.972. Then the mean square, F-value and p-values are all completed just like in the ANOVA example in Chapter 6. Since, the sphericity assumption was met, the "none" correction lines would be followed. The large F-value (29.882) indicates there are changes over time. The effect sizes for eta-squared (0.469) and partial eta-squared (0.769) indicate a large effect over the three time points. There is a between subjects table that will be created in most statistical packages (Table 7.5). The information in it will be just on the error because there is no between group component. In the big picture, it is basic information. Finally, descriptive statistics are provided in Table 7.6. There is a slight difference in standard deviation values across time points and the third stress observation had the highest mean value.

Repeated measures with groups will have all the same information as repeated measures and include the between group source table along with the interaction component between the groups and the time points. Using the previous repeated measures example, we have split the data into two groups, daylight and

Table 7.5. Between Group Analysis for Repeated Measures (One Group).

	Sum of Squares	df	Mean Square	F	p
Residual	60.833	9	6.759		

Table 7.6. Descriptive Statistics Repeated Measures.

	Stress 1	Stress 2	Stress 3
Mean	2.800	5.100	6.600
Median	2.500	5.500	7.000
Standard Deviation	1.619	1.729	1.897
Minimum	1	3	3
Maximum	5	7	9
Shapiro-Wilk W	0.873	0.840	0.942
Shapiro-Wilk p	0.109	0.044	0.573

$N = 10$.

Table 7.7. Mauchly's Test Repeated Measures With Groups.

Tests of Sphericity				
	Mauchly's W	p	Greenhouse-Geisser ε	Huynh-Feldt ε
Stress	0.908	0.714	0.916	1.000

Table 7.8. Repeated Measures With Group.

	Sphericity Correction	Sum of Squares	df	Mean Square	F	p	η^2	η^2_p
Stress	None	73.267	2	36.633	32.806	<0.001	0.469	0.804
	Greenhouse-Geisser	73.267	1.832	39.996	32.806	<0.001	0.469	0.804
	Huynh-Feldt	73.267	2.000	36.633	32.806	<0.001	0.469	0.804
Stress × Group	None	4.200	2	2.100	1.881	0.185	0.027	0.190
	Greenhouse-Geisser	4.200	1.832	2.293	1.881	0.189	0.027	0.190
	Huynh-Feldt	4.200	2.000	2.100	1.881	0.185	0.027	0.190
Residual	None	17.867	16	1.117				
	Greenhouse-Geisser	17.867	14.655	1.219				
	Huynh-Feldt	17.867	16.000	1.117				

night shifts. Table 7.7 shows the Mauchly test, which again shows no sphericity problems. The within analysis (Table 7.8) again follows the "none" correction line. "None" indicates there are changes over time as based on the large F-value and the effect sizes. The Stress by Group has a small F-value indicating little explanation of the variation is coming from the interaction. The small effect size values also indicate this. The between subject analysis shows a moderate sized F-value and moderate to large effect sizes (Table 7.9). Thus, being at work in the morning or night shift is accounting for variation in the stress scores.

Table 7.9. Between Subject Repeated Measures With Groups.

	Sum of Squares	df	Mean Square	F	p	η^2	η^2_p
Group	24.300	1	24.300	5.321	0.050	0.156	0.399
Residual	36.533	8	4.567				

Confidence Intervals and Effect Sizes

The effect sizes and confidence intervals are calculated in a similar manner as previously discussed in t-test, One-Way ANOVA, and factorial ANOVA. In the example in Table 7.8, eta-squared is calculated by taking the sums of squares (correction – none) of 73.267 and dividing it by the total sums (within and between), which is (73.267 + 4.2 + 17.867 + 24.3 + 36.533) = 156.164, which becomes 73.267 / 156.164 = 0.469. Partial eta squared is sum of squares (correction – none) divided by sums of squares (none) + residual (none), which becomes 73.267 / (73.267 + 17.867) = 0.804.

Eta squared for the between group analysis is the group sums of squares / (total between + total within). In this case, that is 24.30 / 156.164 = 0.156. Partial eta-squared is the group sums of squares divided by total between, which is 24.30 / (24.30 + 26.533), and equals 0.399. Partial eta-squared in this example is much higher because it is based on fewer sums of squares. This is why it is important to understand how these are calculated because sometimes only the largest ones get reported and they are not the same. The differences between groups can also be seen in the descriptive statistics in Table 7.10—note the differences in mean values between night and daylight shift.

Table 7.10. Descriptive Statistics Repeated Measures Example.

	Group	A	B	C
Mean	Daylight	2.000	4.600	5.200
	Night	3.600	5.600	8.000
Median	Daylight	1	4	5
	Night	4	6	8
Standard deviation	Daylight	1.732	1.817	1.483
	Night	1.140	1.673	1.000
Minimum	Daylight	1	3	3
	Night	2	3	7
Maximum	Daylight	5	7	7
	Night	5	7	9
Shapiro-Wilk W	Daylight	0.701	0.867	0.956
	Night	0.961	0.881	0.821
Shapiro-Wilk p	Daylight	0.010	0.254	0.777
	Night	0.814	0.314	0.119

$N = 5$ for each group.

Sample Size

Sample size for the traditional power analysis of a repeated measures has more technical issues with it than previous analyses. The sample sizes are often smaller because some power is gained with the repeated observations. An estimated effect size and desired power are required along with number of repeats, number of groups, sphericity correction, and the correlation size of the observations between points. One program, GLIMMPSE, which is funded by the National Institutes of Health and run through the University of Colorado Denver, is a nice program to use for repeated measures. It has a little learning curve, but when you get it down, you will be happy with it. Additionally, there is G*Power (Faul et al.,2009). A simple repeated measure with two groups, power of 0.80, four repeated observations, medium effect size, correlation of 0.50 between observations and a sphericity correction of 0.90 needs a total sample size of 26. We highly recommend reading articles that have used a similar repeated measures as a framework during the design stage of the study.

ANCOVA

Analysis of Covariance, ANCOVA, is a blend between regression and ANOVA (Glass & Hopkins, 1996). ANCOVA has been problematic for decades, not because of the analysis, but how researchers use it. The technique when implemented properly is powerful. As we have already stated, fancy statistics will not save a poor design, and the use of ANCOVA needs to have a very solid design before data collection and analysis occur.

ANCOVA was developed by Eden and Fisher (1927) in an agricultural study, though has been attributed to others. ANCOVA allows for the reduction of error within groups, and this leads to a marked increase in traditional statistical power (Miller & Chapman, 2001). The inclusion of a covariate, sometimes referred to as a nuisance variable or confounding variable, creates the reduction in error. The variable is assumed to be continuous in nature and could not be completely controlled prior or after *random assignment*. Random assignment to groups is expected in this analysis, but there are ways to deal with nonrandomized designs (Cronbach, 1977).

Assumptions

The first assumption is the relationships between the dependent variable and the independent variables (experimental groups and covariates) are linear and not any other relationship. There is some evidence that ANCOVA is relatively robust to the violation (Glass et al., 1972). Errors are assumed to be random and normally distributed and not correlated, independence of errors. As with previous analyses in the ANOVA family, homogeneity of variance is also assumed. The *covariate* is not affected by the treatment. The groups should not differ on the covariate at the start of the study.

Therefore, it is typically better in randomized experiments to stratify on the covariate than to use it as a covariate. In quasi-experiments, when the participants in each group are really different on a covariate, there can be a weird extrapolation where neither group has the actual adjusted mean value. One assumption rarely discussed is the covariate contains no measurement error (Lord, 1960), which never happens. Thus, at a minimum the covariate has to have low measurement error. Finally, the dependent variable is normally distributed.

Cautions to Start With

ANCOVA is misused a great deal (Cronbach, 1977; Glass et al., 1972; Lord, 1960; Miller & Chapman, 2001; Reichardt, 1979). ANCOVA does not magically turn a quasi-experimental design into an experimental one. The analysis can increase power and reduce bias but is not a replacement for randomized experiments, especially balanced designs. And ANCOVA cannot make the same inferences as a randomized experimental design. Unreliability in the covariate will allow for bias to exist. ANCOVA also has issues with the range of data that is covered by the covariate. The values in the covariate do not typically cover all possible values; it is a "restricted range." This means there is part of that potential range that must be assumed to work for the covariate and the dependent variable, for example, not curvilinear. And, as the differences widen between the groups on the covariate, the inferences made become more speculative (Glass & Hopkins, 1995). Thus, the covariate is just an adjustment. It does not substitute for other designs, such as equating of individuals (paired/balanced designs), random selection and random assignment, or multivariable propensity score matching.

Analytic Steps

The actual analysis for an ANCOVA has multiple steps. The first is to test if the groups and the covariate are interacting. This is termed the parallel lines test (Figure 7.10). The ANCOVA is run with the groups, the covariate, and the interaction between the two. Table 7.11 shows the results of simulated data using the body knowledge data. The only line to examine is the interaction (grouping by age in months). The important part is the small F-value indicating the interaction does not play a substantial part in the total sums of squares. The p-value can also be used here and has been traditionally examined with 0.05 as the cutoff. The problem with that is 0.06 might still indicate an interaction. After this decision, the regular analysis without the interaction can be completed.

The results from ANCOVA analysis should include, homogeneity of variance test, normality test of the dependent variable and covariate, along with a residual analysis. Table 7.12 has the homogeneity of variance test, which indicates the variances of the groups are similar (p-value for Levene's test and Bartlett's test is

Table 7.11. ANCOVA Example Source Table With Interaction Test.

	Sum of Squares	df	Mean Square	F	p
Overall model	357.662	3	119.221	5.986	<0.001
Age	340.210	1	340.210	12.342	<0.001
Grouping	8.883	1	8.883	0.322	0.571
Grouping × Age	8.568	1	8.568	0.311	0.578
Residuals	6505.415	236	27.565		

Table 7.12. **ANCOVA, Homogeneity of Variance Test.**

	Statistic	df	df2	p
Levene's	1.218	1	238	0.271
Bartlett's	1.153	1		0.283

Table 7.13. **ANCOVA Example Source Table.**

	Sum of Squares	df	Mean Square	F	p	η^2	η^2p
Grouping	0.411	1	0.411	0.015	0.903	0.000	0.000
AGE (Months)	445.718	1	445.718	16.217	<0.001	0.064	0.064
Residuals	6513.983	237	27.485				

>0.05). The results of the tests of normality for the covariate and the dependent variable are both nonnormal. The researcher would then examine options for transforming the data (Chapter 3) e.g., Shapiro-Wilk (S-W) = 0.962, $p<0.001$. For this example, we are not transforming the data. Table 7.13 has the results of the ANCOVA. The experimental groups are not different. The sums of squares for grouping is very small. And the error sums of squares is quite large (Residuals).

Age does appear to be important given the large F-value and moderate partial eta-squared. But, that was supposed to be the covariate and not the focus of the results. A residual analysis, the comparison of observed outcome with predicted outcome, based on the analysis (see Chapter 8) looks problematic. Figure 7.11 shows multiple residual points not on the line at the top and the bottom. Perfectly normally distributed residuals (error) would all be on the 45-degree line. This may be due to the nonnormality of the data. Figure 7.12

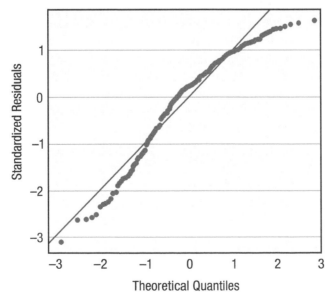

Figure 7.11. Q-Q Plot.

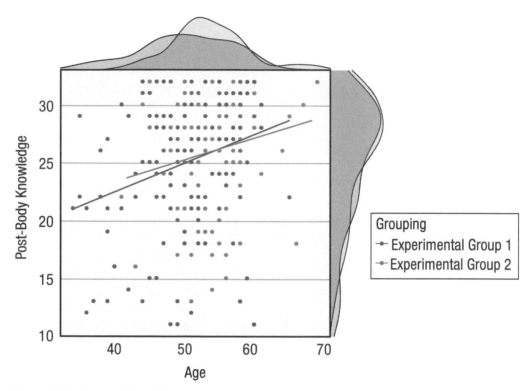

Figure 7.12. Scatterplot of Age in Months by Body Knowledge Separated by Grouping.

displays a scatterplot of body knowledge by age in months separated by experimental group which allows the researcher to see the relationship overall, and within and between groups.

Descriptive statistics are in Table 7.14 and indicate a small difference in age, small difference in post-test knowledge, with some skewness for the knowledge test, but not above historical cut-off value of plus or minus 1. These are the unadjusted means. By that, these are the raw means, for Body Knowledge, not adjusted for age. Some statistical packages will give you one or the other, and sometimes both.

Confidence Intervals and Effect Sizes

The confidence intervals for the means are calculated in the same manner as before. And as with factorial ANOVA, effect sizes for the between group components will be calculated. Additionally, effect sizes for the covariate or covariates will be calculated. If there are more than two groups, Cohen's d is often provided for effect size estimation between each pair of the groups.

Sample Size ANCOVA

Traditional sample size calculations are based on desired power, the p-value cut-off, the number of groups, expected effect size, and the number of covariates. For example, a study with four groups, one covariate, moderate

Table 7.14. Descriptive Statistics of ANCOVA Example.

	Grouping	Age (Months)	Body Knowledge Post	
Mean	Experimental Group 1	50.175	24.923	(CI95 24.00, 25.84)
	Experimental Group 2	53.515	25.763	(CI95 24.74, 26.78)
Median	Experimental Group 1	51.000	27.000	
	Experimental Group 2	53.000	27.000	
Standard deviation	Experimental Group 1	6.528	5.619	
	Experimental Group 2	5.337	5.078	
Skewness	Experimental Group 1	−0.356	−0.841	
	Experimental Group 2	0.541	−0.772	
Kurtosis	Experimental Group 1	−0.354	−0.127	
	Experimental Group 2	0.972	−0.311	

effect size, the cut-off at the traditional 0.05, and power of 0.80 would need about 270 participants. If the expected effect size is small, the sample size needed is over 1,600. A reminder that this is all based on trying to get to $p < 0.05$. We want you to think about accuracy and how many and which participants would make the study stable and believable based on the level of risk concerning the study.

CORE RESULTS SECTIONS

Each analysis has specific information that should be included. This section provides brief results' reports based on the examples in the technical section. A basic check list is provided in the Most Defining Attributes Section. When in doubt, add the information in—more information is better for readers than less.

Results Example: Factorial ANOVA

For the factorial ANOVA results, we are using a fictitious set of data with a simple outcome variable of myocardial functioning and sleep for main effect A (7 or 8 hours) and exercise for main effect B (15 vs. 30 minutes per day).

A 2x2 factorial ANOVA with myocardial functioning score as the outcome was examined. The main effect for sleep was $F(1, 28) = 8.66$, MSe = 2.25, $p < 0.006$ with a partial eta-squared (η^2p) of 0.24. The main effect for exercise was $F(1,28) = 11.66$, MSe = 2.25, $p = 0.002$, with a partial eta-squared of 0.29. The interaction between sleep and exercise of $F(1,28) = 0.125$, MSe = 2.25, $p = 0.73$ with a partial eta squared of 0.004. The Levene's test indicated homogeneity of variance can be assumed $F(3,8) = 1.055$, $p = 0.38$. The mean functioning score for each group is provided in Table 7.15. Those participants who had 8 hours of sleep and 30 minutes of exercise had the highest functioning scores. Compatibility interval values around the dosage groups were large due to the small sample size. Table 7.16 presents the full source table. Finally, residuals were normally distributed based on a Q-Q plot.

Table 7.15. Cross-Tab Descriptives ANOVA Example.

Sleep	Exercise	Mean	sd	n	95% CI
7	15	4.75	1.04	8	3.66–5.84
	30	6.38	1.85	8	5.29–7.46
8	15	6.13	1.81	8	5.04–7.21
	30	8.13	1.13	8	7.04–9.21

Table 7.16. Source Table ANOVA Example.

	Sum of Squares	df	Mean Square	F	p	η²p
Sleep	19.531	1	19.531	8.663	0.006	0.236
Exercise	26.281	1	26.281	11.657	0.002	0.294
Sleep × Exercise	0.281	1	0.281	0.125	0.727	0.004
Residuals	63.125	28	2.254			

ANCOVA

The example below uses the results from the diabetes self-care knowledge example.

An ANCOVA was run with two experimental groups and one covariate, Age. The tests for parallel slopes ($F(1, 237) = 0.311$ $p = 0.58$) and homogeneity ($F(1, 238) = 1.22$ $p = 0.27$) indicated both assumptions were tenable. The normality test indicated nonnormality for both the covariate and the outcome variable. The variables' skewness was not greater then +/- 1 and was not transformed. The main effect for the treatment groups was $F(1,237) = 0.015$, $MSb = 0.411$, $p = 0.90$. The partial eta-squared for treatment groups was 0.00. The covariate results were $F(1,237) = 16.22$, $MSc = 445.72$, $p < 0.001$. Residual analysis indicates problems at the upper and lower end of the outcome variable. Compatibility interval values around the treatment groups were small due to the large sample sizes within groups and the standard error values.

If you have space or there is no limit to tables, we recommend putting in the full source table.

Repeated Measures/Repeated Measures With Groups

For this example write up, we used the repeated measures with groups example (Tables 7.8 and 7.9). The write up are similar with the difference being the addition of between group differences and the interaction of group and time.

A repeated measures ANOVA with two experimental groups (daylight and night shift) and 3 repeats on the outcome variable stress was implemented. The repeated outcome variables were approximately normally distributed with time point 2 having the largest deviation from normality. No outliers were observed in this small data set. Mauchly's test for sphericity did not indicate a problem ($W = 0.91$, $p = 0.71$.). With sphericity assumed, the within-subject results were $F(2, 16) = 32.82$, $p < 0.001$, and a partial eta-squared of 0.80.

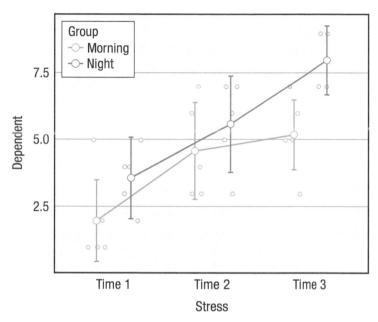

Figure 7.13. Graph of Group by Time for Repeated Measures.

The mean-square error is 1.12, df = 16. The correlations between time points ranged from 0.52 to 0.65. The interaction between the three time points and shift had an $F(2,16) =1.81$, $p = 0.19$, and partial eta-squared of 0.19. The between group analysis had an $F(1,8) = 5.32$, $p = 0.05$, with a partial eta-squared of 0.40.

Note, some statistical packages have a test of linearity across timepoints. In Figure 7.13, we provide a graph to show that even if linearity can be assumed, it does not mean that the lines are perfectly straight, and that is important to know. Note, descriptive statistics for both groups over time along with correlations between each time points would also be included in the narrative. If you have space or there is no limit to tables, we recommend putting in the full source table.

NONPARAMETRIC ANALYSES

There are nonparametric adaptations for these four analyses. They are inherently more technically complicated because the data is either nonnormal and cannot be transformed easily, or the data is ordered categorical. Factorial and longitudinal designs can be analyzed using the R software package (Noguchi et al., 2012). Factorial designs can also be analyzed using an aligned rank test before analysis. Nonparametric ANCOVA (Cangür et al., 2018; Olejnik & Algina, 1985; Tsangari & Akritas, 2004) has begun to be integrated into statistical software packages, but only with one grouping variable (e.g., a One-Way ANCOVA).

MOST DEFINING ATTRIBUTES

Each analysis has specific components that should be included in a results section. Below, we outline the general points for all four analyses, and then for each one's specific needs. Note some of the items in the checklists are not available in certain statistical packages.

Common Across Each

1. Check dependent variable for normality
2. Check dependent variable by group for normality
3. Check for outliers
4. Outliers/missing data and how they were handled
5. Core information to discuss in narrative/tables
    a. Means, sd, and n-size for all groups/categories
    b. Standard errors for all groups/categories

Factorial ANOVA

1. Levene's test for equal variances
    a. Levene's results
2. MSe for each variable (A and B) and the interaction (A x B) at a minimum, degrees of freedom, F-ratio at a minimum
3. descriptive p-value
    a. e.g., $p = 0.17$
4. Type of interaction
5. Contrasts/post hoc
    a. Full details on contrasts, if appropriate
    b. Full details on post-hoc chosen and why, if appropriate
6. CI.
7. Effect size—partial eta-squared, for example
8. Full discussion of residuals
9. ANOVA source table is preferable
10. Observed power

Repeated Measures/Repeated Measures With Groups

1. Normality of the difference between the repeated measures
    a. Same issue in paired t-tests
2. Dependent variable by group for normality if there is a between group component
3. Sphericity test
4. Greenhouse/Huynh-felt tests for within-subjects
5. Linearity examination
6. Between group source table information (if appropriate)

7. Information to also include in narrative
   a. Means, sd, and n-size for both groups and repeats
   b. Standard errors for both groups
   c. Correlation between the repeats–this is rare to see but good for the reader

ANCOVA

1. Check dependent variable by group for normality (within cell outliers)
   a. Unequal group sample sizes due to missing data can be especially problematic
2. Check Levene's test for equal variances for the groups
3. Parallel slopes test
4. Information to discuss in narrative
   a. Means, sd, and n-size for all groups/categories
      i. Main effects for the group differences
      ii. Adjusted marginal means based on the covariate
   b. Standard errors for all groups/categories
   c. Levene's results
   d. Results of parallel slopes test
   e. MSe for the group variable
   f. MSe for each variable (A and B) and the interaction (A x B) at a minimum, degrees of freedom, F-ratio at a minimum
   g. descriptive p-value
      i. e.g., $p = 0.17$
   h. Contrasts/post hoc
      i. Full details on contrasts, if appropriate
      ii. Full details on post-hoc chosen and why, if appropriate
   i. Compatibility intervals
   j. Effect size-- partial eta-squared, for example
   k. Full discussion of residuals
   l. ANCOVA source table is preferable.
   m. Observed power

Finally, if you are in doubt if a piece of information is needed, put it in. It might need to go into an appendix or supplemental materials depending on the journal's manuscript submission rules. As editors and associate editors of journals, we have never been frustrated with too much technical information. We are always frustrated by too little technical information.

SUMMARY

Chapter 7 discussed the conceptual and technical aspects of four very popular analyses. Each analysis within the ANOVA framework has unique components and assumptions. Factorial ANOVA, ANCOVA, and repeated measures with groups all assume random assignment of participants. This is not always the case, and there is a large literature base on nonrandomized designs (Cronbach, 1977; Reichardt, 1979). Factorial ANOVA is best used when two variables of interest have been manipulated, and there is a desire to see if there are differences between the groups and if there is an interaction between the groups. Repeated measures is focused on studies where a variable is measured more than two times. With the additional time points, the analysis has to move from a paired t-test to the ANOVA framework so that the variability over multiple time points can be examined. This change also means that issues related to variability must be examined. Finally, ANCOVA is the most complex from a technical standpoint. It was designed to improve power of experimental designs but has been abused over the years as a way to try and equate nonnormal or naturally occurring groups. Finally, this is an introduction to each of these techniques and as such each could easily be its own chapter or small monograph.

END-OF-CHAPTER RESOURCES

REVIEW QUESTIONS

Answers and rationales for the review questions are located in the Appendix at the end of the book.

1. TRUE or FALSE?

   In a factorial design, when there is an interaction between Factor A and Factor B, the focus of the investigator's discussion should be on the main effects of Factors A and B because the purpose of the study was to look for differences between those groups on the outcome.

2. TRUE or FALSE?

   An investigator wants to determine the effect of a vegetarian diet vs. standard diet and using a food tracking app vs. not using an app on weight loss at 3 months. She finds a disordinal interaction when the vegetarian group who used the app gained weight while the standard group who did not use the app lost weight.

3. TRUE or FALSE?

   In a repeated measures design with two groups, the researcher may find an interaction between the group variable and the variable of time.

4. Which of the following is an example of a research question that would lend itself to statistical analysis using ANCOVA?

   a. What are the changes in functional mobility at 6, 12, and 24 weeks between older adults performing yoga and older adults lifting weights three times a week?

   b. How much difference is there in depression between adolescents who spend ≥4 hours a day on social media compared to those who spend <4 hours?

   c. How much difference is there in anxiety levels at 6 months between the cognitive behavioral therapy group and the medication group after taking into account baseline anxiety?

   d. How much of a difference is there in resting heart rate from baseline to 6 months among participants who join a running group?

5. Which of the following is an example of a hypothesis that would be analyzed using a factorial ANOVA?

   a. Students receiving mindfulness training at the start of their freshman year will report decreasing test anxiety during midterm and final exams weeks over 4 years.

   b. After controlling for heart failure stage, patients who receive an intervention on lowering sodium intake will present to the emergency department less frequently than patients who do not receive the intervention.

   c. Levels of burnout, chronic stress, and insomnia among bedside nurses working 12-hour nightshifts will decrease the longer they work the same schedule.

   d. Among nursing students randomized to high-fidelity simulation or low-fidelity simulation and morning training or afternoon training, students in the high-fidelity simulation morning training will perform better on basic life support skills.

6. A researcher runs a two-way ANOVA looking at the effect of treatment A vs. treatment B on a health outcome and wants to determine the size of the effect of the treatments. In the source table, treatment A has a partial eta^2 of 0.07 while treatment B has a partial eta^2 of 0.20. Which treatment can be said to have a greater effect on the outcome?

7. Describe the unique underlying assumption associated with a repeated measures ANOVA and how you can test for it.

8. Discuss why sample size requirements are usually smaller when conducting a within-subjects repeated measures ANOVA.

9. Which of the following is a common component to be included in the results section for all four designs of factorial, repeated measures, repeated measures with independent groups, and ANCOVA? Select all that apply.

   a. normality testing for the outcome variable

   b. correlations between the measures

   c. normality testing for the outcome variable by each group

   d. Levene's test for equal variances

   e. presence/absence of outlying values

   f. how missing data were handled

   g. Mauchly's Test of Sphericity

   h. descriptives (mean, sd) and sample size for all groups along with standard errors

10. An investigator is carefully considering the covariates (confounding variables) to include in the ANCOVA for his project. Discuss the considerations associated with including a covariate in the model.

 SPRINGER PUBLISHING CONNECT™ | A robust set of instructor resources designed to supplement this text is located at http://connect.springerpub.com/content/book/978-0-8261-6582-4. Qualifying instructors may request access by emailing textbook@springerpub.com.

REFERENCES

Cangür, Ş., Sungur, M. A., & Ankarali, H. (2018). The methods used in nonparametric covariance analysis. *Duzce Medical Journal, 20*(1), 1–6. https://doi.org/10.18678/dtfd.424774

Cronbach, L. J. (1977). *Analysis of covariance in nonrandomized experiments: Parameters affecting bias.* Stanford Evaluation Consortium, School of Education, Stanford University.

Eden, T., & Fisher, R. A. (1927). Studies in crop variation: IV. The experimental determination of the value of top dressings with cereals. *The Journal of Agricultural Science, 17*(4), 548–562. https://doi.org/10.1017/S0021859600018827

Faul, F., Erdfelder, E., Buchner, A., & Lang, A.-G. (2009). Statistical power analyses using G*Power 3.1: Tests for correlation and regression analyses. *Behavior Research Methods, 41*, 1149-1160.

Ferguson, G. A., & Takane, Y. (1989). *Statistical analysis in psychology and education.* McGraw-Hill.

Glass, G. V., & Hopkins, K. D. (1996). *Statistical methods in education and psychology.* Allyn & Bacon

Glass, G. V., & Hopkins, K. D. (1995). *Statistical methods in education and psychology* (3rd ed.). Allyn and Bacon.

Glass, G. V., Peckham, P. D., & Sanders, J. R. (1972). Consequences of failure to meet assumptions underlying the fixed effects analyses of variance and covariance. *Review of Educational Research, 42*(3), 237–288. https://doi.org/10.3102/00346543042003237

Greenhouse, S. W., & Geisser, S. (1959). On methods in the analysis of profile data. *Psychometrika, 24*, 95–112. https://doi.org/10.1007/BF02289823

Huynh, H., & Feldt, L. S. (1976). Estimation of the Box correction for degrees of freedom from sample data in randomized block and split=plot designs. *Journal of Educational Statistics, 1*, 69–82. https://doi.org/10.3102/10769986001001069

Kirk, R. E. (2013). *Experimental design: Procedures for the behavioral sciences* (4th ed.). Sage.

Lord, F. M. (1960). Large-sample covariance analysis when the control variable is fallible. *Journal of the American Statistical Association, 55*(290), 307–321.

Maxwell, S. E., & Delaney, H. D. (2017). *Designing experiments and analyzing data: A model comparison perspective*. Routledge.

Miller, G. A., & Chapman, J. P. (2001). Misunderstanding analysis of covariance. *Journal of Abnormal Psychology, 110*(1), 40. https://doi.org/10.1037//0021-843X.110.1.40

Noguchi, K., Gel, Y., Brunner, E., & Konietschke, F. (2012). nparLD: An R software package for the nonparametric analysis of longitudinal data in factorial experiments. *Journal of Statistical Software, 50*(12), 1–23.

Olejnik, S. F., & Algina, J. (1985). A review of nonparametric alternatives to analysis of covariance. *Evaluation Review, 9*(1), 51–83. https://doi.org/10.1177/0193841X8500900104

Reichardt, C. S. (1979). *Quasi-experimentation: Design & analysis issues for field settings*. Houghton Mifflin.

Schreiber, J. B., & Asner-Self, K. (2010). *Educational research*. John Wiley and Sons.

Stevens, J. P. (2002). *Applied multivariate statistics for the social sciences*. Lawrence Erlbaum Association.

Tabachnick, B. G., & Fidell, L. S. (2007). *Experimental designs using ANOVA*. Thomson/Brooks/Cole.

Tsangari, H., & Akritas, M. G. (2004). Nonparametric ANCOVA with two and three covariates. *Journal of Multivariate Analysis, 88*(2), 298–319. https://doi.org/10.1016/S0047-259X(03)00098-8

CHAPTER 8

Correlation and Regression

CORE OBJECTIVES

- Understand and write questions and hypotheses used with correlation and regression
- Explain magnitude and direction and different types of correlation
- Discuss the three components of causality
- Discuss the use of scatter plots and how to create one
- Discuss and partial and semi-partial correlations
- Explain technical issues related to regression
- Understand questions and hypotheses used in regression
- Explain residual analyses
- Understand dummy coding
- Explain and determine degrees of freedom
- Understand and explain assumptions related to regression
- Explain predictor variable entry methods
- Correctly interpret standardized, unstandardized beta coefficients
- Explain how to calculate t-value
- Explain R-squared, adjusted R-squared, AIC, BIC, and RMSE, and when each is used

INTRODUCTION: ASSOCIATIONS

Correlation and regression are generally interested in association between one or more variables and a specific outcome variable. For example, studies that examine determinants of health typically have multiple independent variables (e.g., eating, sleep, and exercise habits) along with comorbidities and an outcome variable like myocardial functioning or mental health. Correlation and regression are popular because survey data (both research based and administrative data) can be easily used within the analytic framework. For example, there is not an assumption of random assignment to groups. With that ease though, comes a large number of technical and interpretation issues that must be understood for a quality analysis to be completed.

PURPOSE AND QUESTION FOCUS

Correlation

The purpose of a correlation is to examine the relationship between two variables. Given the type of data, that relationship may be assumed to be linear or not. There are different types of correlations based on the data. The research questions related to correlations follow this general format:

Are variables x and y associated?

What is the magnitude and direction of the relationship between variables x and y?

What is the association between x and y after variable z is removed?

The traditional hypotheses are written as:

- $H_0: \rho_{xy} = 0$
- $H_A: \rho_{xy} \neq 0$

The Greek letter **rho** (ρ) is traditionally seen in the literature because it indicates an examination of the population correlation value. If the researcher is discussing the sample, then a small r is utilized like this: $r_{xy} = 0$, where x and y in the subscript indicate the two different variables of interest.

Regression

The purpose of regression (linear regression) is to examine which theoretically driven independent variables account for the variance (the differences in values) of a continuous outcome variable. Therefore, the research questions are centered around the level of association between the independent and outcome variables. The research questions appear at times to be arguing for a causal relationship, but this is typically unfounded since in many studies the data is collected all at once and causality is not possible to determine. Examples of regression research questions are:

- Does engagement in a weight tracking app and exercise in minutes per day lead to weight loss after three months?

- Does the amount of use of a weight tracker predict the amount of weight change?

These examples focus on the associations of the variables. Yet, they miss understanding the size of the associations. For example,

- Is the regression coefficient for weight tracker use smaller or larger than in previous similar studies?

- Do the predictor variables, of age, weight tracker usage, starting weight, and type of job, account for more than 25% of variance in the outcome variable weight loss?

These questions focus on the size of the coefficients and how well the variables account for the differences in the outcome variable. We believe it is important to focus on the size of the coefficients and how well the model works (variance accounted for) than p-values.

The traditional questions focus on the overall relationships, but the traditional null hypotheses focus on the beta coefficients and being different than zero, or nothing. Traditional hypotheses are written as:

$$H_0: \beta_i = 0$$
$$H_A: \beta_i \neq 0$$

Notice the subscript i. Using the subscript lets me have has many beta values in the model without having to write each one out. In a bi-variate regression, this is an independent variable and an intercept. But there can be multiple beta values: for the null there is one for the intercept and one for each independent variable. The same for the alternative hypotheses. Thus, the researcher has,

$$H_0: \beta_{intercept} = 0$$
$$H_0: \beta_{variable\ 1} = 0$$
$$H_0: \beta_{variable\ 2} = 0$$
$$\cdot$$
$$\cdot$$
$$\cdot$$
$$H_0: \beta_{variable\ x} = 0$$

$$H_A: \beta_{intercept} \neq 0$$
$$H_A: \beta_{intercept\ 1} \neq 0$$
$$H_A: \beta_{intercept\ 2} \neq 0$$
$$\cdot$$
$$\cdot$$
$$\cdot$$
$$H_A: \beta_{variable\ x} \neq 0$$

As with all analyses, researchers could test a point estimate instead of the null or alternative. The researcher could test that $H_{p1}: \beta_{variable\ 1} = 1.45$ based on previous research.

GRAPHIC REPRESENTATION

Pearson correlations, aka, product-moment (Pearson, 1907) are an examination of the linear relationship (straight line) between two continuous (e.g., interval or ratio data) variables. Figure 8.1 provides a generic scatterplot to show the relationship between two continuous variables. The first scatterplot is credited to English scientist John Frederick W. Herschel (1833) (Friendly & Denis, 2005, 2008; Friendly & Wainer, 2021).

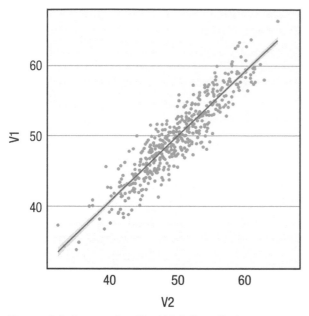

Figure 8.1. Scatterplot Plot With Best Fit Line

Figure 8.1 displays pairs of points for each x and y (variable 1 and 2) pair in the image. The line is a representation of the correlation between the two variables. The line is called a "best fit" line. The value of a correlation, the slope of the line, has two most defining attributes, direction and magnitude. You have actually done this work before, probably a long time ago in algebra with slope, $y = m x + b$ and the slope equation $m = (y2 - y1) / (x2 - x1)$. The direction of a correlation is positive (+) or negative (–) and the magnitude or size is between 0 and 1. Thus, a correlation of –0.56 has a negative direction, indicating as one variable increases the other decreases, and a magnitude of 0.56. In Figure 8.1 the direction is positive, as one increases the other increases. The magnitude is 0.91 and the direction is positive. Figure 8.2 provides a multi-variable scatterplot with best fit lines and the correlations all in one graphic.

LINEAR REGRESSION

Linear regression was actually developed more than 200 years ago (Legendre, 1805) focusing on trying to determine error. Most people have a vague idea about regression and the regression line for a bivariate regression. This comes from algebra and the point slope formula, which is commonly referred to as rise over run, which was discussed previously. In algebra, students are given two points and asked to find the slope and the intercept. This might be a painful memory for some. But the concept is the same in regression, just instead of two points, there are many points typically set up with an independent and dependent variable (x and y).

Graphic Representations

A starting point for learning regression is to look at a scatter plot of two continuous variables. In Figure 8.3 there are 100 pairs of points (Stress, Anxiety) plotted. The scatterplot indicates that higher stress scores are associated with higher anxiety scores, and it appears to be a linear relationship with the

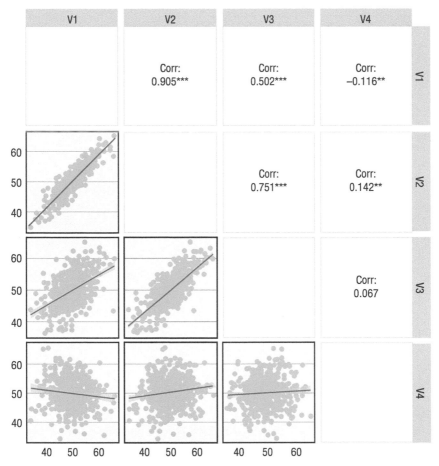

Figure 8.2. Correlation Matrix, Scatterplots, and Best Fit Lines.

data. From here, the researcher might be able to estimate a best fit line, that is a **regression line**. The line might start around zero (in the bottom left corner) and move steeply up and to the right. Going back to Figure 8.1 and comparing, this looks like a correlation value above 0.50 but not as high as 0.90. **Figure 8.4** shows a best fit line, the spot of the intercept (about 0, 34), all of the pairs are not on the line (error/residuals), and the steepness of the line (slope).

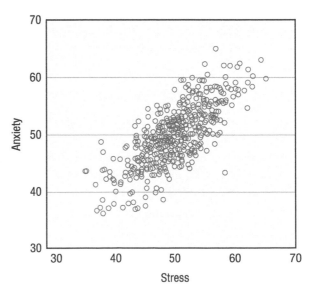

Figure 8.3. Scatterplot of Stress by Anxiety.

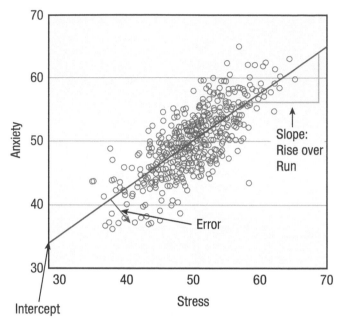

Figure 8.4. Scatterplot With Best Fit Line.

When examining a scatterplot and thinking about regression, the intercept, slope, and error are key attributes to understand. Figure 8.4 highlights those attributes. The slope is the angle of the regression line. In this example, it is positive and the correlation is about 0.62. Each dot (pair of data points) that is not on the line is considered error. The distance from the line to the point is the error. The intercept is the location where the line intersects with the y-axis (Anxiety).

TECHNICAL SECTION

Correlations

For the traditional Pearson correlation, the data are assumed to be normally distributed. The relationship is assumed to be linear, and the data at an interval or ratio level. Though not an assumption, outliers can cause problems with both the magnitude and the direction of the correlation. Finally, rarely discussed, given that the observed correlation is supposed to represent the population correlation, the data are assumed to be *randomly selected* from and representative of the population. This is an argument that applies to all analyses though.

The Correct Correlation by Data

Correlations also need to be calculated by the data type and the normality of the data. Pearson correlations are based on two normally distributed continuous variables. We have only talked about Pearson correlations with normally distributed data. Yet, each type of data (in this case, pairs of data points) has a type of correlation that should be conducted. Specifically,

1. **Spearman rank-order correlation:** both variables are rank-ordered (ordinal)

    a. Works well with nonnormal continuous data,

2. **Biserial correlation:** one variable is continuous and the other is an artificial dichotomy (i.e., a high or low score on a measure) (interval/ratio and ordinal)

3. **Point biserial correlation:** one variable is continuous and the other is a true dichotomy (i.e., a score of right [1] or wrong [0] on a test item) (ordinal data)

4. **Tetrachoric correlation:** both variables are artificial dichotomies (ordinal)

5. **Phi coefficient:** both variables are true dichotomies (ordinal)

6. **Contingency coefficient:** both variables reflect two or more categories (nominal or ordinal)

7. **Correlation ratio, eta:** both variables are continuous, but reflect a curvilinear relationship (interval or ratio)

8. **Kendall's Tau,** which is for nonnormal data and works on a concordant/discordant system by looking at pairs and seeing if their signs (positive or negative) after subtracting each part of the pair ($x1 - x2$ and $y1 - y2$) (Kendall, 1952). The data should be ordinal or continuous and is best if it is monotonic (follows a typical linear pattern either up or down).

The correlation and the type of data are a continual problem in articles. Thus, we recommend paying special attention to the type of data and the correlation being calculated. Finally, there are some general boundaries for correlations. Those less than 0.10 are considered small, 0.30 is considerate medium or moderate, and 0.50 and above are considered large (Cohen, 1988).

Correlations also highlight one of the major problems with p-values; sample size does it all for you to reach the magical 05. In Appendix 8.1, there is a table for determining the 05 two tailed cut-off. Examining the table, it is easy to see that as sample size increases, the magnitude of the correlation needed decreases to hit 05. At 92 participants (df = $N - 2 = 90$) the critical correlation value to reach 05 is 0.204, which is a shared variance of just 4%, or 96% not shared. Between two variables, this is also called the **coefficient of determination.** Examining Figure 8.2, variables 2 and 4 ($v2$ and $v4$) have a correlation of 0.14, a bit lower, but it looks like a circle of dots.

Regression

Regression has many technical components related to the analysis that tend to be overlooked. Regression, and ANOVA and other techniques, are actually mathematical models that are based on an equation. The equation, as you might have seen or figured out by now, has an outcome (Y) and intercept (β_0), and typically one or more variables. There is also the error component (e), which estimates the amount of variability not explained by the model. You will also see this described as residuals after an analysis is run. The bivariate equation, one independent and one dependent variable, for a regression is

$$Y = \beta_0 + \beta_1 (x) + error\ (e).$$

As more variables are included, more **regression coefficients** are added

$$Y = \beta_0 + \beta_1(x_1) + \beta_2(x_2) + \beta_3(x_3) + \beta_4(x_4) + \beta_5(x_5)..... + error\ (e)$$

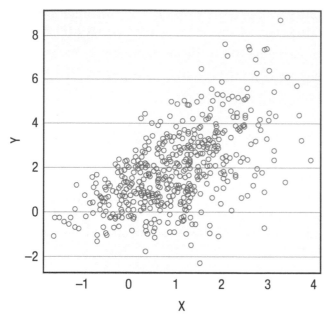

Figure 8.5. Examination for Heteroscedasticity.

And, to save space researchers will often write this as,

$$Y = \beta_0 + \Sigma\beta_i(x_i) + error\ (e)$$

where the summation and the subscript i, tells the reader there are multiple variables that are involved in the equation.

Assumptions

Similar to the previous discussions, the outcome variable is assumed to be normally distributed. This should be tested but again as sample sizes increase, small deviations from normality will indicate a non-normal distribution. Continuous independent variables are also assumed to be normally distributed, but should be tested. Next, for a bivariate regression if both the independent and dependent variables are continuous, their relationship should be linear or approximately linear. If either one or both are not normally distributed, **heteroscedasticity** can occur. If it is equal or close to equal, the relationship is **homoscedastic**. **Figure 8.5** displays an unequal distribution of points that flairs out to the top and bottom right for two continuous variables and indicates potential heteroscedasticity.

For multivariate regression, **collinearity**, how strong are the relationships between the independent variables is the next assumption. Researchers actually want each independent variable to be highly correlated with the dependent variable and <u>not</u> correlated with the other independent variables. **Figure 8.6** provides an example where each independent variable is correlated with the dependent variable but not with each other.

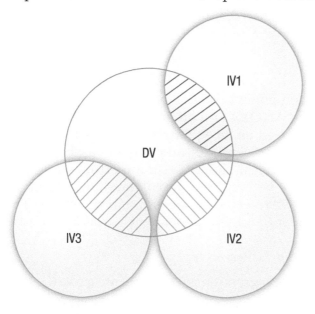

Figure 8.6. Graphic Representation of Noncollinearity.

Thus, examining the relationship between each independent variable using a scatterplot or appropriate correlation is important. Historically, we have noticed that around 0.70, collinearity problems begin to occur. These are tested with collinearity statistics and **variance inflation function** (VIF). VIF of 10 ten is problematic, but overall, once you start to get close to 5 there is a potential problem. In general, values around one are desired. The researcher should have an idea where the problems

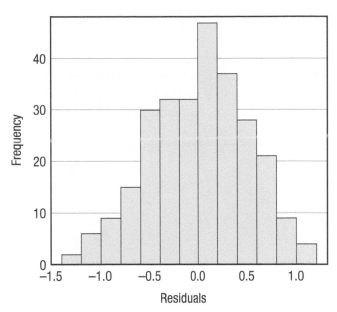

Figure 8.7. Normally Distributed Residuals.

might occur during the design phase based on previous research, but also some logical inference. For example, variables such as age and years of service tend to be highly correlated and have high VIF values.

Specification is another assumption that has not had enough discussion. **Specification** is the assumption that the correct variables are included and the incorrect ones are not. Every regression model is mis-specified to some extent (Box, 1979; Burnham& Anderson, 2002), but this is still a major assumption. With each model, the researchers are making an argument about what is the correct specification, and the inclusion or exclusion of one important variable could drastically alter the results.

The standardized **residuals** should be normally distributed with a mean of zero and a standard deviation of 1, traditionally written as N ~(0, 1). **Figure 8.7** displays a relatively normal distribution of residuals. Residuals are the difference between the observed outcome variable and the predicted outcome based on the regression model Y-$\hat{Y}$, where Y is the original outcome and the $\hat{Y}$ is the predicted value. This provides the researcher with estimates about how much error there is and the distribution of that error. If the error is **homoscedastic**, then the residuals are multivariate normally distributed. In multiple regression, the possibility increases that the residuals are **heteroscedastic** or nonlinear. In **Figure 8.8**, a heteroscedastic residual graph is shown with the outcome variable, Y, compared to the residuals, $Y - \hat{Y}$. The errors are not evenly distributed across the zero-center line.

There are also several different ways residuals that can be calculated. For example, <u>Cook's Distance</u> examines how much one case influences the model. A value of 1 or greater indicates that one case or participant has an over expected amount of influence on the whole model. The values should be around 0. **Mahalanobis distance** (Mahalanobis, 1936) uses a cut-off based on the number

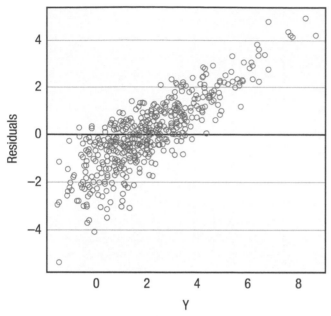

Figure 8.8. A Plot of Nonnormal Residuals.

of variables and a comparison table (Barnett & Lewis, 1978). Not many researchers use the table, but instead use a rule of thumb of 18. **Centered leverage** is based on number of predictors and sample size and is calculated two different ways. The first is $(k + 1) / n$ where k is the number of predictors and n is the number of cases/participants. If the researcher has three independent variables and 100 participants, any value over 0.04 [(3 +1) / 100] would be problematic. Stevens (2002) uses $(3 (k + 1) / n)$. There are also standardized residuals that should be normally distributed and values + or - 3 and higher indicate a problem with a specific case or participant.

Finally, the errors are assumed not to be correlated. This is examined with the Durbin-Watson test. The **Durbin-Watson** value can range from 0 to 4. The basic rule of thumb is less than 1 indicates a positive error autocorrelation problem, around 2 equals no autocorrelation, and greater than 2 indicates negative autocorrelation problem. Many applied studies will have values between 1.5 and 2.5. Note, there is a specific reference table based on sample size and number of variables, which can be found through an internet search.

Table Details

In Table 8.1, regression results are provided for different types of independent variables. Independent variable one has an **unstandardized beta coefficient** of 0.440 and a standard error of 0.088. For every one unit increase in that variable, the dependent variable increases 0.440. There is a small amount of sampling error. Dividing the unstandardized beta coefficient by the standard error provides the t-value (t-value = unst. beta/se). In the case of variable 1, that is 0.440 / 0.088 = 4.976. Note, if calculating by hand, the value may be rounded to 5, since there is a little rounding error from the standard error. The t-value is just a value and traditionally is compared to a t-distribution with the degrees of freedom (df = 94) to obtain the p-value. Most tables are abbreviated and would show the researcher that a large t-value is associated with a p-value less than 0.001. What is important is the beta coefficient and the small standard error.

Table 8.1. Regression Results With Different Types of Predictor Variables.

Predictor	Unstand. Beta	SE	t	p
Intercept	1.918	0.441	4.352	<0.001
Independent 1	0.440	0.088	4.976	<0.001
Independent 2				
1 − 0	1.024	0.344	2.900	0.004
Independent 3				
1 − 0	−0.225	0.369	−0.609	0.544
2 − 0	0.118	0.373	0.317	0.752

ANOVA Table Adjusted R-Squared

Regression analyses produce an ANOVA table with sums of squares for the model (formerly the between sums of squares) and the residuals (formerly the within sums of squares). The table still functions the same way previously detailed. When there is more than one independent variable, there will be a sums of squares for each variable, much like a factorial ANOVA. R-squared is derived from the ANOVA sums of squares that is calculated when a regression is completed. R-squared is the sums of squares of the model (between in ANOVA) divided by the sums of squares total.

$$R - Squared = \frac{(SS_{model})}{(SS_{total})}$$

$$Adjusted\ R - Squared = 1 - \left(\frac{\left(\frac{SS_{error}}{df_{error}} \right)}{\left(\frac{SS_{total}}{df_{total}} \right)} \right)$$

From the bivariate regression example, previously discussed, the ANOVA table is in Table 8.2.

There is an adjustment based on the degrees of freedom which, in this case produces a lower value (0.345 compared to 0.352). If the sums of squares were kept the same, the researcher would need more than 100,000 participants to get the adjusted R-squared to approach being equal to the R-squared value.

Beta Coefficients

The unstandardized beta coefficient is based on the raw data and the standardized coefficient is based on an adjustment; standardization of the underlying variables and can be calculated by hand from the unstandardized beta values. Standardized coefficients can be used to examine which variables are most important within

Table 8.2. Source Table for a Regression.

	Sum of Squares	df	Mean Square	F	p
Model	124.517	1	124.517	52.577	<0.001
Residuals	229.721	97	2.368		
Total	354.238	98			

$$R-Squared = \frac{(124.517)}{229.721+124.517} = \frac{124.517}{354.238} = 0.352$$

$$Adjusted\ R-Squared = 1 - \left(\frac{\left(\frac{229.721}{97}\right)}{\left(\frac{229.721+124.517}{98}\right)} \right) = 1 - \frac{2.368}{3.6146} = 1 - 0.655 = 0.345$$

a study. Two key attributes are important for the standardized beta coefficients. First, if the relationships between the independent variables were 0, the standardized coefficient would simply be the correlation between the independent variable and the dependent (see Figure 8.6). Next, the standardized coefficient *cannot* logically be larger than the correlation between the independent and the dependent variable. It should also be the same direction (positive or negative). When this occurs, a suppressor effect is happening (e.g., Horst, 1941). This effect is being driven by the inclusion of a variable that increases the association of another variable.

Data Types and Scales

In regression, the variables can be on very different scales. In complex regression analyses, this can be problematic. The researcher might have one variable that has a scale of 0 to 4 and another that ranges from 35 to 90. These can lead to very large differences in variance size and cause estimation problems (Kline, 2016). This is a common issue in more advanced linear techniques, yet we have seen this problem in multiple regression analyses.

Data types also have essentially scale issues and coding issues. Dichotomous, binary, or two group variables are easiest to interpret when they are coded using 0 and 1. This is termed **dummy coding** or **design coding**. When the codes are 0 and 1, the coefficient from the results quickly indicates the magnitude and direction of the group coded 1 on the outcome variable and in comparison to the group coded 0. The 0 recode is typically made the reference group. This should be planned in the design phase what to code the groups and which group will be the reference. For example, if the code was 0 for students in grade 2a and 1 for students in grade 2b, then the resulting coefficient after the analysis is the effect of being in grade 2b on the outcome.

When there are more than two groups, the researcher must design or dummy code the variables. The key is you need one less dummy variable than categories. If you have four categories, you need three design codes ($k-1$ categories). For example, in a very old Sesame Street study, there were four groups of children who watched different amounts of the show: 1 = rarely watched the show, 2 = once or twice a week, 3 = three to five times a week, 4 = watched the show on average

Table 8.3. Design Codes for Viewing Groups.

Group	Dummy 1	Dummy 2	Dummy 3
1	0	0	0
2	1	0	0
3	0	1	0
4	0	0	1

more than 5 times a week. Thus, the researcher would need to create three dummy code variables with one as reference. In Table 8.3, Group 1 is the reference group.

You can make any category the reference. The key is the interpretation. For example, if letter memory was the dependent variable and after the analysis, the beta coefficient for dummy coded Group 4 was 1.23, this would be interpreted as Group 4 scored 1.23 points higher than the children in the other groups. What this does from the regression model is take what seems like one variable and makes it three so it can be analyzed properly, for example,

$$Y = \beta_0 + \beta_1(Dummy\ 1) + \beta_2(Dummy\ 2) + \beta_3(Dummy\ 3) + \beta_4(x_4) + error\ (e).$$

Finally, some scales or items that are used in regression are reversed coded, typically with higher values indicating a lower level of the phenomenon. For example, "Today, I feel great" where 1 = strongly agree and 5 = strongly disagree. Therefore, when interpreting the coefficients, the researcher needs to remember the coding of the variable and its relationship with the other variables.

Variable Entry

In the multiple regression example earlier, we ran all the independent variables at the same time; this is called the traditional method of variable entry. We are partial to the traditional method of letting all the variables in the analysis at the same time. Other researchers are not. When the researcher allows the variables to enter the analysis at the same time, the resulting beta coefficients are an estimate of the unique relationship between the independent variables and the dependent (Figure 8.9). Other methods, such as step, block or hierarchical, do not do that.

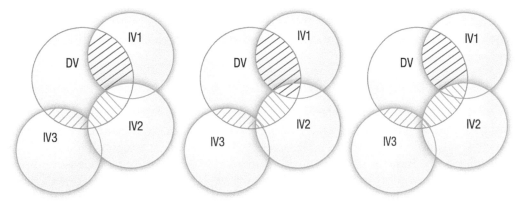

Figure 8.9. Traditional, Step, and Block Variable Entry.

In **simultaneous** (enter/traditional) regression, each variable is shown with its unique relationship with the DV (far left figure). In **block/hierarchical** and **step**, this is not the case. The relationships for block/hierarchical are overlapping, specifically IV1 and IV2 and IV3 and DV. Depending on the interrelationships of the variables, this can lead to very biased estimates. For the step entry, the largest relationship is kept. Notice in the middle, that IV1's complete relationship is kept even though part of it is actually shared with IV2. The same with IV2 and IV3. In the step, forward or backward, approach variables are entered or removed based on their meeting 05 criterion generally, though you can switch that value. Some researchers like this approach because the added shared variance increases the coefficient and therefore increases the possibility of meeting the 05 threshold for a few of the variables. It also makes the coefficients hard to interpret because of the overlap of variance. Since the coefficient of IV1 is actually a mix of shared variance of IV1 and IV2 and both variables have a relationship with Y, what does the resulting beta coefficient really mean? In general, do not use stepwise entry, with one caveat for predictive or exploratory purposes in new research areas. If the researcher is considering step, forward or backward entry, backward tends to reduce **suppressor** effects. Suppressor effects occur when an independent variable, which is not related to the DV, has an effect on the dependent variable once the other variables are held constant. The suppressor variable improves the model. This can sometimes be examined by looking at the raw correlations between the DV and the IVs. If one of the IV's correlation is smaller than the standardized coefficient, then a suppressor effect may be occurring. Finally, remember, the goal is to obtain the most accurate beta value ("how much"). Step and block tend to not accomplish that, but are sometimes excellent at absorbing variance and increasing the R-squared value.

Some researchers use block to control for specific variables that have commonly been observed to be important in previous empirical studies and then use a second block for new variables. Yet, by doing this, the blocked variables can absorb all of the relationship and, specifically the overlapping relationships, with the new variables of interest. This can lead to decisions that the new variables are not important. Notice in the Block entry, IV2 and IV3 are blocked first and then IV3 enters. This makes IV2 look potentially larger than it really is after accounting for other variables. If the researcher uses this entry pattern, use the block approach, at a minimum you should run the model with traditional entry and see what occurs.

Partial and Part Correlations

To dive deeper into understanding the relationships between the dependent and independent variables, analyzing part and partial correlations with the dependent variable is completed. This used to be the system to calculate regression coefficients by hand and is a foundation of regression. These two techniques provide an examination of an independent variable and a dependent variable while controlling for other independent variables. A **part**, or **semi-partial**, correlation is the correlation between an independent variable and the dependent variable after the linear effects of the other independent variables have been removed from the independent variable only. A **partial** correlation is the correlation between an independent variable and the dependent variable after the linear effects of the other variables have been removed from both the independent variable and the dependent variable. One way to understand this is through **Figure 8.10**, where part A is the semi-partial correlation between variable 1 and the dependent variable after the linear effect of variable 2 is removed. It is essentially the pure relationship between independent variable 1 and the

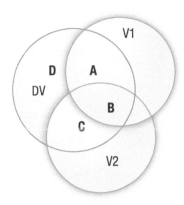

Figure 8.10. Semi-Partial Separation.

dependent variable. Part B is the shared variance of both independent variables and helps to explain the variance in the dependent variable. Part C is a semi-partial correlation between independent variable 2 and the dependent variable with the linear effects of independent variable 1 taken out. And part D, is the variance that is not explained by either independent variable, that is the error or unexplained variance.

The semi-partial correlation, for example $r_{1(2.3)}$, is the relationship between variables 1 and 2 where 3 is partialed out only from variable 2. To calculate it, this equation is used:

$$r_{1(2.3)} = \frac{r_{12} - r_{13}r_{23}}{\sqrt{1 - r_{23}^2}}$$

Where there are three correlations needed: 1) between variables 1 and 2, 2) between variables 1 and 3, and 3) between variables 2 and 3. In this example, variable 1 would be the dependent variable. You could conceptually rewrite this as, using **Figure 8.10**:

$$r_{DV(IV1.IV2)} = \frac{r_A - r_C r_B}{\sqrt{1 - r_B^2}}$$

Partial correlations are the removal of (partial out) a third variable from both of the variables in the correlation of interest. The partial correlation is $r_{12.3}$ where variable 3 is being removed from the correlation between 1 *and* 2. Using this equation,

$$r_{12.3} = \frac{r_{12} - r_{13}r_{23}}{\sqrt{1 - r_{13}^2}\sqrt{1 - r_{23}^2}}$$

You will notice that the numerator is the same, but the denominator is added into the correlation between variables 1 and 3.

Sample Size

Regression has generally needed less participants or cases to reach the "magical 05." Again, we think the focus on accuracy and not reaching 05 is more important. The old rule thumb for a regression was 50 to start and then take the number of independent variables, multiple that by 8 and add it to the 50, thus

$$\text{Sample size needed} = 50 + 8 \times (\text{Number of IVs})$$

Using free software programs such as G*Power, with a moderate effect size (R-square), power of 0.80 and the traditional 05, similar results compared to the equation above would be obtained.

This, though, is still focused on reaching 05, and the researcher needs to weigh how precise the results need to be, the accuracy of the measures, and the risk related (e.g., disease) to the outcome. If the results must be very precise and the dependent variable is a high risk topic, the sample size and representativeness of the sample should be the driving force of the sample size needs.

Correcting for Unreliability

Though rarely done, regressions should technically be corrected for unreliability in the data, that is measurement error (e.g., Davey Smith & Phillips, 1996; Riggs et al., 1978). There is a long history of research in this area beginning essentially with Pearson (1904) and adjusting correlation coefficients for measurement error. Most statistical software do not provide an easy way to do this, and more specialized software is typically used.

CORE RESULTS

These next sections provide detail on examples for bivariate (one independent and one dependent variable) and multivariate regression (multiple independent variables and one dependent variable). The core results for a correlation are relatively straight forward, the magnitude and direction of the correlation, sample size or degrees of freedom, tests of normality if it is a Pearson correlation, and, if needed, p-value.

Bivariate Regression: Core Results

Bivariate regression is not common in the literature, but is a good launching point for understanding the technique, the assumptions, and issues that occur. The traditional narrative for a bivariate regression contains multiple key elements: 1) R-squared, 2) unstandardized and standardized beta coefficients, 3) discussion of outliers and normality, 4) residual analysis, 5) any changes that were made to the data or the model, and 6) the regression equation.
The typical narrative would read as such:

> Results of the ordinary least squares regression indicate the model has a R-squared value of 0.35 and adjusted R-square of 0.34 with $F(1,98) = 52.98$, MSe = 2.74, $p < 0.001$. The independent variable had an unstandardized

beta of 1.60 (se = 0.46, t = 3.52, p <0.001) and standardized beta of 0.59. There were no outliers, normality (S-W = 0.994) multivariate normality, or heteroskedasticity concerns. A residual analysis indicated one participant was very far off the 45-degree line in the Q-Q plot and had the highest Cook's value and was removed. A second analysis with the one participant removed, did not meaningfully change the results. The prediction equation is outcome = 12.54 + 1.60 × (independent variable) and indicates that each unit increase in the independent variable creates an 1.60 increase in the dependent variable.

Tables

The core tables to be included are descriptive with both variables of interest (Table 8.4) a correlation table (Table 8.5), and the regression results table (Table 8.6). In the correlation table, it is common to have the upper half of the matrix be the covariances and the bottom half be the correlations. Or, if there are two groups, the upper and lower half the correlation matrix are the correlations for each group. Table 8.4 shows that there are no missing data, the mean for each group along with other key information such as skewness and kurtosis. Table 8.5 shows the correlation between the variables. Table 8.6 provides the regression results. The intercept is 1.74 and is the starting point (refer to the technical section). Notice that in a bivariate regression, the standardized beta value is

Table 8.4. **Descriptive Statistics.**

	Dependent	Independent
N	99	99
Missing	0	0
Mean	4.613	5.032
Median	4.793	5.008
Standard Deviation	1.901	1.976
Minimum	0.792	0.494
Maximum	9.006	10.337
Skewness	−0.041	0.019
Std. Error Skewness	0.243	0.243
Kurtosis	−0.441	0.115
Std. Error Kurtosis	0.481	0.481

Table 8.5. **Pearson Correlation Matrix.**

Correlation Matrix		
	Dependent	Independent
Dependent		–
Independent	0.593	–

Table 8.6. Regression Results Table.

Model Coefficients - V1					
Predictor	Unst. beta	se	t	p	Stand. Beta
Intercept	1.743	0.425	4.101	<0.001	
Independent Variable	0.570	0.079	7.251	<0.001	0.593

the same as the correlation value. In a bivariate regression with continuous variables, this is always the case. This is a key piece of information because the standardized value should never be above the correlation value, and that is the same for multivariate regression. Finally, the unstandardized beta value divided by the standard error gives the researcher the t-value.

Multivariate: Core Results

Multivariate regression is essentially the same with more variables, but there is also an increase the number of assumptions and technical issues that must be addressed. In general, they will look similar. The core information in a multivariate regression are: 1) Type of variable input, 2) R-squared, 2) unstandardized and standardized beta coefficients, 3) discussion of outliers and normality, 4) residual analysis, 5) multicollinearity, 6) any changes that were made to the data or the model, and 7) the regression equation.

The typical narrative would read as such:

Results of the traditional ordinary least squares regression indicate the model has a R-squared value of 0.41 and adjusted R-square of 0.39 with $F(4, 94) = 16.41$, MSe = 2.20, $p < 0.001$. Independent variable 1 had an unstandardized beta of 0.44 (se = 0.08, $t = 4.98$, $p < 0.001$) and standardized beta of 0.46. Independent variable 2 is a binary grouping where group 0 is the reference and had an unstandardized beta of 1.02 (se = 0.34, $t = 2.98$, $p = 0.004$). Outcome scores are 1.02 points higher for Group 1 compared to Group 0. Independent variable 3 has three categories with the reference group as 0. Group 1, compared to Group 0, had lower scores with an unstandardized beta of –0.23 (se = 0.37, $t = -0.61$, $p = 0.54$) and a standardized estimate of –0.12. Group 2, compared to Group 0, had higher scores with an unstandardized beta of 0.19 (se = 0.37, $t = 0.317$, $p = 0.004$) and a standardized estimate of 0.06.

There were no outliers, normality (S-W = 0.990), multivariate normality, or heteroskedasticity concerns (Breusch-Pagan = 0.84). A residual analysis indicated one participant was very far off the 45-degree line in the Q-Q plot, had the highest Cook's value, and was removed. A second analysis with the one participant removed, barely changed any of the results. The prediction equation is outcome = 1.92 + 0.44 × independent 1 + 1.02 × independent 2 + –0.23 × independent 3 : 1 – 0 + 0.19 × independent 3 : 2 – 0.

Table 8.7. Correlation Matrix.

		DV	IV1	IV2
Dependent	Pearson's r	–		
	Kendall's Tau-B	–		
Independent 1	Pearson's r	0.593	–	
	Kendall's Tau-B	0.370	–	
Independent 2	Pearson's r	0.492	0.488	–
	Kendall's Tau-B	0.395	0.392	–
Independent 3	Pearson's r	0.139	0.189	0.099
	Kendall's Tau-B	0.104	0.152	0.093

Table 8.8. Multiple Regression Results-Coefficients.

Model Coefficients				
Predictor	**Estimate**	**se**	**t**	**p**
Intercept [a]	1.918	0.441	4.352	<0.001
Independent 1	0.440	0.088	4.976	<0.001
Independent 2				
1 – 0	1.024	0.344	2.980	0.004
Independent 3				
1 – 0	−0.225	0.369	−0.609	0.544
2 – 0	0.118	0.373	0.317	0.752

Tables

The Correlation Matrix will need to have different types of correlations and an indicator of those differences. Table 8.7 has the correlation matrix using Pearson and Kendall Tau-B correlations to highlight the differences in values and the differences in data types. For Independent 1 and the dependent variable, Pearson is the correct correlation. For the other comparisons, Kendall Tau-B would be the more appropriate correlation. Most researchers typically create just a Pearson Correlation Matrix. Rarely do we see the adjustments made or indicated. Part of this issue is due to the options that statistical software packages offer to the researcher. Table 8.8 provides the regression analysis results. Note the unstandardized beta coefficient divided by the standard error (se) equals the t-value. There are two tables that are not typically included, ANOVA and fit table, but some of the information is provided in the narrative (e.g., R-squared, and mean square error (MSE).

Effect Sizes

The effect sizes are slightly different in regression. The overarching effect size is really *variance accounted for* (R-squared or R^2) in the outcome variable. That is, how much of the variability in the dependent measure do the independent

Table 8.9. Fit Values for Regression.

Model	R	R^2	Adjusted R^2	AIC	BIC	RMSE	Overall Model Test			
							F	df1	df2	p
1	0.593	0.352	0.345	370.282	378.068	1.523	52.577	1	97	<0.001
2	0.641	0.411	0.386	366.726	382.296	1.452	16.410	4	94	<0.001

variables account for; or as some say explain. For the multivariate example, it is about 41%, or 39%, with the adjusted R-square (see Technical Section).

When a researcher is comparing regression models, the **AIC, BIC,** and **RMSE** are commonly used. *AIC* is the *Akaike's Information Criteria,* developed by Japanese Statistician Hirotugu Akaike (Akaike, 1970). The AIC penalizes, that is increases the AIC value, in more complicated models. Thus, the more variables, the worse the score. Researchers are looking for the lowest AIC value when comparing models. The lower the AIC, the better the model. *BIC* is the *Bayesian information criteria* that works the same way as the AIC. The difference is there the penalty is stronger than the AIC penalty. There are times when the BIC is lower than the AIC and that is a good indicator that model is best comparatively. The *root mean square error* (RMSE) is the standard deviation of the residuals. The RMSE gives the researcher how dispersed the residuals are. The smaller the value, the closer the residuals are to the regression line.

For example, the bivariate and multivariate models are based on the same simulated data. Though in general, AIC works for simpler models, both AIC and BIC penalize for more complex models (that is more variables). The lower the value the better for AIC, BIC, and RMSE. In Table 8.9, AIC and RMSE are lower for Model 2 indicating that Model 2 is better fitting than Model 1. But BIC is a little higher. This is because BIC has a stronger penalty. In this case, with both AIC and RMSE lower, with R-squared being higher, Model 2 is a better fit. Now, with that, this does not mean that Model 2 is correct, just that Model 2 has a better fit.

Compatibility Intervals

The traditional 95% Compatibility Intervals are based on the unstandardized beta coefficients or the standardized coefficient, instead of the means of the groups like ANOVAs. For example, if the standardized coefficient is 0.34 and the standard error is 0.6, the lower bound is $0.34 - (1.96 \times 0.6) = 0.22$, and the upper bound is $0.34 + (1.96 \times 0.6) = 0.46$.

NONPARAMETRIC

Nonparametric correlations were discussed earlier and include such options as Spearman and point-biserial. Nonparametric regression is separated into a few types of regressions. There is logistic regression (Chapter 11), **polytomous/ multinomial regression**-an extension of logistic, **Poisson** for dependent variables that follow a Poisson distribution, and a family of nonparametric regressions that use a data smoothing technique, kernel, nearest neighbor, or spline

(Long, 1997). These are out of the scope of the book, but it is important to know that nonlinear regression analyses exist.

MOST DEFINING ATTRIBUTES—WHAT SHOULD I LOOK FOR?

As in every chapter with analyses, there are key attributes you should look for or include with writing up the results for correlation and/or regression.

Correlation/Bivariate/Multiple Regression

1. Check normality of each variable
2. Check Pearson correlation for continuous variables and heteroscedasticity
3. Outliers, multivariate outliers, large residuals, missing data, and how handled
4. Dichotomous or categorical (e.g., dummy coded) predictors normality discussed for each group.
5. Core information for narrative
   a. R-squared, adjusted R-squared
   b. Sum of squares for regression (model) and error
   c. Intercept, unstandardized beta, se, t-ratio, and standardized beta, and descriptive p-value
      i. Tables work the best here with more explanation in the narrative
   d. Independent variable, raw beta, se, t-ratio, and standardized beta, *and* p-value
   e. Durbin-Watson and multicollinearity
   f. Residuals- center leverage, Mahalanobis, Cook's, etc. (check for heteroscedasticity also)
   g. If space allows, providing scatter plots, histograms, and so on of the variables and residuals is useful
6. Discuss any changes made related to residuals. If a problematic case(s) is removed and the analysis rerun, discuss both results. This is a key component of transparency in regression.
   a. You are answering, What happens to the results with these changes?
      i. Do the coefficients really change?
      ii. Would your conclusions change?
7. Prediction equation (nicely placed at the bottom of a coefficients table)
8. Covariance/correlation matrix with means and standard deviations integrated

CAUSALITY, SPURIOUS CORRELATIONS, AND REGRESSION

Causality is difficult to truly ascertain in regression because most of the data are collected all at the same time. Even when the dependent variable is collected later, making a causal argument can be difficult. There are many stories about smoking and lung cancer. For instance R. A. Fisher (yes *p*-value Fisher) argued that lung cancer caused smoking and pushed that there was genetic component to those who smoked and got lung cancer (Stolley, 1991) while also being funded by the tobacco industry. The key is the amount of evidence appropriately weighed when arguing for causality, especially with regression. Researchers are trying to avoid spurious correlations–that is associations that appear there but really are not.

For researchers, a causal statement has two components: a cause and an effect (Kenny, 1979). Three commonly accepted conditions must hold for a scientist to claim that A causes B:

- **Time precedence:** For A to cause B, A must precede B.

- **Relationship:** There is a functional relationship between A and B.

- **Nonspuriousness:** A third variable or more removes the association between A and B.

SUMMARY

Linear regression is a popular analytic technique because of the wide variety of data that can be used. Additionally, experimental and nonexperimental studies can use regression. With this flexibility, there are a large number of assumptions that must be examined and many details with which to contend. It is not as simple as put the data in and hit enter, though it is often treated that way. Finally, remember that it is a mathematical model, one of many possible models and most likely is not specified correctly because not all relevant variables are probably in the model.

END-OF-CHAPTER RESOURCES

REVIEW QUESTIONS

Answers and rationales for the review questions are located in the Appendix at the end of the book.

1. TRUE or FALSE?

   If a Pearson correlation between two variables is 0.81, this means there is a strong positive relationship between the variables such that as one variable increases, the other variable decreases.

2. TRUE or FALSE?

   Linear regression cannot normally determine if there is a causal relationship between the independent and dependent variables because the data are often collected at one point in time.

3. Which of the following is an example of a question that would be addressed using a linear regression analysis and captures how well the variables account for differences in the outcome?

   a. What is the difference in skin breakdown between patients on a specialty air mattress and a conventional hospital mattress?

   b. Is the correlation coefficient stronger between minutes of weekly vigorous activity and blood pressure or minutes of weekly moderate activity and blood pressure?

   c. Do LDL cholesterol levels, mean systolic blood pressure, and C reactive protein account for at least 30% of the variance in myocardial infarction incidence among men age >50?

   d. Is the regression coefficient for the relationship between dietary self-monitoring and 6-month weight loss stronger or weaker than in research from the past 5 years?

4. The correlation between average hours of sleep per night and episodes of heart palpitations is $r = 0.21$. What should the investigator conclude about the size of the correlation?

5. Which of the following is the best first step for conducting a linear regression analysis between two continuous variables?

   a. generate a correlation matrix

   b. examine a scatterplot of the variables

   c. calculate the effect size

   d. fit the regression line

6. An investigator is examining the bivariate relationship between number of medication errors and number of nurse interruptions that occurred as medications were being administered. She finds that the variable number of nurse interruptions is not normally distributed. What type of analysis should she perform?

7. A study to examine the association age in years, BMI, and number of daily steps walked with hemoglobin A1c in patients with type 2 diabetes found the following:

Results of a multiple linear regression using ordinary least squares revealed the model has a R^2 value of 0.39 and adjusted R^2 of 0.35 with $F(3, 96) = 17.81$, MSe = 1.39, $p < 0.01$. Age had an unstandardized beta of 0.54 (se = 0.10, $t = 3.95$, $p < 0.001$) and standardized beta of 0.57. BMI had an unstandardized beta of 0.34 (se = 0.16, $t = 1.99$, $p < 0.01$) and standardized beta of 0.38. Daily steps walked had an unstandardized beta of 0.10 (se = 1.90, $t = 0.98$, $p = 0.25$) and standardized beta of 0.12.

What is the interpretation associated with the adjusted R2 in this study?

8. Using the above study of hemoglobin A1c in patients with type 2 diabetes, interpret the analysis of age and its association with hemoglobin A1c.

9. Which of the following are underlying assumptions that must be met before conducting a multiple linear regression analysis? Select all that apply.

    a. dependent variable has a normal distribution

    b. there is true correlation between independent variables

    c. independent variables have a normal distribution

    d. error terms do not have to be normally distributed

    e. the observed data points are independent of each other

    f. no multicollinearity among the independent variables

    g. there is multivariate normality among the residuals of the model

    h. homoscedasticity (residuals have constant variance at each point in the model)

    i. there is a linear relationship between all continuous independent variables and the dependent variable

10. Describe under what circumstances you would choose to use a simultaneous (traditional), stepwise (forward or backward), and hierarchical linear regression model.

A robust set of instructor resources designed to supplement this text is located at http://connect.springerpub.com/content/book/978-0-8261-6582-4. Qualifying instructors may request access by emailing textbook@springerpub.com.

REFERENCES

Akaike, H. (1970). Statistical predictor identification. *Annals of the institute of Statistical Mathematics*, 22(1), 203–217.

Barnett, V., & Lewis, T. (1978). *Outliers in statistical data*. Wiley.

Box, G. E. (1979). Robustness in the strategy of scientific model building. In R. L. Launer & G. N. Wilkson (Eds.) *Robustness in statistics* (pp. 201–236). Academic Press.

Burnham, K. P., & Anderson, D. R. (2002). *Model selection and multimodel inference: A practical information-theoretic approach* (2nd ed.). Springer-Verlag.

Cohen, J. (1988). *Statistical power analysis for the behavioral sciences* (2nd ed.). Erlbaum.

Davey Smith, G., & Phillips, A. N. (1996). Inflation in epidemiology: "The proof and measurement of association between two things" revisited. *British Medical Journal*, 312(7047), 1659–1661. https://doi.org/10.1136/bmj.312.7047.1659

Friendly, M., & Denis, D. (2005). The early origins and development of the scatterplot. *Journal of the History of the Behavioral Sciences, 41*(2), 103–130. https://doi.org/10.1002/jhbs.20078

Friendly, M., & Denis, D. (2008). *Milestones in the history of thematic cartography, statistical graphics, and data visualization.* York University.

Friendly, M., & Wainer, H. (2021). *A history of data visualization and graphic communication.* Harvard University Press.

Herschel, J. F. W. (1833). On the investigation of the orbits of revolving double stars. *Memoirs of the Royal Astronomical Society, 5,* 171–222.

Horst, P. (1941). The role of predictor variables which are independent of the criterion. *Social Science Research Council, 48*(4), 431–436.

Kendall, M. G. (1952). *The advanced theory of statistics* (5th ed.). Charles Griffith & Company.

Kenny, D. A. (1979). *Correlation and causality.* John Wiley and Sons.

Kline, R. B. (2016). *Principles and practice of structural equation modeling* (4th ed.). The Guildford Press.

Legendre, A. M. (1805). *Nouvelles méthodes pour la détermination des orbites des comètes.* F. Didot. There is an English version you can read for free online.

Long, J. S. (1997). *Regression models of categorical and limited dependent variables.* Sage.

Mahalanobis, P. C. (1936). Mahalanobis distance. *Proceedings National Institute of Science of India, 49*(2), 234–256.

Pearson, K. (1907). *On further methods of determining correlation* (No. 16). Dulau and Company.

Riggs, D. S., Guarnieri, J. A., & Addelman, S. (1978). Fitting straight lines when both variables are subject to error. *Life Sciences, 22*(13–15), 1305–1360. https://doi.org/10.1016/0024-3205(78)90098-x

Stevens, J. (2002). *Applied multivariate statistics for the social sciences.* Lawrence Erlbaum Associates.

Stolley, P. D. (1991). When genius errs: RA Fisher and the lung cancer controversy. *American Journal of Epidemiology, 133*(5), 416–425. https://doi.org/10.1093/oxfordjournals.aje.a115904

FURTHER READING

Fisher, R. A. (1921). On the 'Probable Error' of a coefficient of correlation deduced from a small sample. *Metron, 1*(4), 1–32.

Spearman, C. (1904). The proof and measurement of association between two things. *The American Journal of Psychology, 15*(1), 72–101.

Stigler, S. M. (1986). *The history of statistics: The measurement of uncertainty before 1900.* Harvard University Press.

Szucs, D., & Ioannidis, J. (2017). When null hypothesis significance testing is unsuitable for research: A reassessment. *Frontiers in Human Neuroscience, 11,* 390. https://doi.org/10.3389/fnhum.2017.00390

APPENDIX 8.1

Sample Size	df	Correlation Table	
		Two-Tailed	
		0.05	0.01
3	1	0.997	0.999
4	2	0.95	0.99
5	3	0.878	0.959
6	4	0.811	0.917
7	5	0.754	0.874
8	6	0.707	0.834
9	7	0.666	0.798
10	8	0.632	0.765
11	9	0.602	0.735
12	10	0.576	0.708
13	11	0.553	0.684
14	12	0.532	0.661
15	13	0.514	0.641
16	14	0.497	0.623
17	15	0.482	0.606
18	16	0.468	0.59
19	17	0.456	0.575
20	18	0.444	0.561
21	19	0.433	0.549
22	20	0.423	0.537
23	21	0.413	0.536
24	22	0.404	0.515
25	23	0.396	0.505
26	24	0.388	0.496
27	25	0.381	0.487
28	26	0.374	0.479
29	27	0.376	0.471
30	28	0.361	0.463
31	29	0.355	0.456
32	30	0.349	0.449
42	40	0.304	0.393
52	50	0.273	0.354
62	60	0.250	0.325

(continued)

	Correlation Table		
		Two-Tailed	
Sample Size	df	0.05	0.01
72	70	0.232	0.303
82	80	0.217	0.283
92	90	0.205	0.267
102	100	0.195	0.254

CHAPTER 9

Logistic Regression

CORE OBJECTIVES

- Explain main difference between logistic and traditional regression
- Explain and calculate odds ratios from 2x2 tables
- Interpret Wald statistic values
- Calculate and interpret the coefficient, Wald test, and exponentials
- Interpret and calculate pseudo R-squared values
- Explain the classification table
- Explain and calculate sensitivity and specificity
- Describe how ROC curves work
- Describe sample size needs based on expected odds-ratio

INTRODUCTION: OUTCOMES ARE GROUPS

Many research studies have a dependent variable that is not normally distributed such as, ordinal or categorical. Studies that focus on outcomes such as mortality, spread of Sars-COV-2, behavior change, physical health, risky behaviors, or weight change are just some of the examples where the dependent variable can be ordinal or categorical. Logistic regression is a specific analytic technique for use when the dependent variable is naturally dichotomous such as yes/no or survived/died or has been coded to be dichotomous (Long, 1997).

PURPOSE AND QUESTION FOCUS

The purpose of logistic regression is to examine independent variables that can classify group membership in one category or the other of the binary outcome variable, for example, smoker/nonsmoker. Logistic regression is also used in experimental and nonexperimental studies and with prospective and retrospective data sets. Since the outcome is a binary group, many of the research questions tend to using wording such as classify or predict. Thus, generic questions would read as:

Does variable X accurately predict the groups in Y?

Do variables Q, R, and S correctly classify membership in Y?

Are variables Q, R, and S associated with membership categories in Y?

Probability based questions generally read as:

What is the probability of an event given a specific level of X?

A more specific question might read as:

Do change in eating times, days walking, and text reminders predict weight loss or no weight loss over a 6-month time period?

GRAPHIC REPRESENTATION

The best place to start with representing logistic regression is a 2x2 table. This is also an excellent time to learn about a Chi-square table, which is a nonparametric analysis when the outcome is binary, and the independent variable is binary. Chi-square and 2x2 tables are the foundation of logistic regression and provide a concrete introduction to the topic. Chi-square tables can be larger than 2x2, but the key is to understand this table.

Table 9.1 shows example data where birth weight has been dichotomized at 2,500 grams and number of cigarettes per day has been recoded as zero for smoking no cigarettes per day, and one for smoking at least one cigarette per day. This has been coded with both "ones," in the upper left corner. This organization scheme makes analysis and interpretation a bit easier.

Table 9.1. Contingency Table for Chi-Square.

Contingency Tables			
	Smoking (Yes/No)		
Birth Weight Grams	1	0	Total
1 <2,500	356	2,646	3,002
0 ≥2,500	2,252	27,238	29,490
Total	2,608	29,884	32,492

There are three key pieces of information to be determined from the table, 1) Chi-square (χ^2) value, 2) Phi-coefficient, and 3) OR. The Chi-square value can be calculated by hand but is typically calculated in a software package. The Chi-square value for these data is 65.80. That is a large value and would be interpreted traditionally as important. But this value only indicates there is a deviance in the pattern. Deviance in this case means that the frequency count in each cell is not even. If the counts were all even, the Chi-square would be 0. Thus, all this analysis indicates is something is going on among the frequencies but does not indicate the size of the association. For that, the Phi-coefficient is needed. The Phi-coefficient is calculated using the Chi-square value and the sample size.

The Phi-coefficient for this 2x2 is 0.045, quite small. The value is interpreted like a correlation value and ranges from 0 to 1. This indicates that although there is great deviance in the frequency counts, the association between smoking and birth weight under 2,500 grams is small. Lastly, the odds ratio (OR) (Cornfield, 1951), usually used in a case control type of study, is a measure of association between exposure (smoking) and event (birth weight less than 2,500). ORs are grouped by size categories:

■ 1.0 (or close to 1.0) indicates that the odds of exposure among positive cases (patients) are the same as, or similar to, the odds of exposure among non-positive cases (e.g., control group). Thus, the exposure is not considered to be associated with the event (e.g., disease).

■ Greater than 1.0 indicates that the odds of exposure among positive cases (patients) are greater than the odds of exposure among nonpositive cases (those with no disease). Thus, the exposure might be a risk factor for the event.

■ Less than 1.0 indicates that the odds of exposure among positive cases (patients) are lower than the odds of exposure among nonpositive cases (those with no disease). Thus, the exposure might be a risk factor for the event. This is usually termed a protective factor against the event.

■ Note: how the data were coded and then analyzed can change the interpretation.

The OR for smoking at least one cigarette per day and a birth weight less than 2,500 is 1.63. This is interpreted as the OR of having a baby with an initial birth-weight under 2,500 grams is 1.63 times greater if the mother smoked at least one cigarette per day. ORs are also discussed as a strength of association indicator because the value is not upper bounded–the value can go from 0 to infinity. The larger the OR, the stronger the association. Finally, there are arguments about when and how to interpret ORs in health research (e.g., Holcomb et al., 2001; Nurminen, 1995).

Ogive Curve

In addition to the 2x2 table another foundational piece of logistic regression is the Ogive curve (Hosmer & Lemeshow, 1989). Since the outcome is binary, if one of the independent variables is continuous, the Ogive curve is needed because the relationship between the outcome and continuous, variable cannot be linear in nature (see Chapter 8 on linear regression). The x-axis can be thought of as your continuous variable of interest, such as age. The y-axis is the probability of being categorized in one of the two groups of interest, usually coded as a 1 and 0. For this example, birth weight less than <2,500 is coded 1. In the Ogive curve, as age increases the probability of a birth less than 2,500 increases. In Figure 9.1, an Ogive curve moves along an s-shape where lower income values are associated with a lower probability. As the age increases, the curve increases. At the $P = 0.5$, the curve is at the value where age value changes from being below 50% (in one group) to above 50% probability of being in the other group. That change occurs around age 30 in this simulated data. The steeper that slope,

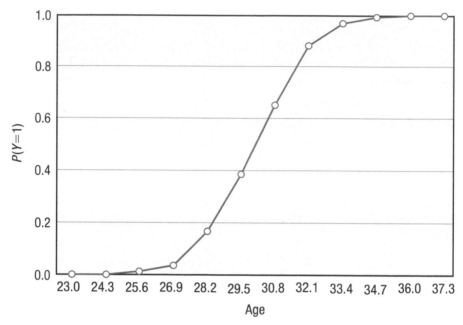

Figure 9.1. Ogive Curve Example.

the more easily it is to determine which group the person is in, based on the score. If a specific age, such as 35, was a perfect separator, then a flat line from the lowest age to 35 at the bottom left of the graph would be shown, a vertical line at 35 from zero to one would be shown, and then a flat line from 35 to the highest age at the very top of the graph would be shown.

TECHNICAL SECTION

In logistic regression, there are three key assumptions that need to be examined by the researcher. The three assumptions are:

- The relationships between continuous variables and the outcome need to be examined for linearity. The linearity is based on a log transformation and is part of the previous discussion on the Ogive curve.

- Errors are not correlated, like linear regression. The cases/participants in the data set are not related.

- No multicollinearity between predictors; just as in linear regression.

A major concern, but not an assumption, is the cell frequency. Basic crosstabulations to examine if there are five or more participants in each cell are important. With five or fewer cases in a cell, it can cause analytic problems. For example, the researcher had two age groups, Under 60 and Over 60 (two categories), by three postcardiac surgery rehabilitation techniques (three categories), there are a total of 6 cells (2×3). Each cell should contain at least five cases to complete the basic analysis. Logistic regression though, has always been a sample size heavy analytic technique, requiring a fairly large number of participants. Finally, like all the previous analyses, there is an assumption the sample is randomly chosen from the population, which is rarely the case.

Equations

Linear regression's basic equation from Chapter 8 is

$$Y = \beta_0 + \beta_1 \times (IV) + error,$$

This is a probability model, such that it is typically written as

$$E(y \mid x) = \beta_0 + \beta_1 \times (IV) + error,$$

which is interpreted as the expected value of y given x. And in general, that is what the researcher wants to know. What is the value of y if the researcher knows x or several values—what is the value of y given the knowledge of different independent variables? For logistic regression this is translated to,

$$P(Y = 1) = \beta_0 + \beta_1 \times (IV) + error$$

as the probability that $Y = 1$, given the equation because of the nature of the outcome. Because of that 1/0 nature, the equation cannot stay as is. A log transformation of the outcome is needed, which looks like this:

$$ln\left(\frac{\hat{p}}{1-\hat{p}}\right) = \beta_0 + \beta_1 \times (IV),$$

and is interpreted as the regression equation is the natural log (ln) of the predicted probability of being in one group divided by the predicted probability of being in the other group. This is not easy to deal with, ln (natural logs), thus the natural log is removed by using e^x, which results in,

$$\hat{p} = \frac{e^{\beta_0 + \beta_1 \times (IV)}}{1 + e^{\beta_0 + \beta_1 \times (IV)}},$$

Thus, to determine a predicted probability ($\hat{p}$) of being in a group, the results needed are the intercept coefficient β_0, the predictor coefficient β_1, and a value for the IV. This looks complicated, but it works just like regression once the beta coefficients are calculated.

For example, if β_0 (intercept coefficient) = −4.189 and β_1 (drinks coefficient) = 0.709. Substituting those values results in,

$$= \frac{e^{-4.189 + .709 \times (IV)}}{1 + e^{-4.189 + .709 \times (IV)}}.$$

Now if choosing 1 as the IV value (indicates at least one drink per day), this becomes,

$$= \frac{e^{-4.189 + .709 \times (1)}}{1 + e^{-4.189 + 0.709 \times (1)}}$$

$$= \frac{0.02}{1 + 0.02}$$

$$= 0.019.$$

Therefore, one drink a day or more is associated with a two percent chance of a low birthweight baby in this data set.

Fit Indices/Effect Size

Just as in linear regression, the effects sizes are set up to examine how well the model worked—an overall model fit. In linear regression, we had R-squared, and in logistic regression, we have *pseudo-R-square* values. These cannot be a traditional R-squared value because the outcome is dichotomous. The interpretation is essentially the same, the closer to one the better, the closer to 0 the worse the fit. Two fit indices, Cox and Snell (1989) and Nagelkerke (1991) are often used for logistic regression. You may also see values proposed by McFadden (1974) and Tjur (2009), among others. The calculations provided vary by software used. Each of these fit indices is based on a likelihood value that compares the model with only the intercept to the model with the independent variables. Thus, the researcher is comparing nothing against something. Something should be better, but how much is the key. The likelihood value can be thought of as the mean square error, the amount of error in the model, and the effect size calculation is amount that is explained.

Cox and Snell is calculated as a ratio of the baseline or null model (only the intercept) and the model of interest. The equation is

$$\text{Cox \& Snell pseudo-}R^2 = 1 - e^{\frac{(-2ll_{k\,model} - (-2ll_{baseline})}{n}}.$$

The subscript k model contains the independent variables, and the baseline only has the intercept. As the lower the value $-2ll_k$ (negative log likelihood for the desired model) approaches zero, the values for the Cox & Snell will approach 1, leaving everything else the same. If, for example, the $-2ll$ is 5072.27 for the baseline and for a one independent variable model is 5027 model, with a sample size of 32,492 the pseudo R-squared will be extremely close to zero. The Cox and Snell (C & S) R-squared is computed as follows:

$$\text{Cox \& Snell pseudo-}R^2 = 1 - e^{\frac{(-2ll_{k\,model} - (-2ll_{baseline})}{n}},$$
$$= 1 - e^{(5027 - 5027.27)/32,492}$$

$$= 1 - e^{(0.27)/32,492}$$
$$= 1 - e^{0.0000083}$$
$$= 1 - 1.0000083 = 0.0000083$$

This is essentially zero for the purposes of interpretation. The one variable model does not do much to help understand the difference between the two outcome groups.

Nagelkerke is the adjusted the Cox & Snell R-squared value because it cannot reach 1.0. The adjustment allows the value to reach one.

$$\text{Nagelkerke pseudo-}R^2 \; \frac{C \& S \, R^2}{1 - e^{\frac{-(-2ll_{baseline})}{n}}},$$

$$= \frac{0.0000083}{1 - e^{(-5072.27/32,492)}},$$

$$= \frac{0.0000083}{1 - e^{(-0.156)}},$$

$$= \frac{0.0000083}{1 - 0.86} = 0.0000574$$

The statistical software packages will let the researcher use a different number of decimal places or will change very small numbers such as this to scientific notation. Now, these values are not always the best indicator. When there is sparse data, not all cells have high frequency counts or it is a smaller data set, the deviance statistic (−2ll) is not distributed as Chi-square. Again, sparse data occurs when one or more of the cells (e.g., 2x2) have few observed values (and therefore few expected values) in the cells formed by crossing all of the values of all of the predictors. This often occurs when the phenomenon being studied is a rare event case, for example, apraxia or idiopathic pulmonary fibrosis. The Hosmer-Lemeshow fit test is designed to correct for this as long as there are continuous predictors. Hosmer and Lemeshow (2000) do not recommend the use of this test when there is a small n, around 400 and below. Logistic regression has always depended on relatively large sample sizes. As the expected OR decreases, the sample size need increases.

ORs are also used as effect sizes in logistic regression. The OR is equal to e^b where (b) is the unstandardized coefficient and is the exponent in e^b. Thus, if a weight gain variable has a beta coefficient of −0.056, the researchers raises the exponential e to that value which equals $e^{(-0.056)} = 0.946$. This is close to 1, so there is little relationship between the independent variable and dependent variable. The interpretation of the OR is affected by the coding of the variables (see Data Coding section). It is common in narrative reports to also see this written as, exp(B), the Greek symbol Ψ (psi, pronounced sigh), or simply "OR." Finally, researchers might discuss the unstandardized coefficient b from the OR, or use the log of the OR, $ln(e^b)$ the log odds. The variety can be confusing, but focus on the fact it is all a discussion of the OR.

Estimation

In linear regression, the analysis was run on least squares, which is easy to accomplish, even by hand, and fit can be estimated from the source table. Due to the nature of the outcome variable, least squares is not possible, so a different estimation technique is needed to obtain the coefficient values and other parameter estimates (beta, se, etc.). Logistic regression uses maximum likelihood (ML). ML is a mathematical technique for obtaining the smallest possible *deviance* between the observed and predicted values based on derivatives (aka calculus). ML tries to solve the smallest possible deviance by creating different solutions until it determines no better solution exists at this time with this data—that is, smallest deviance. That smallest deviance is termed the negative two log likelihood or just –2ll (Cohen et al., 2003). Historically, –2ll has also been indicated by D, for deviance (e.g., Hosmer & Lemeshow, 1989). Interpretation is pretty easy, the higher the value, the worse the situation. Using variables in the model should reduce this value, and the more deviance reduces, the better the model. Thus, this is why the effect sizes are based on the –2ll, the log likelihood.

Compatibility Intervals

Compatibility Intervals are commonly created for the exponential (ORs) values. In the example within the core results section, there are 95% compatibility intervals for the ORs. Note that the "true" population odds ratio may not fall in the CI. All of these results are based on the data at hand. The odds ratio and the related confidence (i.e., compatibility) intervals are important pieces of information from that table because they provide evidence of "how much." The calculations for confidence intervals on the odds ratios are a bit more complicated for logistic regression due to the exponential function aspect of the model, and the hand calculations are not shown here.

Data Coding

Based on how the data is coded, OR of 0.5 indicates that the outcome would be half as likely with an increase of an independent variable by one unit. For example, in Figure 9.1, because smoking and weight <2,500 grams were both coded one, an OR less than one would have indicated a decrease in births under 2,500 gm with smoking. As discussed earlier, an OR less than one also generally indicates a negative relationship between the independent variable and dependent variables. An odds ratio of 1.0 indicates there is no relationship between the independent variable and dependent variable.

Interpretation of ORs in reference to the coding is one of the largest problems we see in logistic regression manuscripts. This is why we recommend setting

**Table 9.2. Formatting
Chi-Square Table.**

	DV	
IV	1	0
1	11	10
0	01	00

up the coding for the variables based on what the researcher is interested in (Table 9.2) using a 1,1, format. The table is organized such that the IV, for example, medical test result, is organized by row, and the resulting DV, for example, disease or no disease, is organized by column.

Continuous Variables

Continuous variables are special in logistic regression because you must examine their linearity with the outcome, a technical assumption. To test this assumption, you need to:

1. Create a log version of your continuous variable, that is, transform it into a new variable. You will have a log version and the original variable.
2. Run a logistic regression with the original continuous variable and an interaction between the log version and the original.
3. Check the results table. Most researchers use the 0.05 cut off, but I think that is not taking time to look at what is going on. I also graph the variables, especially if the p-value is between 0.05 ad 0.20

Multiple Groups

If a variable has multiple categorical groups, a dummy code has to be created or the software program has to create them. For example, mother's education can be collected as a multi-group categorical variable. Some software programs do this automatically if you have coded the variable as categorical. Others you must create dummy codes with a reference level. The reference level in mother's education could be assigned to Group 1, less than 8th grade education, or the highest value. The key for the researcher is to choose the reference group of most interest and to make sure the inferences from the results are in reference to the that group.

Technical Component of the Results Table

The main results table for logistic regression is organized like the one from linear regression. First there are the unstandardized coefficients and the standard error (se) of the estimate. Those values are used to calculate the Wald Statistic or Z-statistic, just as it is needed to calculated the t-value in linear regression.

The Wald Statistic follows a Chi-square distribution, and the value is compared to the Chi-square distribution, just as the t-value was compared to the t-distribution. The formula is

$$\text{Wald} = \left(\frac{\hat{\beta}}{se\hat{\beta}} \right)^2$$

where the unstandardized beta coefficient is divided by the standard error of the estimate. That value is then squared. If the Z-value is calculated, then the Z-value is just the unstandardized beta coefficient divided by the standard error and is compared to the normal distribution. Finally, the odds ratios for the intercept and each variable are provided. The OR is the exponential value of unstandardized coefficient (e^b).

Residuals

Software programs have a variety of residuals analysis options. Examining the residuals should be a major component of any analysis because it is important for making good decisions. Residuals, again, are the difference between the observed values to the expected values based on the model. The larger the difference, deviance, of the original raw observed values from the predicted values, the worse the fit of the model and the larger the residuals. Some of the common options for residual analysis for logistic regression are Pearson, Dfbeta, C, Cbar, DIFDEV and DEFCHISQ, Cook's D, and centered leverage. Since analysis software have different options, it is important to take time to understand which ones are available.

Pearson residuals are important if the researcher wants to identify individual observations the model poorly explains. Dfbeta tells the researcher if an individual variable is affecting the parameter estimates. Dfbeta is good for determining which observations cause instability in each coefficient. C and CBAR are scalar versions of DFbeta and are similar to Cook's D in linear regression. DIFDEV and DIFCHISQ highlight ill-fitted observations that contribute heavily to the difference between the observed data and the predicted values. DIFDEV specifically shows what happens to the deviance value if a specific individual observation is deleted. DIFCHISQ does the same but with the change in the Pearson chi-square statistic. Cook's D (or distance) examines the effect of large residuals. Cook's values show the leverage on the outcome, that is the distortion of results. Centered leverage will give the researcher the same information as Cook's through a different process.

Prediction Accuracy Tables

In coordination with the residual analysis, a careful examination of the classification table is warranted. The classification table compares the observed to the predicted, thus the original to how the model would classify each participant or case. This provides an overall accuracy picture of the model. Table 9.3 provides the classification table for the example in the core results section. Notice that the software program put the 1,1 group at the bottom left.

Table 9.3. Classification Table.

	Predicted		
Observed	0	1	% Correct
0	32,003	0	100
1	489	0	0.00

As can be seen, this one variable did not classify the outcome variable of low, birth weight very well. There were 489 low weight births, yet the model predicted zero. The percentage might look good, but in reality, this one variable model did not work well.

In addition to the classification tables, there are other evaluative indictors; correct and incorrect, sensitivity, specificity, false positive, and false negative. *Correct* and *incorrect* are simply whether the prediction matches the original classification for each participant, case, or event. *Sensitivity* is the ratio of the number of correctly classified **events** (low birth weight) divided by the total number of events and is often called the true positive rate. *Specificity* is the ratio of the number of correctly classified **nonevents** divided by the total number of total number of events, and is often called the true negative rate. These indicators provide evidence concerning how well the model works and makes correct classifications. In our experience, having both sensitivity and specificity be high has been rare in research studies we review. If sensitivity is near 1, specificity will likely be low. This is part of the tradeoff in design of which one you want to focus on.

A **false positive** are those observations that are negative but were predicted to be events. **False negatives** are those observations that are positive but were predicted to be negative. Table 9.4 provides the traditional framework.

Based on the data from the example (Table 9.5), specificity and sensitivity are:

Table 9.4. Inference Categories for Correct Predictions.

		Observed		
		Positive	Negative	
Predicted	Positive	A True Positive	B False Positive	Total Predicted Positive
	Negative	C False Negative	D True Negative	Total Predicted Negative
		Total Observed Positive	Total Observed Negative	

Table 9.5. Birth Weight and Smoking Contingency Table.

Smoking Yes/No	Birth Weight Grams		
	1 <2,500	0 ≥2,500	
1 = Yes	356	2,252	2,608
0 = No	2,646	27,238	29,884
Total	3,002	29,490	32,492

$$\text{False positive} = (B/ (B + D)) = 2{,}252 / 29{,}490 = 0.076$$

$$\text{False negative} = (C / (A + C)) = 2{,}646 / 3{,}002 = 0.88$$

$$\text{Sensitivity} = A \text{ (true positive)} / A + C \text{ (true positive + false negative)}$$

$$= 356 / (356 + 2{,}646) = 0.12$$

$$\text{Specificity} = D \text{ (true negative)}/ B+ D \text{ (false positive + true negative)} =$$

$$27{,}238 / (2{,}252 + 27{,}238) = 0.924$$

The results from the analysis provide sensitivity and specificity values based on the model prediction. Now based on the results from the prediction model (Table 9.6), we see:

Table 9.6. Actual vs. Predicted Values.

Predicted	Actual	
	1	0
1	0	0
0	489	32,003

$$\text{Sensitivity} = A \text{ (true positive)} / A + C \text{ (true positive + false negative)}$$
$$= 0 / 489 = 0$$

$$\text{Specificity} = D \text{ (true negative)} / B + D \text{ (false positive + true negative)}$$
$$= 32{,}003 / (32{,}003 + 0) = 1.00$$

These results for sensitivity and specificity are due to the fact none of the low weight babies were predicted to be low weight.

ROC Curves

Finally, **ROC**, receiver operating characteristic, curves visualize the predictive accuracy of a logistic results for Sensitivity and Specificity (Figure 9.2). The ROC curve from the multivariable model shows that the ROC curve (in red) is above the 45-degree line (blue) which is good, but it is not far above it and dips below at the higher end which indicates low/poor predictive accuracy, that is, not able to classify well. It is not separating the signal from the noise. The 1-specificity is the false positive rate.

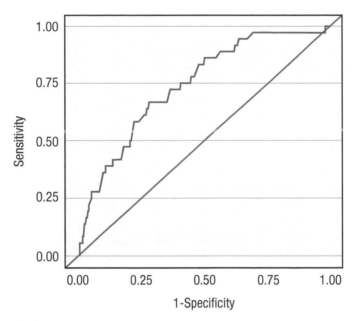

Figure 9.2. ROC Curve.

At the end of all this information, the results indicate that the independent variable or variables for both examples do not do a great job of predicting the outcome variable. The residuals are not problematic, and the accuracy paints a picture of the model working, but taking in all the information, the model does not work well. The key is the summary of all of this information, not just those that appear to be good.

Cut-Values, Input, Linearity Test

There are a few technical components that do not get enough attention; cut-values, input of variables, and test of linearity for continuous predictors. **Cut-values**, or points, are the probability value for deciding if an observation represents an event or a nonevent. If the researcher were to choose that all observations with predicted probabilities over zero count as an event, then all observations will be classified as event. Thus, the sensitivity is one and specificity is zero and not very interesting. The default cut-value in programs is 0.50. As the cut-point is changed, specificity and sensitivity will change. One way to understand cut-points is the discussion with a patient about blood pressure. At what point does the nurse begin to talk to the patient about reducing blood pressure, 120/80, 125/85, 130/90? If the cut-off value is switched to 0.1 in the smoking data, accuracy becomes 0.85, specificity is 0.91, and sensitivity is 0.14. You can change this value in most programs and compare what happens. In general, we rarely see researchers test or change the cut-value.

Logistic regression, like linear regression, allows for different input patterns of the independent variables, traditional, step, and block. It is much more common to see forward or backward step input than all-at-once. This is the same topic as in traditional linear regression. In general, stepwise creates some of the same issues as in linear regression. Backward step input might be the most popular, using the Wald Statistic or Z as the cut-off for keeping a variable in the model, that is inclusion. In a traditional backward step, all of the variables are included, and then the "worst" variables are removed one at a time based on the a priori size of the Wald or Z or p-value cut-off choice. If the area is new and there is little prior knowledge, a forward step or even backward step might be a suitable starting point. But the results can indicate very different models, that is, model specification problems. The researcher must then determine which is best, usually using a Chi-square AIC or BIC value, and the theoretical arguments. But the decision and the value used for it also has its own requirements. The researcher can block some of the variables first, but this is essentially a forward step type of model

Discussed previously, but worthy of stating again because it is rare to see it examined in articles, is the linearity test. The test is used with continuous predictors and involves using the original continuous variable and the natural log of the continuous variable as an interaction predictor. If the natural log of the interaction reaches a p-value less than the traditional 0.05 (or even if close), a different analysis may be necessary or some recoding of the continuous variable may be required.

Sample Size

Based on the traditional null hypothesis significance testing and $p < 0.05$ framework, logistic regression is a large sample size technique. The expected odds-ratio is a key driver of the sample size. The examples in the chapter have been quite large, but if the researcher expected an OR of 1.25, traditional 0.05 for the cut-off, 0.80 for power, and 30% of the cases are 1,1: (for example, true positive), the sample size needed is 795. If the outcome variable is considered a rare event, this situation can be worse, and a larger sample is needed along with other technical adjustments that must be made (King & Zeng, 2001). Finally, as with linear regression and the other techniques, the focus needs to be on accuracy and risk related to the topic at hand.

CORE RESULTS

Results narratives and tables can vary widely with logistic regression articles—possibly the most variability that we see. We believe there should be more information included in the narrative and more tables. And, if not in the narrative or tables, it should be included in the supplemental materials. More journals are allowing supplemental materials to be able to be accessed electronically, though they will not be with the print edition of the article.

Bivariate

Below is an example narrative for a bivariate logistic regression results section. The narrative covers major components that should be included in the results.

A logistic regression was used to examine one categorical predictor (Tables 9.7–9.11, Figures 9.3–9.4). Table 9.9 provides beta coefficients, z-statistics, p-values, ORs, and compatibility intervals. Drinking one drink per day doubled the probability of a birth less than 1,500 grams with an OR of 2.033 CI95% (.95, 4.34). There were two cases that were considered outliers in the prediction model and were

Table 9.7. Fit Measures.

Model	Deviance	AIC	R^2_{McF}	R^2_{CS}
1	5,072	5,076	5.40e-4	8.43e-5

Table 9.8. Likelihood Test.

Omnibus Likelihood Ratio Tests			
Predictor	χ^2	df	p
Drinks	2.74	1	0.098

Table 9.9. Model Coefficients.

						95% Compatibility Interval	
Predictor	Estimate	se	Z	p	Odds ratio	Lower	Upper
Intercept	−4.189	0.0459	−91.27	<0.001	0.0152	0.0139	0.0166
Drinks							
1 − 0	0.709	0.3865	1.84	0.066	2.0329	0.9531	4.3361

Note: Estimates represent the log odds of birth weight 1,500 = 1 vs. birth weight 1,500 = 0

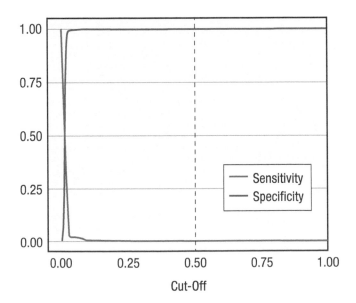

Figure 9.3. Cut-Point Plot.

removed. The Cox & Snell *R*-squared was 0.00008, indicating very little difference in outcome being accounted for by the drinking variable. The logistic model had an accuracy of 98% of the cases, with a specificity of 1.00 and a sensitivity of 0.00. The model essentially predicted no births under 1,500 grams (Table 9.10) and given the comparatively few births under 1,500 grams and the mother drank at least one drink a day, this accuracy is biased upwards. The cut-off value for a case was left at the default of 0.50. The area under the curve (AUCROC) was 0.504, indicating essentially no predictive accuracy (Table 9.10, Table 9.11, and Figure 9.4).

Table 9.10. Accuracy/Classification and Original Data Table.

	Predicted		
Observed	0	1	% Correct
0	32,003	0	100
1	489	0	0.00

	Drinks		
Weight	0	1	Total
>1,500	31,776	227	32,003
≤1,500	482	7	489
Total	32,258	234	32,492

Table 9.11. Predictive Measures.

Accuracy	Specificity	Sensitivity	AUC
0.985	1.00	0.00	0.504

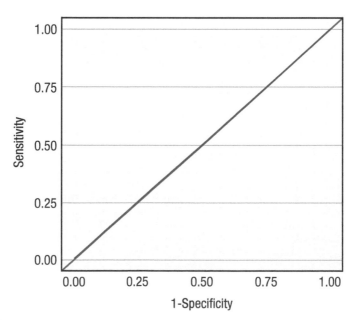

Figure 9.4. ROC Curve.

Multivariate

Multivariate logistic regression, like multiple linear regression is the use of more than one predictor variable. With multiple variables, more complicated models can be examined with a wide variety of data types, along with interactions between two variables (e.g., age and health status). Below is an example narrative for a multivariate logistic regression results section. The narrative covers major components that should be included in the results.

A multivariate logistic regression was used to examine one continuous predictor and two categorical predictors (Tables 9.12–9.16, Figures 9.5–9.6). Linearity between continuous predictor and the dichotomous outcome was examined and can be assumed ($Z = 1.85$, $p > 0.05$). The continuous variable did not have outliers and was approximately normal. In addition, all predictor variables were not highly correlated and did not create a collinearity problem (Table 9.14). A traditional enter-all-at-once method was used for the predictors. Table 9.13 provides beta coefficients, z-statistics, p-values, ORs, and compatibility intervals. Weight gain appeared to be an important predictor indicating increased maternal weight is associated with not having a birth weight less than 1,500, but the OR is near one. Cigarette smoking appears to decrease the probability of a low-birth-weight child, but this appears to be an artifact of the data or an indicator of a potential interaction. Mother's education, comparing each level to the lowest education category, does not appear to be predictive of the outcome. The model overall had a very small Cox & Snell value (.009). There were only 36 babies in this data set with a birth weight under 1,500 grams (Table 9.15). Residuals were normally

Table 9.12. Fit Measures.

Model	Deviance	AIC	R^2_{McF}	R^2_{CS}	R^2_N
1	359.163	373.163	0.067	0.009	0.071

Table 9.13. Model Results.

Predictor	Estimate	se	Z	p	Odds ratio	95% Compatibility Interval Lower	Upper
Intercept	−2.630	0.767	−3.427	<0.001	0.072	0.016	0.324
Weight Gain	−0.056	0.014	−3.951	<0.001	0.946	0.920	0.972
Cigarettes							
1 − 0	−0.678	0.617	−1.099	0.272	0.508	0.151	1.700
Mother's Education							
2 − 1	−0.090	0.853	−0.106	0.916	0.914	0.172	4.864
3 − 1	0.198	0.761	0.260	0.794	1.219	0.274	5.417
4 − 1	−0.254	0.803	−0.317	0.752	0.776	0.161	3.743
5 − 1	−1.134	0.878	−1.291	0.197	0.322	0.058	1.800

Note: Estimates represent the log odds of "<1,500 = 1" vs. "≥ 1,500 = 0"

distributed with no outliers. The accuracy appears to be quite high, but this is an artifact of the small number of low weight births and the fact the model is simply predicting all births are over 1,500 grams (Table 9.15, Table 9.16, and Figure 9.5).

Table 9.14. Collinearity Statistics.

	VIF	Tolerance
wtgain	1.005	0.996
cigsbinary	1.015	0.986
meduc_rec	1.005	0.995

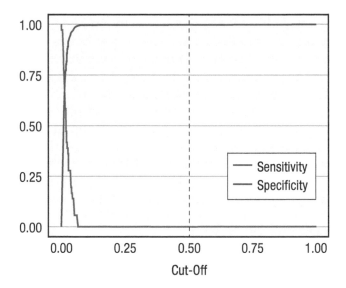

Figure 9.5. Cut-Off Plot.

Table 9.15. Classification Table – Weight 1,500.

	Predicted		
Observed	0	1	% Correct
0	2,763	0	100.000
1	36	0	0.000

Note: The cut-off value is set to 0.5.

Table 9.16. Predictive Measures.

Accuracy	Specificity	Sensitivity	AUC
0.987	1.000	0.000	0.741

Note: The cut-off value is set to 0.5.

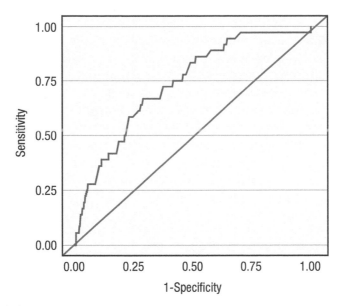

Figure 9.6. ROC Curve.

MOST DEFINING ATTRIBUTES—WHAT SHOULD I LOOK FOR?

When reading, or writing, a logistic regression results section, there are key attributes that should be included. They include:

1. Adequacy of expected frequency
2. Explanation of design/dummy codes if appropriate
3. Linearity of continuous predictors
   a. Means and standard deviations of predictors by the outcome variables
   b. Multicollinearity
   c. Outliers/missing data
   d. Testing of linearity
4. Method for predictor variable input
5. Explanation of each variable with parameter estimates
6. ORs and compatibility intervals
7. Evaluation of overall model
8. Evaluation of model without predictors
9. Classification or prediction table
10. Residual analysis/incorrect prediction analysis

We have observed that logistic regression analyses tend to have the least detail related to key attributes compared to the other analysis techniques discussed in this book. Given the health-related nature of many logistic regression analyses examining patient outcomes, there should be much more detail.

SUMMARY

Logistic regression is used when the outcome variable of interest is binary in nature, such as yes/no, smoker/nonsmoker, or survived/did not survive. Categorical and continuous variables can be used as independent variables. The binary outcome variable causes the analysis to be more complicated than linear regression and thus more computationally complex. Therefore, to estimate the parameters (e.g., beta coefficients) ML has to be implemented. Additionally, there are more complex assumptions related to linearity of continuous independent variables and the outcome variable. Logistic regression also produces several more pieces of evaluative information than regression, such as accuracy, ROC curves, and sensitivity and specificity.

END-OF-CHAPTER RESOURCES

REVIEW QUESTIONS

Answers and rationales for the review questions are located in the Appendix at the end of the book.

1. TRUE or FALSE?

   In looking an outcome with three categories (underweight, normal weight, overweight), a researcher can use binary logistic regression.

2. TRUE or FALSE?

   Independent variables that are continuous or categorical may be included in a logistic regression model.

3. TRUE or FALSE?

   An investigator could use logistic regression to analyze data for the research question, "Do barriers to healthy eating and self-efficacy for following a low-fat diet predict <5% weight regain or ≥5% weight regain at one year post weight loss?"

4. Which of the following is needed to determine the size of the association in a contingency table?
   a. Odds ratio
   b. Chi-square
   c. Phi-coefficient
   d. Compatibility interval

5. A nurse manager is trying to determine if being a nonsmoker is associated with being discharged after CABG surgery in less than 7 days. Which of the following Odds Ratio reflects that nonsmokers are more likely to be discharged in <7 days?

   a. 0.80

   b. 1.80

   c. 1.0

   d. 0.90

6. Which of the following tests is used to determine if an independent variable is significant in the logistic regression model?

   a. Cox & Snell R^2

   b. Nagelkerke R^2

   c. beta coefficient

   d. Wald test

7. Research question: Is daily sodium intake associated with having hypertension? What is the Chi-square from the following contingency table?

Daily Grams of Sodium	Hypertension (Yes/No)		
	1	0	Total
1 <2,000	340 (1763.7)	2,855 (1431.2)	3,195
0 ≥ 2,000	3,400 (1976.2)	180 (1603.7)	3,580
Total	3,740	3,035	6,775

8. Describe the assumptions that must be checked prior to using logistic regression.

9. In linear regression, the R^2 statistic measures the amount of variance in the outcome variable that can explained by the predictors in the regression model. What does the *pseudo R^2* value represent in logistic regression?

10. Describe what residuals are in a logistic regression model and why they are important to examine.

11. Describe sensitivity and sensitivity in relationship to logistic regression.

12. Describe a receiver operating characteristic (ROC) curve and why it matters.

A robust set of instructor resources designed to supplement this text is located at **http://connect.springerpub.com/content/book/978-0-8261-6582-4.** Qualifying instructors may request access by emailing **textbook@springerpub.com.**

REFERENCES

Cohen, J., Cohen, P., West, S. G., & Aiken, L. S. (2013). *Applied multiple regression/correlation analysis for the behavioral sciences.* Routledge.

Cornfield, J. (1951). A method of estimating comparative rates from clinical data; applications to cancer of the lung, breast, and cervix. *Journal of the National Cancer Institute, 11*(6), 1269–1275. https://doi.org/10.1093/jnci/11.6.1269

Cox, D. R., & Snell, E. J. (1989). *The analysis of binary data* (2nd ed.). Chapman and Hall.

Holcomb, W. L., Jr., Chaiworapongsa, T., Luke, D. A., & Burgdorf, K. D. (2001). An odd measure of risk: Use and misuse of the odds ratio. *Obstetrics & Gynecology, 98*(4), 685–688.

Hosmer Jr, D. W., & Lemeshow, S.(1989). *Applied logistic regression.* John Wiley & Sons.

Hosmer Jr, D. W., & Lemeshow, S. (2000). *Applied logistic regression* (2nd ed.). John Wiley & Sons.

King, G., & Zeng, L. (2001). Logistic regression in rare events data. *Political Analysis, 9*(2), 137–163. https://doi.org/10.1093/oxfordjournals.pan.a004868

Long, J. S. (1997). *Regression models for categorical and limited dependent variables.* Sage.

McFadden, D. (1974). Conditional logit analysis of qualitative choice behavior. In P. Zarembka (Ed.), *Frontiers in Economics.* Academic Press.

Nagelkerke, N. J. D. (1991). A note on the general definition of the coefficient of determination. *Biometrika, 78*(3), 691–692. https://doi.org/10.1093/biomet/78.3.691

Nurminen, M. (1995). To use or not to use the odds ratio in epidemiologic analyses? *European Journal of Epidemiology, 11*(4), 365–371.

Tjur, T. (2009). Coefficients of determination in logistic regression models—A new proposal: The coefficient of discrimination. *The American Statistician, 63*(4), 366–372. https://doi.org/10.1198/tast.2009.08210

FURTHER READING

Belsley, D. A., Kuh, E., & Welsch, R. E. (2005). *Regression diagnostics: Identifying influential data and sources of collinearity.* John Wiley & Sons.

CHAPTER 10

Introduction to Bayesian Analysis

CORE OBJECTIVES

- Understand differences between Bayesian analysis and Fisher/Frequentist analyses
- Explain different probabilities, such as joint and conditional
- Calculate a conditional probability
- Explain why Bayes analyses are used
- Explain key terminology for Bayes analyses
- Explain the differences between prior, likelihood, and posterior
- Understand differences between informative and noninformative priors

INTRODUCTION

Bayesian analysis is philosophically and fundamentally different than the Fisher based statistics used in the previous chapters (Aldrich, 2008; Efron, 1986; Morey et al., 2016). Bayesian analysis is based on beliefs and, more important, belief adjustment. People have beliefs, or technically hypotheses, about how the world works. There is generally more than one belief for a phenomenon, which is called a candidate hypothesis. These candidate hypotheses are on a continuum from plausible to not plausible. If we encounter some data that aligns with or is consistent with the belief, it gets stronger. If we encounter data that is inconsistent, it decreases our belief. This chapter is a very brief introduction to Bayesian analysis and thus does not mean one can run a Bayes analysis after reading it. But the chapter does provide a foundational understanding that will let you begin a journey that will lead to using Bayes. We provide references for reading about Bayes; some are more mathematically oriented than others.

GRAPHIC REPRESENTATION

When Jim is working in Dublin, Ireland, he always carries an umbrella. Why? His belief is it will rain at some point in the day. It will rain, or it will not, but the belief is that it will rain. That belief is termed a *prior* in Bayesian analysis. But, we need to get a bit more specific. How much does it actually rain

Table 10.1. Prior Distribution Chart.

Hypothesis	Degree of Belief
Rains	0.52
Does Not Rain	0.48

Table 10.2. Initial Probabilities of Carrying Umbrella.

Hypothesis	Remembers	Does not Remember
Rains	0.80	0.20
Does Not Rain	0.70	0.30

Table 10.3. Joint Probabilities of Rain and Remembering to Carry an Umbrella.

	Remembers	Does Not Remember
Rains	0.80 × 0.52 = 0.42	0.20 × 0.52 = 0.10
Does Not Rain	0.70 × 0.48 = 0.34	0.30 × 0.48 = 0.14

Table 10.4. Checking the Row Summations.

	Degree of Belief
Rains	0.42 + 0.10 = 0.52
Does Not Rain	0.34 + 0.14 = 0.48

in Dublin during the year? Well, we can look that up (https://www.dublin.climatemps.com/precipitation.php) where it shows that there are 191 days per year with more than 0.1 mm of rain in Dublin. Thus, it rains 52% and does not rain 48%. If we belief this, then we can create this prior distribution chart (Table 10.1). $P(h)$ means probability of the hypothesis, so P(Rain) = 0.52.

Well, this is wonderful. We have priors, and we can collect data and make adjustments. But we need a bit more information about Jim. What is the probability of Jim carrying an umbrella in Dublin when he is working there? Well, it is pretty high, but not perfect. On rainy days he remembers his umbrella about 80% of the time, and on days it does not rain about 70% of the time. So, he is a little lucky with the proportions (Table 10.2).

Table 10.2 sets up the ability to make conditional probabilities. That is what is likely to happen, given a certain circumstance. Conditional probabilities are very important and are how we negotiate most of our life. Most people understand general probability. What is the probability of seeing a tail when flipping a coin? Well, over the life of the flip, it is 0.50. Some people remember joint probabilities, which is understanding two things together. What is the probability that it is raining *and* Jim brought his umbrella? Joint probabilities are a first step in understanding Bayesian analysis. In our scenario, that would be P(Rains, remembers umbrella) = P(Both) × P(Rains). Well, P(Both) is 0.80 (see Table 10.2) and P(Rains) is 0.52, see Table 10.1, which makes the joint probability 0.80 × 0.52 = 0.42. We now have worked with prior knowledge about Jim and the likelihood it actually rains (Table 10.3). And if we sum the values across, we get back to Degree of Belief (Table 10.4).

Isn't this great? We have merged what we know from previous research on raining days in Dublin with what we believe! We can also add in the columns and get a full table. The totals are termed *marginal probabilities* because they are on the margins of the table (Table 10.5).

Thus, the probability that Jim remembers, regardless of rain status, is 76% and does not remember is 24%. This was a specific example, but most of Bayes analyses are written with a symbolic system. The first start of abstracting is

Table 10.5. Marginal Probabilities.

	Remembers	Does Not Remember	Total Rows
Rains	0.80 × 0.52 = 0.42	0.20 × 0.52 = 0.10	0.52
Does Not Rain	0.70 × 0.48 = 0.34	0.30 × 0.48 = 0.14	0.48
Total Columns	0.76	0.24	1.00

in Table 10.6. Now we can make this look more mathematical by removing the words and using the generic symbols (Table 10.7). The chart can be adjusted more formally with hypotheses and data (Table 10.8).

Table 10.6. First Level of Symbolic Representation of the Rain Example.

	Remembers	Does Not Remember	Total Rows
Rains	P(Remembers, Rains)	P(Does Not Remember, Rains)	P(Rains)
Does Not Rain	P(Remembers, Does Not Rain)	P(Does Not Remember, Does Not Rain)	P(Does Not Rain)
Total Columns	P(Remembers)	P(Does Not Remember)	

Table 10.7. Second Level of Symbolic Representation of the Rain Example.

	Remembers	Does Not Remember	Total Rows
Rains	P(Re, Ra)	P(DRe, Ra)	P(Ra)
Does Not Rain	P(Re, DRa)	P(DRe, DRa)	P(DRa)
Total Columns	P(Re)	P(DRe)	

Table 10.8. Full Symbolic Representation of the Rain Example.

	D_A	D_B	Total Rows
H_A	$P(H_A, D_A)$	$P(H_A, D_B)$	$P(H_A)$
H_B	$P(H_B, D_A)$	$P(H_B, D_B)$	$P(H_B)$
	$P(D_A)$	$P(D_B)$	

TECHNICAL COMPONENTS

The previous example sets the base or prior information for Bayes theorem (Morey et al., 2016). Bayes theorem is what links prior knowledge to current knowledge. Let's imagine a typical day for Jim. He is carrying an umbrella and that makes sense. But what numbers should we put in? What is missing? Let's start with basic information in Table 10.9. The total for carrying has to be 1 because Jim is carrying

Table 10.9. Updating Probabilities.

	Carrying	Not Carrying
Rains		0
Does Not Rain		0
Total Columns	1	0

an umbrella, and the column for not carrying has to be 0. Here is where the strength of Bayes comes in because you can update your probabilities with this information in Table 10.9.

We can use the Bayes formula (Bayes, 1763), a conditional probability, to answer these two probabilities. It is formally written with this equation:

$$P(h \mid d) = \frac{P(d \mid h) \times P(h)}{P(d)}$$

This means, for our example, the probability of h given d is equal to the probability that d given h * probability of h divided by d. This vertical symbol | means "given." Now, this can be confusing. In our example, that is the probability that it rains given Jim is carrying an umbrella equals the probability Jim is carrying an umbrella given it is raining times the probability it is raining. That quantity is then divided by the probability that Jim is carrying an umbrella. But it appears that in Table 10.5, we have the probabilities of Jim carrying an umbrella (0.76) and of it raining (0.52), but there is nothing for the probability of Jim carrying and umbrella given it is raining ($P(d \mid h)$). Well, that is easily solved because $P(d \mid h) = P(h,d)/P(h)$, where $p(h,d)$ is the joint probability (both together, like the overlap in a Venn diagram). We do know $P(h,d)$, that the joint probability of Jim carrying an umbrella and it rains is 0.42. Now we can put all of this together.

We are looking for $P(h \mid d)$. It rains given Jim is carrying an umbrella. We have:

$P(h)$, the probability it rains, 0.52
$P(d)$, the probability Jim is carrying an umbrella, 0.76
$P(h,d)$, it is raining and Jim is carrying an umbrella = 0.42

$$P(h \mid d) = \frac{P(d \mid h) \times P(h)}{P(d)}$$

Substituting in $p(d \mid h)$,

$$P(h \mid d) = \frac{\frac{P(d,h)}{P(h)} \times P(h)}{P(d)}$$

Putting in our numbers,

$$P(h \mid d) = \frac{\frac{0.42}{0.52} \times 0.52}{0.76}$$

Cancelling those same numbers in the numerator and denominator, we are left with

$$P(h \mid d) = \frac{0.42}{0.76} = 0.55$$

Thus, the probability of it raining, given Jim is carrying an umbrella, is 0.55. This probability is a posterior probability (Table 10.10)

Table 10.10. Conditional Probabilities for P(h|d).

	Carrying	Not Carrying
Rains	0.55	0
Does Not Rain	0.45	0
Total Columns	1	0

Bayes Versus Fisher

Bayes and Fisher (Bayesian vs. Frequentist) analyses have key differences in how statistical inferences are positioned and analyzed (Christensen, 2005; Efron, 1998; Lambert, 2018).

1. Fisher/Frequentists believed that you worked with the data at hand and only that data. Thus, prior information does not matter.

2. Bayes requires prior information that is used in conjunction with the information at hand.

A great example of this is from an interview between Brian Cox and Sir David Spiegelhalter, using a pool table from the Bayes thought experiment. The key is what is included. The first step is to roll the cue (white) ball and determine where it lands. While Sir David is not looking, Brian Cox rolls the cue ball, and when the ball stops, he removes it, remembering the line (Figure 10.1).

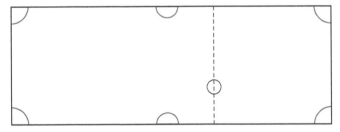

Figure 10.1. Cue Ball Rolled and Stop Location.

Then Brian rolls five balls at once, randomly, and when the balls stop Sir David asks him to tell him how many landed to the left of the line and to the right. The split was 3 to the left and 2 to the right. Fisher would argue that the line is 2/5th of the way down the table, Bayes would argue it is 3/7ths and move that line a bit toward the center (Figure 10.2).

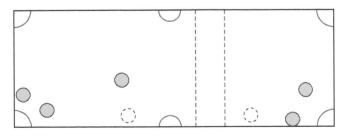

Figure 10.2. Five Rolled Balls and Their Location.

Therefore, Fisher would use the data about the split: 2 out of the five balls, 2/5th. Bayes takes into account the randomly rolled first ball, and you get 2 + 1/3 + 2 or 3/7th because the ball could be on either side.

3. Fisher did not use or believe in alternative hypotheses. The results met his threshold of $p \leq 0.05$ or they did not. It is essentially a contradiction method of science. Does the data at hand contradict the null hypothesis?

4. Bayesian analyses work with both null and alternative hypotheses; specifically, the results provide an argument to which one is more plausible along a continuum and not a specific cut off. It also treats the null and alternative hypotheses equally.

5. Frequentists assume that the events occur with probabilities that represent long-run frequencies over an infinite series of experiments or studies, thus repetitions. Frequentists assume this probability actually exists and is fixed.

6. Bayesians do not assume fixed probabilities or parameters but rather distribution of possible outcomes, some more probable than others.

7. Bayesians also do not believe in repetitions of a study or experiment in order to define and specify a probability. A probability is just a measure of certainty of a particular belief.

8. Frequentists assume the data to be random and that results from sampling are fixed and defined by a population distribution. Any differences from the population are just an artifact of the sampling variation. Pick a different sample and get different results.

9. Bayesians, since the data is observed, assume that the data is fixed and does not vary. Bayesians do not need to imagine an infinite number of studies. Bayesians don't assume to ever perfectly know a value of a parameter (e.g., mean, or probability, of a coin landing heads up). One way Bayesians view an unknown parameter is as truly fixed in some absolute sense, and our beliefs are uncertain, and that uncertainty is expressed using probabilities. Thus, our sample may be "noisy." Or, one can suppose that there is no true value for the parameters, and we should get slightly different results with each sampling. These are different ways of viewing uncertainty, but the mathematics do not change and that is important!

10. Inference making by Fisher/Frequentists based statistics and Bayesian have to deal with probability calculations around the hypotheses. Frequentists assume the hypothesis is true and calculate the probabilities of obtaining the observed data (sample). If the probability is small, the assumption is that it is unlikely and should be rejected. This is actually the opposite of what researchers hypothesis is true, this is actually the opposite of what researchers want. Bayes works around that by inverting the Frequentist probability to get the probability of the hypothesis given the actual data observed (sample).

Lambert (2018) has a great example of Bayesian versus Frequentist analyses. We have adapted that example here. Suppose there are two radar control workers who have to scan for enemy fighter planes during World War II. The first follows a Frequentist mode of analysis and the other a Bayesian. They work in the same room but are from different counties in the country. They both see an enemy plane that has entered the airspace of their country. They know they have to make a decision on how many intercept planes to send up and where to send them, thus there are costs to sending them to the wrong place. The unknown is where this enemy is headed. The Frequentist takes the current location of the plane and inputs it into the model, which compares it to historical enemy plane data. A result is immediate, that the plane is headed to city X. The Frequentist orders 10 planes from his county to meet the plane at city X. The Bayesian knows from experience that the enemy has used three different attack paths during the war. He gives these paths a high probability (density) for his prior and, with the plane's location, feeds this into the same model program that the Frequentist used. The output is different because of the prior, and instead of just a single location, there are three, with one having clearly the highest probability, city X, but there are two other cities, Y and Z, that could be the destination for the enemy jet. The Bayesian decides to send four planes to intercept at city X, and two planes each for cities Y and Z. The enemy was headed for city Y and was intercepted.

WHY USE BAYES

There are four main reasons to use a Bayesian analysis (van de Schoot & Depaoli, 2014). The first is that prior or background information can be included in the analysis. This allows for the inclusion of uncertainty into the analysis, specifically a parameter, such as the variance of a group. Thus, everything that is known based on previous publications can be used to add in "informative priors." This allows for updated information to be examined to see if it "disagrees" with the new data. This conflict is important for learning and seeing new things. Fisher/Frequentist statistics have no way to deal with this. The second reason is the definition of probability. In the Frequentist-based confidence intervals, for example, the confidence interval is based on the quite large assumption of a very large number of repeated samples from the population. Bayesian analysis creates a credibility interval that is based on a distribution of possible values for the parameter. There is no assumption of repeated data collection. The third reason is that Bayes is not based on large samples (that is getting to $p < 0.05$). The more precision you specify prior to the new data, the smaller the sample size needed for the analysis. Finally, some complex models cannot be used with Fisher/Frequentist-based statistical analysis along with solving issues when the data are multilevel and complex (e.g., random slopes with observed categorical data).

Change in Technology

The technology for running Bayesian analyses has radically changed over the past decade. At one point, it was too computationally expensive to run Bayesian analyses; now these options are built into many statistical programs: SPSS, SAS, JAMOVI, and JASP to name a few along with running Bayes analyses in R and R-Studio. The analyses in this book have options. Thus, the key issue now is the gathering of prior information from research studies, the development of the prior information to be used in the analyses, or the decision to use a specific prior distribution in the analyses.

KEY TOPICS

There are key topics that have to be discussed before examples, like a Bayesian *t*-test, can be shown. The three key topics are likelihood, priors, and posteriors, as well as several key terms (Table 10.11). In Bayesian inference, the likelihood is the $P(d\,|\,h)$ from the equation

$$P(h\,|\,d) = \frac{P(d\,|\,h) \times P(h)}{P(d)}.$$

This, as a reminder, is the probability of the data, given the hypothesis. It is also commonly written as $P(d\,|\,\theta)$. The symbols change depending on who wrote it, but the meaning is the same. Bayesian analyses are trying to represent uncertainty for the unknown quantities, such as a mean difference between two independent groups from a sample. Thus, $P(d\,|\,\theta)$ gives the researcher the probability of generating a particular sample of data if the parameters in the model are equal to θ. Flipping a coin is a good starting point to understanding the likelihood function.

If we have a coin that we flip and write down the outcome, and we ignore previous flips. Assuming the coin is fair, the probability of landing heads or tails is $\theta = 1/2$. If the researcher flips the coin twice, the options are HH, TT, HT, and TH. The probability of each is:

HH ½ × ½ = ¼

TT ½ × ½ = ¼

HT ½ × ½ = ¼

TH ½ × ½ = ¼

Thus, these are the likelihoods of the outcomes. The distribution of outcomes for heads is in Figure 10.3. This provides a likelihood distribution of possible outcomes.

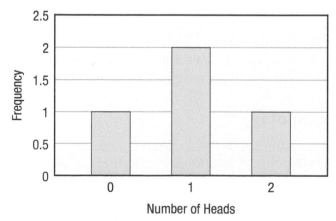

Figure 10.3. Frequency of Heads With Two Tosses.

Table 10.11. Key Terms.

Background Knowledge	Previous knowledge about a population parameter, such as a *t*-value, regression coefficient, and so on, which can be obtained by using prior research, previous analyses, or expert opinions.
Credibility Interval	This is the Bayesian version of the confidence/compatibility interval previously discussed. The difference is the researcher can state that the probability that the population parameter is between the upper and lower boundaries, such as 95%.
Hyperparameters	The specific parameters for a prior distribution. If the researcher believes the *t*-distribution should be used, the mean and variance parameters of this *t*-distribution prior are termed *hyperparameters*. The values used control the amount of uncertainty or certainty incorporated into the model.
Likelihood Function	This is the representation of the observed data likelihood. This will be used to weigh the prior distribution in the analysis to get to the posterior distribution where decisions can be made.
MCMC (Markov Chain Monte Carlo)	This is this simulation system for drawing samples from a distribution that creates a Markov chain, which will represent the posterior distribution.
Parameter	A fixed but unknown feature of the model that is estimated by Frequentist or Bayesian methods
Posterior	The distribution that is obtained after combining the prior and likelihood functions.
Posterior *p*-Value	This is a *p*-value that is based on the posterior distribution after a Bayesian analysis.
Precision	This is the amount of information incorporated into the prior distribution. The more information, the more certainty.
Prior	A statistic distribution that can be used to capture the amount of certainty or uncertainty in a population parameter.

Source: Adapted from van de Schoot, R., & Depaoli, S. (2014). Bayesian analyses: Where to start and what to report. The European Health Psychologist, 16(2), 75–84..

Priors, What Are They?

Priors, *P(h)*, are a researcher's beliefs about a situation or phenomenon (Depaoli, 2021; Lambert, 2018; van de Schoot et al., 2014). This is also the part of Bayes analyses that is the most controversial. One way to think about this is the alternative hypothesis. The vast majority, >95%, of research has a belief about what will happen. That belief has to come from somewhere, usually previous research. With the Bayesian analysis framework, prior information, typically with a belief about the distribution of the phenomenon, is the starting point. A concrete example is a good entry into priors.

Using the traditional red ball example, imagine there is a bag with five balls in it and you are trying to understand how many are red. We need to start out with a prior belief (Table 10.12). If there is no "belief," a flat or **uniform** prior can be used (Aldrich, 2008; Efron, 1986; Morey et al., 2016). This uniform distribution is also known as a *noninformative prior*. **Figure 10.4** shows a uniform distribution where the belief shows the numbers of balls are all equally likely.

Table 10.12. Red Ball Using a Bayesian Approach.

Number of Red Balls	Prior Distribution	Likelihood Distribution	Prior × Likelihood	Posterior $(\frac{prior \times likelihood}{p(data)})$
0	1/6	0	0	$=\frac{0}{(\frac{1}{2})}=0$
1	1/6	1/5	1/30	$=(\frac{2/30}{1/2})=1/15$
2	1/6	2/5	2/30 = 1/15	$=(\frac{2/30}{1/2})=2/15$
3	1/6	3/5	3/30 = 1/10	$=(\frac{3/30}{1/2})=3/15$
4	1/6	4/5	4/30 = 2/15	$=(\frac{4/30}{1/2})=4/15$
5	1/6	1	5/30 = 1/6	$=(\frac{5/30}{1/2})=5/15$
	1	3	P(red ball) = 15/30 = 1/2 or 0.5	1

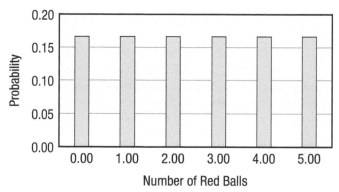

Figure 10.4. Uniform Prior.

Likelihood

The likelihood is the probability of generating the particular sample of data based on parameters of the statistical model (Figure 10.5). Think of this as the distribution of outcomes a researcher assumes about the data. Our likelihood in the example of 5 red balls is 1.

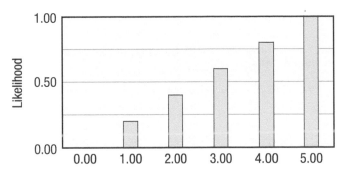

Figure 10.5. Likelihood.

Posterior

This is the goal, to get to the posterior distribution, $P(h\,|\,d)$ (Aldrich, 2008; Efron, 1986; Morey et al. 2016). This is completed through the heart of Bayesian analysis: prior times likelihood equals posterior. The researcher wants to know what the probability distribution is around the parameter estimate. The distribution summarizes the uncertainty about the parameter estimate with a distribution. Wider distributions indicate more uncertainty, and narrow distributions indicate more certainty (**Figure 10.6**).

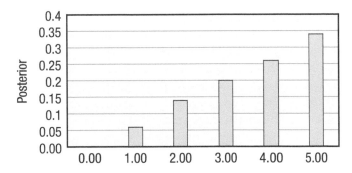

Figure 10.6. Posterior.

In the ball example, a uniform or noninformative prior was implemented. What if the researcher uses a different previous experience, a simulation, or previous research? **Table 10.13** displays a prior that is more normally distributed.

Notice how the posterior adjusts based on the change in the prior. As information changes, the posterior changes. If the model is very strong, the posterior distribution will not change much regardless of prior distribution change.

Table 10.13. Revised Prior for Ball Example.

Number of Red Balls	Prior Distribution	Likelihood Distribution	Prior × Likelihood	Posterior ($\frac{prior \times likelihood}{p(data)}$)
0	1/12	0	0	$=\frac{0}{(\frac{1}{2})}=0$
1	1/6	1/5	1/30	$=(\frac{2/30}{1/2})=1/15$
2	¼	2/5	2/20 = 1/10	$=(\frac{2/30}{1/2})=2/15$
3	¼	3/5	3/20	$=(\frac{3/30}{1/2})=3/15$
4	1/6	4/5	4/30 = 2/15	$=(\frac{4/30}{1/2})=4/15$
5	1/12	1	1/12	$=(\frac{5/30}{1/2})=5/15$
	1	3	P(red ball) = 15/30 = 1/2 or 0.5	1

BAYES INDEPENDENT t-TEST EXAMPLE

The independent t-test is a good place to begin understanding the integration of Bayes into an analysis. Different software packages have different options, but all have the ability to use noninformative priors or informative priors. Priors are statistical distributions that are used to capture the amount of uncertainty in a population parameter. This is used to weigh the sample data to get the posterior. We use the posterior information to make decisions.

Noninformative priors are priors that are general in nature and typically do not alter the results compared to a traditional t-test very much.

Informative priors are prior information that can be used to improve the analytic process and the inferences from the results. The more information you put in, the more accurate the results are; this is termed *precision* in Bayes analyses. Bayes also allows for the comparison of the alternate hypotheses against the null hypotheses, alternative models against the null, or model versus model. Frequentist-based analyses cannot do this.

Traditional Independent t-Test

Tables 10.1 and 10.2 have the traditional information from a traditional independent t-test. For this example, simulated data related to general happiness from an ongoing study in the Middle East is used. There are two groups: a control and an experimental group. There are 34 participants in each simulated group.

Table 10.14. Descriptive Statistics.

Outcome	Group	Mean	Median	sd
Happiness	Control	17.912	19.000	4.129
	Experimental	23.971	24.000	3.252

Table 10.15. *t*-Test Results.

Independent Samples *t*-Test							
		Statistic	df	p	Mean Difference	se Difference	Effect Size
Happiness	Student's *t*	-6.721	66	<0.001	-6.059	0.901	Cohen's d -1.63

The mean, median, and standard deviation by group are in Table 10.14. The student's *t*-value is large, and Cohen's *d* is also large (Table 10.15). These values are negative because the higher scores (experimental) were subtracted from the lower scores (control).

Normality and homogeneity are assumed based on the test results. The results are easily interpreted within the Frequentist framework and Null-Hypothesis Statistical Test (NHST). Traditionally, the null would be rejected due to the *p*-value. This does not tell the researcher how much weight should be given to the alternative hypothesis, just that the null is rejected. With an effect size of 1.63, the researchers would be very happy because that effect size is quite large and indicates a large separation of the two distributions.

Bayesian Analysis

Tables 10.16 and 10.17 display the basic results for a Bayesian analysis with a limited-informative prior and a Cauchy distribution as the default. The Cauchy distribution is similar to the normal distribution with fatter tails. Technically, Cauchy is a *t*-distribution with one degree of freedom. The Bayes factor is quite large in this example. The Bayes factor provides a numeric indicator of the weight toward the null or toward the alternative hypothesis. This is different than a *p*-value that can only give an inference of rejecting or not rejecting the null. BF_{10} over 100 is considered extreme evidence toward the alternative hypothesis (Figure 10.7; Kass & Raftery, 1995).

Table 10.16. Bayes With Informative But Limited Prior.

Bayesian Independent Samples *t*-Test		
	BF_{10}	Error %
Happiness	1,767,312.364	0.000

Table 10.17. Group Descriptive Statistics

		N	Mean	sd	se	95% Credible Interval	
	Group					Lower	Upper
Happiness	Control	34	17.912	4.129	0.708	16.471	19.353
	Experimental	34	23.971	3.252	0.558	22.836	25.105

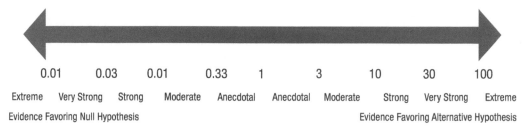

Figure 10.7. Scale of Bayes When BF_{10} Is Being Used.

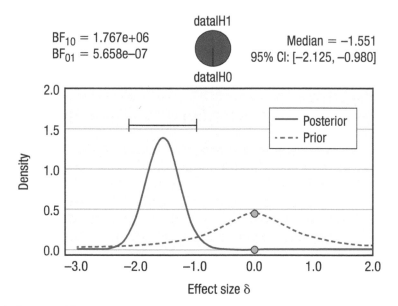

Figure 10.8. Prior and Posterior Results.

The BF_{10} value is 1,767,312.364, which is quite a distance from 100. **Figure 10.8** has the prior and posterior graph where the prior is shown with a dashed line and is the Cauchy distribution set at 0 with a 0.707 width. The width indicates where 50% of the distribution falls. The larger the width value, the more uncertainty you have about the prior.

The Cauchy distribution has two main parts: a scale parameter (λ) and a location parameter (x_0).

- The location parameter (x_0) tells us where the peak is.

- The scale parameter is half the width of the probability density function at half the maximum height.

In other words, the location parameter x_0 shifts the graph along the x-axis, and the scale parameter λ results in a shorter or taller graph. The smaller the scale parameter, the taller and thinner the curve.

The descriptive statistics for the groups are provided in **Table 10.17**. At the right end of the table, notice it states, Credible Interval. The researcher can state that there is a 95% chance that the mean value for the control group is between

16.47 and 19.35. The researcher cannot do that with a compatibility (confidence) interval from previous analyses in this book. Both are dealing with uncertainty but in very different ways. The previous compatibility interval (Frequentist) is based on the assumption of an infinite number of exactly repeated experiments trying to understand the true value of the X across all of these repeated experiments. Thus, the uncertainty with a compatibility is with the interval itself (Lambert, 2018). In a Bayesian analysis, the data is perceived as fixed, and the parameters vary.

Figures 10.10 and 10.11 provide information about the quality of the results. Table 10.10 is a robustness check based on the Cauchy prior width. The burgundy dot with black edging is where the default width was set for this analysis. There are three priors used in the graph. The issue is all three overlap; thus, regardless of prior width (uncertainty), the results are the same. Additionally, there are the indicators where the researcher should make a decision about the evidence. In this example, the evidence is extremely strong for the alternative (H1) hypothesis and not the null (H0). Finally, the fully red circle indicates that evidence supports the alternative. A fully yellow circle would indicate support for the null hypothesis. Some examples of in-between values are in **Figure 10.9**.

Notice in **Figure 10.11** there is a BF_{10} and BF_{01}. These (BF_{10} and BF_{01}) are inverses of each other due to the mathematics of Bayes factors. For example, if the BF_{01} is 3, the BF_{10} is $1/3$ and would indicate that evidence points toward the null hypothesis. This is also important to understand because different software packages will give different BF results, and the researcher must pay attention to which one is being used.

Figure 10.11 has a sequential analysis, which provides evidence for H1 or HO as sample size changes along with the change in Bayes factor values. Again, three priors are provided. As sample size increases in the simulation, the Bayes factor increases and the evidence for the alternative hypothesis grows.

Change Prior

If the researcher has previous knowledge from other studies or previous data analyses, the prior can be changed to that new information. For example, maybe the researcher knows that, from previous studies, the width of the prior should be smaller (tighter), or the effect of being in the two groups has an effect size of

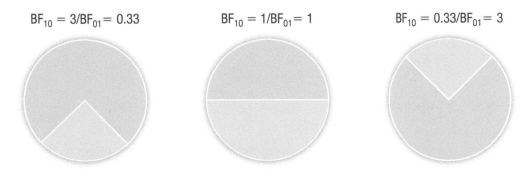

$BF_{10} = 3/BF_{01} = 0.33$ $\qquad$ $BF_{10} = 1/BF_{01} = 1$ $\qquad$ $BF_{10} = 0.33/BF_{01} = 3$

Figure 10.9. Bayes Factor Values Reference Graphic.

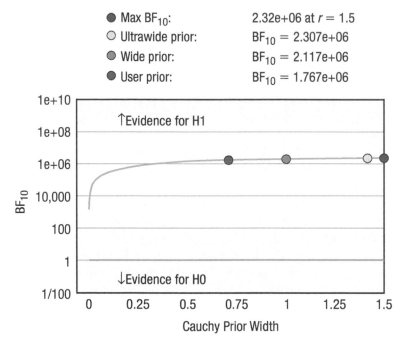

Figure 10.10. Bayes Factor Robustness Check.

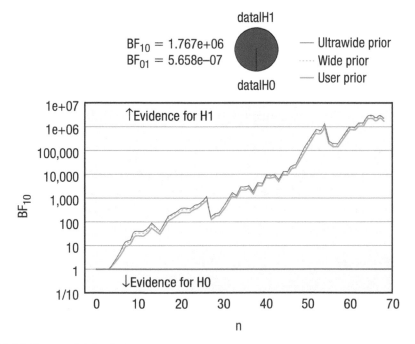

Figure 10.11. Sequential Analysis.

−1.5. For example, this information could change the prior to reflect that effect size with a normal distribution centered at −1.5 with a width of 0.707. Again, the width just indicates the level of uncertainty. A smaller width would indicate more certainty on the part of the researcher. The change will alter the posterior results and would be considered an informative prior and a very strong informative prior. **Figure 10.12** has a demonstration of that change.

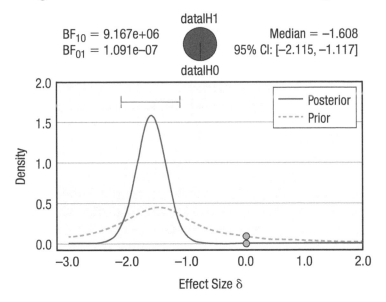

Figure 10.12. Prior and Posterior.

Notice with the change the increase in Bayes factor, now 9166622.97. For illustration purposes, maybe the researcher has information that the difference was in the other direction previously—the control participants were better than the experimental participants. Changing the prior to 1.5 with the same width produces a much smaller Bayes factor because the prior is very different than the current data (**Figure 10.13**), thereby creating a smaller Bayes factor and reducing the effect size. The median difference is closer to 0.

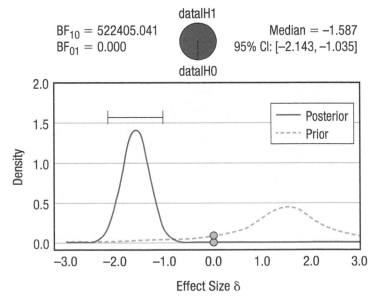

Figure 10.13. Prior and Posterior With Change in Prior.

WHAT YOU NEED TO KNOW TO IMPLEMENT BAYES

As stated previously, Bayesian analysis is complicated and understanding all of the details is imperative. The mathematics involved in Bayes are more complicated than most of the analyses in this book. Thus, this chapter is an introduction to the basic concepts and how it works. To implement Bayesian analyses correctly, we strongly recommend that you read extensively in the area. Two readings to start with are Lambert (2018) and van de Schoot and DePaoli (2014). We have also provided additional references in a Further Reading list after the Reference section.

SUMMARY

Bayesian analyses are philosophically and technically different than the previous analytical techniques in the book. The largest difference is the addition of prior information in the analysis. Frequentists do not include prior information into the analysis and Bayesians do. Another major difference is Frequentists assume the data to be random and results from sampling are fixed and defined by a population distribution. Any differences from the population are just an artifact of the sampling variation that would be corrected by an infinite number of studies. Pick a different sample and possibly get different results. Bayesians, because the data is witnessed, assume that the data are fixed and do not vary. Bayesians do not need to imagine an infinite number of studies. If the researcher is thinking about a Bayes or traditional analysis, the researcher must decide what they believe about that data and the importance of using prior information in the analysis.

RESOURCE

https://royalsociety.org/about-us/programmes/people-of-science/david-spiegelhalter-bayes-fisher/

END-OF-CHAPTER RESOURCES

REVIEW QUESTIONS

Answers and rationales for the review questions are located in the Appendix at the end of the book.

1. Discuss how Bayesian analysis differs from Fisher/Frequentist analysis.

2. Describe the three key aspects of a Bayesian analysis.

3. Consider the following information on patients presenting to the emergency department:

	Chest Pain (CP)	No Chest Pain	(Totals)
Hypertension (HTN)	20	5	40
No HTN	5	50	60
(Totals)	25	75	100

Using Bayes' Theorem, what is the probability that a person with chest pain has HTN?

4. TRUE or FALSE?

The Bayes factor within the Bayesian framework is different than the *p*-value is the Fisher framework.

5. TRUE or FALSE?

The Credibility Interval in Bayesian analysis represents the same thing as the Compatibility (Confidence) Interval in a Fisher/Frequentist analysis.

6. TRUE or FALSE?

In determining to use a Bayesian approach, the researcher believes including previous information in the analysis is vital and that the collected data are fixed.

A robust set of instructor resources designed to supplement this text is located at http://connect.springerpub.com/content/book/978-0-8261-6582-4. Qualifying instructors may request access by emailing textbook@springerpub.com.

REFERENCES

Aldrich, J. (2008). RA Fisher on Bayes and Bayes' theorem. *Bayesian Analysis, 3*(1), 161–170. https://doi.org/10.1214/08-BA306

Bayes, T. (1763). An essay towards solving a problem in the doctrine of chances. *Philosophical Transactions of the Royal Society, 53*, 370–418. https://doi.org/10.1098/rstl.1763.0053

Christensen, R. (2005). Testing fisher, Neyman, Pearson, and Bayes. *The American Statistician, 59*(2), 121–126. https://doi.org/10.1198/000313005X20871

Depaoli, S. (2021). *Bayesian structural equation modeling*. The Guilford Press.

Efron, B. (1986). Why isn't everyone a Bayesian? *The American Statistician, 40*(1), 1–5. https://doi.org/10.2307/2683105

Efron, B. (1998). RA Fisher in the 21st century. *Statistical Science, 13*(2), 95–114.

Kass, R. E., & Raftery, A. E. (1995). Bayes factors. *Journal of the American Statistical Association, 90*(430), 773–795.

Lambert, B. (2018). *A student's guide to Bayesian statistics*. Sage.

Morey, R. D., Romeijn, J. W., & Rouder, J. N. (2016). The philosophy of Bayes factors and the quantification of statistical evidence. *Journal of Mathematical Psychology, 72*, 6–18. https://doi.org/10.1016/j.jmp.2015.11.001

van de Schoot, R., & Depaoli, S. (2014). Bayesian analyses: Where to start and what to report. *The European Health Psychologist, 16*(2), 75–84.

van de Schoot, R., Kaplan, D., Denissen, J., Asendorpf, J. B., Neyer, F. J., & Van Aken, M. A. (2014). A gentle introduction to Bayesian analysis: Applications to developmental research. *Child Development, 85*(3), 842–860. https://doi.org/10.1111/cdev.12169

FURTHER READING

Depaoli, S., & Van de Schoot, R. (2017). Improving transparency and replication in Bayesian statistics: The WAMBS-Checklist. *Psychological Methods, 22*(2), 240. https://doi.org/10.1037/met0000065

Depaoli, S., Rus, H. M., Clifton, J. P., van de Schoot, R., & Tiemensma, J. (2017). An introduction to Bayesian statistics in health psychology. *Health Psychology Review, 11*(3), 248–264. https://doi.org/10.1080/17437199.2017.1343676

CHAPTER 11

Quality Improvement

CORE OBJECTIVES

- Explain the background of two key individuals in the development and QI
- Explain a Shewart Chart
- Discuss the Theory of Change model
- Discuss both the PDCA and PDSA cycles
- Explain Deming's four components of profound knowledge
- Describe differences between area of concern, symptom, and problem
- Explain clinical reasoning and PDSA cycle
- Describe other QI models such as Lean and Root Cause Analysis

INTRODUCTION: IMPROVEMENT AND CHANGE

Most people have at some point wanted to try an improve something in their personal lives or at work. This desire for improvement involves changing something that is supposed to lead to improvement. The key components are the current state, the change, and the results, which hopefully improve. But these three components have important questions with them:

Why is the current state not acceptable? We don't want to change just for change.

What options are there for change? There is rarely one option for a change.

What counts as improvement? Improving a product, but it doubles the cost may not be considered improvement.

Basic History

Improvement, or improvement science, has a long history that began in the manufacturing industry, and specifically manufacturing processes and products. There are two individuals who are commonly identified as the main developers and promoters of improvement sciences, Walter Shewart and W. Edwards Deming.

Walter Shewart was essentially a combination of physicist, engineer, and statistician, but formally had a Ph.D. in Physics for the University of California, Berkeley. In 1918, he joined the Western Electric Engineering Company, which was the precursor for Bell Laboratory where he worked until his retirement. He began working on electrical line production inspection and in the first few years at the company, he had developed his quantitative production improvement model of assignable and chance causes (Shewart, 1931). Assignable (common) causes are those that are part of the normal variation in production. Shewart (1931) wrote,

> "The practical situation, however, is that in the majority of cases there are unknown causes of variability in the quality of a product which do not belong to a constant system. This fact was discovered very early in the development of control methods, and these causes were called *assignable.* The question naturally arose as to whether it was possible, in general, to find and eliminate such causes." Page 14.

This led to his third postulate that, assignable causes can be found and eliminated. Chance causes (special) are those that are outside the normal variation in production. Chance variation can be a computer crashing or errors created by a newly trained employee that is still learning the job. If the only variation occurring is chance, then the system is in "statistical control" for Shewart. He developed this model while working in the inspection department and wrote a memorandum about what he saw and included what became the Shewart Chart. The chart displays when the system is within statistical control. An example of the Shewart Chart is in **Figure 11.1**.

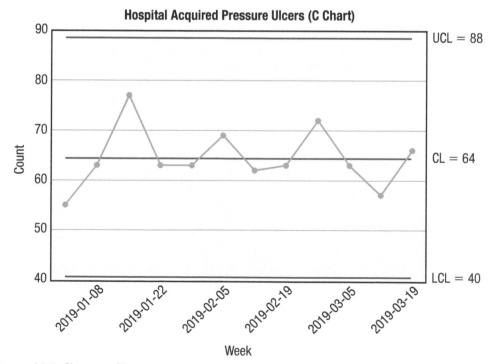

Figure 11.1. Shewart Chart.

The Statistical Control Chart contains upper and lower control limits (UCL, LCL), which define the natural variation observed in the process. The UCL and LCL are three standard deviations from the mean or CL, control line. These are now commonly referred to as sigma limits, such as 3, 4, 5, or 6 sigmas. Thus, the control lines are determined in relation to the desired improvement level. There may be other rules implemented that direct the behaviors of investigation, such as one data point over the 1 sigma level is not investigated, but two or more are. The charts x-axis is based on time, and the time samples could be minutes, hours, days, months, and so on. The time is simply a choice based on the data needed. For example, health-based options in new watches and activewear collect data from continuously to user pre-set timings. The y-axis is the output or outcome variable of interest, such as a production size or amount produced. Shewart also discussed in detail the issues with precise measurement and the need to understand errors of measurement and sampling, as a pair. Specifically, he focused on good data and acknowledged that good data are expensive, but the cost of making an efficient analytical study of the data is small.

Finally, the Shewart Cycle, which was a Plan, Do, Check, Act system, was an iterative process that is more commonly known now as the PDSA cycle by Deming (1989). Deming earned a doctorate from Yale in 1928 in mathematical physics and went to work for the United States Department of Agriculture (USDA). It was his time at Yale that changed his life. During 1925 and 1926 he spent 4 months each summer working on transmitters at the famous Western Electric Hawthorne Plant in Chicago. There he saw the inhuman conditions people had to work under, both of these affecting his views of organizations later. While at USDA, one of his superiors, Charles Knusman, thought that it would be good for Deming to meet Shewart. In the fall of 1927, he began to work intermittently with Shewart (Kilian, 1992). Their relationship grew from there. In 1939 Deming joined the Census and had an impact on the collection of data, the sampling, for the 1940 Census. Deming left the Census in 1946 and an odyssey in consulting began post World War II in Japan where they were excited about his idea of quality control. Deming returned to Japan multiple times in the 1950s. He had a clear impact on Japanese production that would not be recognized in the United States until the 1980s when Japanese manufacturing was clearly out-performing U.S. manufacturing in consistent quality (Kilian, 1992).

PURPOSE AND QUESTION FOCUS

The purpose of quality improvement (QI) studies is to enact some desired change that should cause an improvement in a process, product, or end state. The questions are not the traditional research questions, but can appear similar. For example, the generic QI question would be:

■ Does the implementation of X process lead to a decrease in errors?

More specifically,
  • Do more BSN trained nurses, lead to fewer medical errors?

- Does implementing a bundle of care interventions reduce falls among hospitalized older adults?
- Does administering weight-based antibiotic therapy preoperatively reduce the number of postoperative infections?
- Does a chemical change in the tube creation process lead to longer usage (or less degradation)?

THEORY OF CHANGE

A core component QI is change, and essentially what is meant by change. Therefore, there needs to be theory of change that is the foundation of the QI process. Theory of Change (ToC) is a comprehensive description and illustration of how and why an expectation of change should happen within a context given specific parameters. It is the explanatory mechanism between what is currently occurring, how a change works and how this will specifically lead to the desired outcomes. ToC has been attributed to Weiss (1995) and is housed within the family of theory driven evaluations (Schreiber & Asner-Self, 2011). The focus is typically on a long-term outcomes or outcomes through a sequence of steps or outcomes (Vogel, 2012). An initial step is to determine the long-term goal of an outcome and work backward, or backward mapping and then work on the process of change that must occur to reach that goal; sometimes these are mapped onto an outcomes framework (Anderson, 2006).

A major component of this process is to identify all of the assumptions being made and the assumptions about what needs to be in place for this to work. During this process, the *assumptions* are about what needs to be in place. Often not central, but need to be, are the context factors that will affect the ToC. For the ToC to occur, the assumptions need to be made explicit as well as the *contextual* factors that influence the ToC. In addition to the contextual factors, the ToC must be developed with stakeholders through a variety of participatory opportunities. This will also allow for the development of stakeholders who were not initially identified (Sullivan & Stuart, 2006). Finally, ToC do not create a prescribed design related to the goals, such as an ethnography or randomized controlled trial.

PDCA

Shewart PDCA cycle is the precursor to the QI models of today. PDCA, stood for Plan, Do, Check, Act. Specifically,

1. Plan: Recognize an opportunity and plan a change.
2. Do: Test the change. Carry out a small-scale study.
3. Check: Review the test, analyze the results, and identify what you've learned.
4. Act: Take action based on what you learned in the study step. If the change did not work, go through the cycle again with a different plan. If you were successful, incorporate what you learned from the test into wider changes. Use what you learned to plan new improvements, beginning the cycle again.

The four cycles are part of the continuous improvement philosophy and a heavy focus on the checking component of the model. Different versions have added that the organization should also add on O at the beginning, for Observing what is currently occurring. This is similar to baseline measurements in research so that you understand levels of the outcome of interest. This has also been called the Shewart Cycle, Deming Cycle, and control/circle/cycle wheel. It actually has roots much older than Shewart, such as Bacon's hypothesize-experiment-evaluate in Novus Organum or even Aristotle's argument of we learn by doing.

PDSA

Deming, though a fan of Shewart, thought that the checking part over analysis was too much. His view morphed into what is commonly referred to as the PDSA cycle. To begin to understand the PDSA you must understand three core questions:

- What are we trying to accomplish?
- How will we know that a change is an improvement?
- What change can we make that will result in an improvement?

With these questions as a focal point, there is the actual cycle of:

Plan:

- What is the objective?
- What are the predictions about the change?
- Who, what, where, when, of carrying out this cycle?
- Plan for data collection.

Do:

- Carry out the plan.
- Document the problems/unexpected outcomes or consequences/observations.

Study:

- Complete the analysis of the data.
- Compare data to prediction.
- Summarize what was learned.
- Build new knowledge of the observed system.

Act:

- What changes are to be made?
- What will occur in next cycle?
- Head back to plan stage.

On the surface, this appears easy and simple to accomplish, but it is not. There is a great deal of information that must be developed, and people organized to make PDSA cycles create information that is useful and helps the organization build knowledge and improve.

PDSA CYCLE EXAMPLE

The first step is to develop a charter. A Charter is designed to answer the question, "What are we trying to accomplish?" The charter is written and then submitted to stakeholders who are involved in the work or the outcome. These people may also be part of the PDSA team during the cycle phases. An example initial charter is:

Initial Charter

> Reduce the number of coding errors in the electronic health record (EHR) database of the office. Consistent errors should be identified and processes improved to reduce these errors.

This is a broad charter and is just a starting point. As the stakeholders return comments, it will be refined to more detailed information for example:
The system to be improved: The coding of medical information into the EHR.

Setting/Population/Sample: All patients

What is expected to happen: Reduction in coding errors, which should lead to better patient care and fewer medical billing errors.

Time Frame: within next 6 months

Performance Goals: Reduce errors from 10 a week to <5 a week

Guidance: Potential activities are to interview nurses and staff doing the coding.

> Using a case to see how the coding occurs and compare to what should happen.

> Consider second coder during times of high office traffic

> Consider changing end of day process to double check coding

The charter now has more details and ideas of how to start the first PSDA cycle. The stakeholders typically have a great deal of information that can be used to develop the PDSA cycle.

Now, the group can start the DO phase, and implement this first cycle. As they implement the process, they are collecting the data and looking for problems, such as the staff are confused about certain codes—which is data they can use during the analysis phase. Once in the analysis phase, problems that arose and the data gathered can be analyzed to make preliminary conclusions, but more importantly to feed into what to do next. With the data analyzed, the team can Act and make decisions on what changes need to be made and plan for the next stage.

Quantitative Goal

The doctor's office example is based on numeric goals because PDSA is a quantitative system. The original Shewart charts and the derivatives from them are all numeric based. Additionally, numeric goals help the team and organization answer "How will we know that a change is an improvement?" With that, there are a few caveats, because numeric goals can have unintended consequences and simply be abused (Muller, 2019).

For example, Jim once worked in a company that had metal as core input for the product. Each division was told to reduce costs. Purchasing did just that, by buying less expensive metal and were rewarded for their cost reduction. The problem came when the production machines jammed and the product could not be consistently made. This is an issue of understanding the system that you are in, also known as appreciation of a system. This is discussed in more detail later. There are also hundreds of examples of unintended consequences that are just adjustment to the definition of the number being examined. For example, what counts as an application for admissions to a graduate program. If you count everyone who submitted any information, and you accept the same number each year, your admission rate will be much lower than if you only used complete applications. Some of these issues should also be worked out over the PDSA cycle. The numeric goals have to be connected to the method used to reach the goals. One way to achieve that is to ask stakeholders what they think would need to happen to reduce errors to some specified level, or how to increase sales some percentage. Jim was involved in a team to raise graduation rates, and a leader in the higher education field was brought it. The members of the team wanted a 10% increase in a few years, Jim and another member did not think that was realistic. The consultant actually stated it would take 10 to 15 years of sustained work to get the graduation rate that high. Finally, as hard as it is, the current system needs to be removed as an option. Current systems are like black holes sucking everyone back into them and kill creativity and innovation. If change, and large change, is needed, the current system has to be removed as an option.

In small system changes, it is relatively easy to watch numeric changes over time. The most basic is to start with the baseline of the system, such as number of error rates per day. Then implement the new system and track the errors per day. Shewart Charts (**Figure 11.1**) are an important tool for change. In **Figure 11.1**, the first time point can act as a baseline with the time frame on the x-axis and the frequency of errors on the y-axis. More complex changes that are in more complex systems will need to more data collected, the different measures and different data types. In the doctor's office example, there may be data such as billing errors, patient complaints, time lost, and even job satisfaction–yes, if you are not dealing with consequences of errors a great deal the job is typically more satisfying. Yet, keep the number of measurements as small as possible, around 5, because it can become overwhelming and not helpful to reaching the goal.

The Shewart Charts help to develop information related variation discussed earlier. Variation is natural, but understanding natural variation and problematic variation is critical. Without understanding the variation, it is impossible to improve.

There are also three different measurements that should be considered, outcome, process, and balancing. Outcome measures are the ones replated directly to the system that is being studied. These measures should document the evidence that the change has occurred. Process measures provide evidence the activity has occurred, such as a protocol checklist. This is commonly implemented to see if the PDSA cycle occurred as planned. Balancing measures are used to make sure that as one measure improves, other measures do not indicate a reduced or negative performance. From the metal example, the costs were reduced but production suffered greatly.

Appreciate a System

It is imperative that a QI process appreciate the system where it is housed. Systems are interdependent components that work together to reach the goals of the organization (Deming, 1989). The organization has to have an aim to be to be able to function and needs an aim that can be managed. The key part of this management is to understand the cooperative components. If the different components do not cooperate, such as becoming competitive with each other, there will be destructive elements that occur (Deming, 1989). Those destructive elements will decrease the productivity of the organization and reduce the possibility of the QI process working.

A key factor of the system is to make sure that it is a system and not a grouping of independent running components after their own ends. If there is a clear aim, this helps create a system. Short-term thinking is the demon of a working system. Short-term thinking creates a loss of the long-term aim.

Understanding the dynamic aspect of a system is included in understanding it. To help see the dynamic aspects of a system, to the creation of flow charts of materials, people, and processes is necessary. The flow chart can also be used to examine where friction possibilities exist between different components of the system.

Profound Knowledge

The PDSA cycle should lead to development of knowledge, specifically profound knowledge (Deming, 1989), which in turn leads to being able to manage the system and work in a continuous improvement way. Deming (1989) discussed four components related to profound knowledge, 1) Understanding Variation, 2) Appreciation of a System, 3) Theory of Knowledge/Theory of Change, and 4) Psychology. Understanding variation, as discussed earlier, is trying to determine what is natural variation, but this is where some problems can occur. The first is mistaking an outcome as a special cause when in actuality, it is part of the normal variation and the reverse of this. This is why it is critical to understand the variation in the system. Relatedly, if the system is in statistical control, the variation is understood and the future is predictable. For example, retention rates from first year to second year at our institution are 84% to 86% over the past 8 years, which is stable. If it was unstable, trying to manage it and everyone involved without understanding the system would lead to calamity. Reacting to this stable system as an unstable system can lead to short term decisions, which can create chaos and the mismanagement of people and processes.

The system, as stated earlier, must be understood and the traditional management by objective can in fact lead to one division destroying another if they are only focused on their objectives. The system is interdependent. Deming uses an orchestra to highlight the interdependence of a system. The Pittsburgh Symphony Orchestra (PSO) is composed of 101 world class musicians. The PSO is judged not as much by each single musician but by how they work together to create the music. The conductor (aka manager) has to build cooperation among the musicians of this system to produce a high-quality musical experience the audience will enjoy. Thus, an orchestra has a high degree of interdependence.

Those in charge of the QI need a theory of knowledge/change. Certain changes or behaviors should predict specific outcomes. Knowledge is built of theory and the ability to predict. Additionally, you must have data that can be used for the prediction and the inferences made from that experiment or test add to the development of knowledge. We have information, and a massive amount of information at our fingertips all day long. But information is not knowledge. Without knowledge, the information cannot be used in a temporal fashion to predict what will happen. As Deming used to say, the dictionary we use has information, but it will not write this paragraph or critique it.

The fourth component related to profound knowledge, psychology, gets left behind a great deal in QI projects. For us, it binds the other three components of profound knowledge together. People are different and for a QI system to be in place, you have to understand the people involved, how people interact, and how they learn. People are born with the natural inclination to learn. Over time, many "processes" and "rewards" in our systems destroy that inherent inclination. Deming was quite clear in his writing concerning destructive forces (Deming, 1989). He stated that we begin life born with a natural desire to learn, self-esteem, curiosity, intrinsic motivation, and a joy in learning. If you have watched a baby see something happen and try and replicate it while giggling, you have witnessed what Deming meant. Soon, though you see reward systems being put in place that decrease all of these natural inclinations. At an early age, there are gold starts, and sometimes forced distribution of grades (aka grading on a curve). Then come state mandated tests. Next are the competitions where children begin to be judged, grouped, separated, and put into slots. As you get older and in the work force there is "merit" pay based on a tyranny of metrics (Muller, 2019), and numerical goals without methods in place to get there. And Deming argued this leads to sub-optimal performance for every person, group, and division. Additionally, he argued that this leads to fear, humiliation, and self-defensiveness. Most importantly, it crushes the joy of learning and innovation and leads to doing things for extrinsic motivators. Deming argued it was imperative to understand the people performing the work, to spend time with them and understand their intrinsic and extrinsic motivations along with understanding what each employee was looking for, such as recognition for work, or extra time to work on a project, or flexible working hours, or even time for personal development such as a university course.

For profound knowledge to be developed in a continuous QI system, all four of these areas must be tended to by those in charge. Thus, for an organization to get the most out of their PDSA cycle, not only must the PDSA cycle be focused on, these components must also part of it.

Original N-P

What is interesting about Shewart Charts and Deming's PDSA is the fact the Null Hypothesis Statistical Testing from Neyman-Pearson (1933) is essentially these two ideas. The Neyman-Pearson model was a long-run idea. The Neyman–Pearson approach, with alpha, beta, power, Type 1 and Type II errors is designed to work efficiently (Neyman & Pearson, 1933) in the context of long-run repeated testing (exact replication). Just like control charts are about long run repeated testing. This is not overly shocking given they were all working in the same time frame and were probably reading each other's papers or listening to talks by each other. Essentially, Neyman and Pearson developed *a reasoning-free inductive behavioral rule* (Szucs & Ioannidis, 2017) which was simply a choice between two actions: accepting or rejecting H0. This is regardless of the researcher's actual belief about whether H0 and H1 are true or not (Neyman & Pearson, 1933).

AREAS OF CONCERN, SYMPTOMS, PROBLEMS

Problems are not problems at the beginning of a QI project. They are **areas of concern** that come from our engagement within the system we work. We call them problems, but at the start of systematic and intentional inquiry (Moss, 1998; Schreiber et al., 2007), these are just areas of concern. The concern comes from something that appears incorrect, is incorrect, is taking too much time and so on. That appearance is a clue or symptom related to something else (Cunningham et al., 2005; Schreiber, 2021). This is an **abductive reasoning** process (Cunningham et al., 2005; Schreiber, 2021; Schreiber & Ferrara, 2016) where the person or team is trying to identify the actual problem based on the clues and symptoms. They are developing a scenario which should lead to a theory. This theory is a formalization of what the problem potentially is. From this, a theory of change can be developed. This abductive process is the core of clinical reasoning, (Schreiber et al., 2020). The healthcare worker reasons through clues and symptoms to develop a scenario, theory about what the problem is, that is what is occurring. The nursing clinical reasoning model (NCRM), for example, has five major areas (Muntean et al., 2015): Recognize cues, generate hypotheses, judge hypotheses, take action, and evaluate outcomes (**Figure 11.2**).

As argued by Muntean et al., nurses must recognize cues, pieces of information or signs, within the clinical problem space (Reed, 1972) to get to the next stage of hypothesis generation, this is the abductive process. Additionally, this

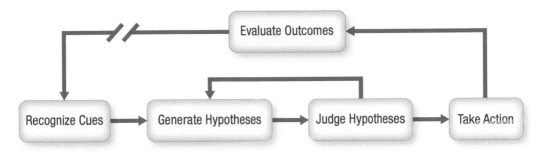

Figure 11.2. Nursing Clinical Reasoning Model.

is analogous to the PDSA planning stage, and the model overall is analogous to the PDSA cycle.

During this abductive process, the healthcare worker or PDSA Team are weighing evidence, building scenarios to potentially act on, and prioritizing those actions. At the point of hypothesis or hypotheses generation in the NCRM, nurses have to rank these developed scenarios with the criteria according to how well they explain the cues, or the probability, that is, likelihood that the diagnosis explains the cues (Tversky & Kohler, 1994). This is a focus on probabilistic thinking and not deterministic thinking (Cahan et al., 2003; Licata, 2007). The team has moved from area of concern to problem identification. From this point, a theory of change can be developed. The behaviors related to the theory of change can then be implemented (take action in the NCRM, DO in the PDSA cycle). The actions may be simple or more complex depending on the situation. Once actions are taken, the theory of change is being tested, the data are being gathered and eventually analyzed (Evaluate Outcomes in NCRM and Study in PDSA). The results obtained from testing let the team or healthcare worker make a conclusion, or reengage in the abductive process because the expected results were not obtained, and more knowledge is built. The team might enter a state of doubt. When that doubt occurs, a re-engagement with the cues and the new knowledge, and abductive reasoning will occur. The system for both then moves to the next cycle. The healthcare worker is making decisions on what to do next and so is the PDSA team in the Act phase.

LEAN

Lean is the by-product of the **Toyota Production System** (TPS) and is very popular across multiple industries. Lean was originally developed within the Japanese car industry. The system can be traced to Sakichi Toyada's 1924 loom system and an automatic stopping device to halt the creation of a defective product. The basis of Lean is the just-in-time manufacturing system that focused on creating a continuous flow so that the completion of the process before produces what is needed for the next process. Combining Just in Time with jidoka, the concept of automation with human touch, which allows for the stopping of production when a problem occurs, thus preventing defective products being produced, creates the TPS, preventing defective products from being produced. The basic process of jikoda is

1. A machine detects a problem and communicates it,
2. A situation occurs the deviates from the normal workflow,
3. The line is halted,
4. Manager or Supervisor removes cause of problem, and
5. Improvements are incorporated into the standard workflow.

As the continuous improvement process moves forward, the flow perfected, the system reaches a point where any human operator can use the line to get the exact same result.

Respect for the Customer

In healthcare, the Lean system is focused on the patient, thus the patient is central to all activities, aims, goals, and objectives (Shortell et al., 2018; Smith et al., 2020). With the patient in the center of the goals, the aims then become focused on eliminating or reducing activities that do not "add value" to the patient. This improvement is achieved by applying Lean's operational principles, which involve five steps for continuous improvement (Jones et al., 2021), but this does not work for everyone (Kaplan et al., 2014).

1. Defining what is value-adding to patient care and recovery.
2. Mapping value streams (pathways that deliver care).
3. Making value streams efficient by removing waste, delay, and duplication from them.
4. Allowing patients to essentially direct resources and staff toward them so care meets each patient needs.
5. Pursuing perfection as an ongoing goal.

Therefore, Lean is about creating needed value with fewer resources and less waste. To do this, continuous experimentation and improvement must occur. Thus, it is a practice and a thought pattern happening simultaneously. The starting point of Lean is always with the customer or patient.

OTHER QI MODELS

There are several other QI techniques in addition to PDSA and Lean and some that are specific to healthcare. The first is **Clinical Micro Systems** are small groups of individuals in an organization who provide care to a specific group of patients (Godfrey et al., 2010; Mohr & Batalden, 2002; Nelson et al., 2002). The philosophy of this method is that the quality, safety, and centering the patient are determined mainly by what happens in the micro-system around the patient. Clinical microsystems use a 5-p model: patients, people, patterns, processes, and purpose. Evaluating each of the five leads to opportunities for improvement.

Experience based co-design is a United Kingdom based system within the National Healthcare System (NHS) (Bate & Robert, 2006, 2007). In this method, patients and staff create working groups to design systems that improve patient experience. The focus is to determine touch points in the system that are emotionally significant. This is a person intensive system to determine the touch points and develop improvements.

Model for improvement is used to decide upon, test, and refine QIs and works the best when 1) a procedure or process or systems needs changing, 2) one system tested is against other versions, and 3) there is an outcome that can be measured. Performance benchmarking focuses on the utilization of national, or international benchmarks to compare to the current process or product (and outcomes) in an organization. This works best when there are clear established performance targets which have clear meaningful measurable data that can be collected. For this to work effectively, accessible key performance indicators that allow for monitoring and benchmarking must be available and used. This may mean creating these indicators as options in the database or adjusting current data options. Any action plans that are created related to performance need to have clear targets and time frames related to the action.

Process mapping is the following of patient trajectories through the healthcare system to determine where there are improvement opportunities. Process mapping is successful when implemented for patient trajectories that are complicated and there are many inefficiencies. The mapping process should illuminate any unnecessary steps, duplication or people or processes, gaps, and variation that should not be occurring. Done well, the process will provide opportunities to generate ideas to improve the system.

Root cause analysis is traditionally implemented after an adverse event to identify the causes of the event. Root cause analysis can also be used to examine potential problems that might occur in a system as the process is examined, thus a risk assessment. "Fishbone" diagrams are commonly used to map out the factors that led to the adverse events, such as patients, staff, task, equipment, and training factors that could have contributed to event. The diagram looks like a fish with the tail as the start point, each bone a different factor, and the head is the adverse event.

SAMPLING

How much is enough? That is the question we commonly get asked. In reality, most people who ask this question, are really asking, "What is the minimal sample size needed that will cost the least and still provide the answers needed?" And like good methodologists and statisticians, we also say it depends. But it depends based on very specific factors.

Power Versus Accuracy Versus Time

In traditional research this discussion has focused around power—as previously discussed the desired to have a large enough sample that the association or difference can be detected at $p < 0.05$. This is very different than focusing on accuracy and being very confident in the results (Trafimow & McDonald, 2017).

If the team or person wants to be very confident, more data are required. If there is a time element, such as improvement over time, then the sample size needed becomes the length of time needed to show a stabilized change. Depending on the topic being examined, that will vary greatly.

Unit of Analysis

Unit of analysis is the level of the data and sometimes the nested nature of the data, such as patients nested within floors, department, or a hospital. The unit of analysis be seconds, hours, days, weeks, and so on. In a year where data are collected daily, there are 365 data points. But, if the data are only collected quarterly, then there are four. Thus, the unit of analysis can affect how long to collect data and how much data.

Risk

The level of risk affects both the amount of data and the time needed to collect data. The higher the risk if the change is made, more time and data may be required to make sure the change is a stable improvement. Lower risk changes may require less time and data to make a decision about the expected level of improvement.

Pecuniary Value/Cost

The value gained/cost of a change has to also be considered. Changes that make a small improvement but are significantly more costly are not, on balance, helpful to the organization. That is, costly changes affect the whole system. Gosset spent a great deal of time in the early 1900s at Guinness working to improve production process, and the final product and had a deep focus on the pecuniary value and cost of changes (Schreiber, 2021). This also drove a great deal of creativity (e.g., inventing the t-test) to try and deal with all of the issues in the most efficient way possible. The enterprise had this focus, which is why the company also gave sabbaticals to employees to go develop new skills.

PICO(T)

PICO(T) stands for patient/problem, intervention, comparison, outcome, and (sometimes) time. The PICO(T) process begins with a case scenario, and the question is phrased to elicit an answer. PICO(T) are commonly patient-based and very parameterized, which means they do not generalize very far. A first step is developing the PICO(T) (Table 11.1).

Once the core PICO(T) is set up, then a detailed protocol will need to be created for examining the literature base, creating the sampling process of people or processes, the data collection instrument, the data collection process, and analyses will need to be completed. A key factor, as discussed in Chapter 2, is the quality of the measurement. Without a high-quality data collection instrument, the results will be suspect, and to repeat, a fancy or not so fancy statistical technique will not save bad data.

Table 11.1 PICO(T) Example.

Patient/Problem	What group/person/problem are we interested in studying?	Patients with a BMI > 35 kg/m² experience higher rates of post-knee replacement infections than patients with a BMI <35.
Intervention	What is the action we are taking or going to take	Administer 2 gm of antibiotic pre-operatively to patients with a BMI >35.
Comparison	What other action or intervention are we comparing it to?	Standard of care of administering 1 gm of antibiotic to everyone.
Outcome	What do we expect to see occur?	Reduced infections among the patients receiving 2 gm of antibiotic.
Time	How long will this take?	After 6 months of the intervention being in place

Data Collection

Collecting the data, and the difficulty collecting the data, all depends on that is systems in place. Electronic health record records (EHR) store the data the is collected on patients as they enter and exit the healthcare system. That data can be extracted from the data base and used relatively easily. The data must be examined and checked for correct coding. Data that are not within a system such as an EHR, can be collected digitally, such as an online system or it can be collected by "hand," which is more time- and resource-intensive.

Analyses

Depending on the project, there are a variety of analyses that may occur. The most common are visual representations of the data over time. Shewart Charts, discussed previously (Figure 11.1), are always popular because changes over time can be examined. There are also projects that only focus on a baseline, an intervention or change, and a post examination of the results. This is the pre-posttest design that would use a dependent t-test in the analysis phase. There can also be extensions where more post timepoints are collected to see if the observed change is maintained. The analysis would then change to a repeated measures design, for example. If there are multiple changes or interventions that need to be compared, a repeated measures ANOVA will allow for the analysis of multiple groups (i.e., different interventions), and examine the differences in changes over time across and within each group.

HEALTHCARE QI DIMENSIONS

The key with healthcare QI is defining what is meant by quality. One way to operationally define healthcare quality is using three dimensions: 1) clinical effectiveness, 2) patient safety, and 3) patient experience (Department of Health,

2008). Clinical effectiveness is the utilization of the current evidence that has been observed to improve health outcomes. Patient safety is the care delivered so that harm and risk are avoided for each patient. Patient experience is giving the patient a positive experience related to care and recovery. This also included being treated with compassion, dignity, and respect. Within these, three more operational definitions are needed. For example, patient safety can be anything from walking in the hospital, to incorrect drug or dosage administration, to surgical errors. Once the definitions are stable, it becomes easier to design what data are to be collected and which QI Method to use.

SUMMARY

QI is the norm in organizations worldwide. The QI field has a long history, and multiple methods of QI exist. PDSA cycles and Lean are two common approaches for QI. Both PDSA and Lean are not only methods, but ways of thinking, and there is an implicit expectation that they are embedded in the culture of the organization. PDSA focuses on developing profound knowledge. Lean focuses on perfecting the flow of the system. In addition to the focal points of different models, during the design phase of a QI process, there are key issues to be covered which include sampling, unit of analysis, and the analytic approach, along with cost and risk. Finally, QI in healthcare has three focal areas: 1) clinical effectiveness, 2) patient safety, and 3) patient experience.

END-OF-CHAPTER RESOURCES

REVIEW QUESTIONS

Answers and rationales for the review questions are located in the Appendix at the end of the book.

1. TRUE or FALSE?

   Chance causes of variation within a production improvement model represent normal variation and can be pin-pointed and stopped.

2. TRUE or FALSE?

   The Plan, Do, Check, Act cycle is often limited to one iteration.

3. TRUE or FALSE?

   When using a Theory of Change, a common approach is to work backward by first identifying the long-term objective and then backward mapping the process to achieve that goal.

4. A nurse practitioner working in a federally qualified health center wants to improve the clinic's referral of patients to mental health services. Recognizing the importance of engaging all the stakeholders in the process, she knows she must first develop a:

   a. Plan

   b. Charter

   c. Goal

   d. Theory of Change

5. Appreciation of the system in which the QI project will occur is essential, and a tool for identifying potential points of obstruction to the project is a:

   a. Process map

   b. Prediction model

   c. Protocol checklist

   d. Organizational flow chart

6. Which of the following is the reason to include balancing measures in a QI project?

   a. so the work of a project is equal among team members

   b. so the costs of the improvement are equal to the savings

   c. so the unplanned consequences are identified and eliminated to the extent possible

   d. so there is a balance in the amount of time required for each stage of the project

7. A nurse manager notices that the number of patient falls occurring on night shift has increased in the last few weeks. Describe how the manager would use the Nursing Clinical Reasoning Model (NCRM) to address this concern.

8. The nurse manager wishes to use the PDSA cycle with the goal of building profound knowledge about how to decrease the number of patient falls on night shift. Discuss the four components of profound knowledge as applied here.

9. The director of the cardiac cath lab observes that patient discharges have been delayed post-procedure, and patient satisfaction is dropping. Describe how the director could implement the Lean system to improve patient satisfaction.

A robust set of instructor resources designed to supplement this text is located at http://connect.springerpub.com/content/book/978-0-8261-6582-4. Qualifying instructors may request access by emailing textbook@springerpub.com.

REFERENCES

Anderson, A. A. (2006). *The community builder's approach to theory of change. A practical guide to theory development*. The Aspen Institute Roundtable on Community Change.

Bate, P., & Robert, G. (2006). Experience based design: From designing services around patients to co-designing services with patients. *Quality and Safety in Health Care 15*(5), 307–310. https://doi.org/10.1136/qshc.2005.016527

Bate, P., & Robert, G. (2007). *Bringing user experience to healthcare improvement: the concepts, methods and practices of experience-based design*. Radcliffe Publishing.

Cahan, A., Gilon, D., Manor, O., & Paltiel, O. (2003). Probabilistic reasoning and clinical decision-making: Do doctors overestimate diagnostic probabilities? *QJM: An International Journal of Medicine, 96*(10), 763–769. https://doi.org/10.1093/qjmed/hcg122

Cunningham, D. J., Schreiber, J. B., & Moss, C. M. (2005). Belief, doubt and reason: CS Peirce on education. *Educational Philosophy and Theory, 37*(2), 177–189.

Deming, W. E. (1989). *The new economics for industry, government, and education* (2nd ed.). MIT Press.

Department of Health. (2008). *High quality care for all: NHS next stage review final report*. Health and Social Care Act 2012.

Godfrey, M., Nelson, D., & Batalden, P. (2010). *Supporting microsystems. Assessing, diagnosing and treating your microsystem*. http://clinicalmicrosystem.org/knowledge-center/ workbooks

Jones, B., Kwong, E., & Warburton, W. (2021). *Quality improvement made simple*. The Health Foundation.

Kaplan, G., Patterson, S., Ching, J., & Blackmore, C. C. (2014). Why Lean doesn't work for everyone. *BMJ Quality and Safety, 23*, 970–973. https://doi.org/10.1136/bmjqs-2014-003248

Kilian, C. S. (1992). *The world of W. Edwards deming* (2nd ed.). SPC Press, Inc.

Licata, G. (2007). Probabilistic and fuzzy logic in clinical diagnosis. *Internal and Emergency Medicine, 2*(2), 100–106. https://doi.org/10.1007/s11739-007-0051-9

Mohr, J., & Batalden, P. (2002). Improving safety on the front lines: The role of clinical microsystems. *BMJ Quality and Safety, 11*, 45–50.

Moss, C. M. (1998). *Teaching as intentional learning: In service of the scholarship of practice*. CASTL, Duquesne University.

Muller, J. Z. (2019). *The tyranny of metrics*. Princeton University Press.

Muntean, W. J., Lindsey, M., Betts, J., Woo, A., Kim, D., & Dickison, P. (2015). *Evaluating clinical judgment in licensure tests: Applications of decision theory*. The annual meeting of the American Educational Research Association, Chicago, IL.

Nelson, E. C., Batalden, P. B., Huber, T. P., Mohr, J. J., Godfrey, M. M., Headrick, L. A., & Wasson, J. H. (2002). Microsystems in health care: Part 1. Learning from high-performing front-line clinical units. *The Joint Commission Journal on Quality Improvement, 28*(9), 472–493. https://doi.org/10.1016/s1070-3241(02)28051-7

Neyman, J., & Pearson, E. S. (1933). On the problem of the most efficient tests of statistical hypotheses. *Philosophical Transactions of the Royal Society of London. Series A, Containing Papers of a Mathematical or Physical Character, 231*(694–706), 289–337. https://doi.org/10.1098/rsta.1933.0009

Reed, S. K. (1972). Pattern recognition and categorization. *Cognitive Psychology, 3*, 382–407. https://doi.org/10.1016/0010-0285(72)90014-X

Schreiber, J., & Asner-Self, K. (2011). *Educational research: The interrelationship of questions, sampling, design, and analysis*. John Wiley & Sons.

Schreiber, J. B., & Ferrara, L. N. (2016, April). *Six modes of peircean reasoning and crime scene investigation education* [Paper presentation]. The American Educational Research Association, Washington, DC.

Schreiber, J. B., Glasgow, M. E., & Dreher, M. (2020). Changing the NCLEX-RN to the clinical judgement measurement model: Educational, legal, and ethical implications. In M. E. Smith Glasgow,

H. M. Dreher, M. Dahnke, & J. Gyllenhammer (Eds.), *Legal and ethical issues in nursing education: An essential guide.* Springer

Schreiber, J. B., Moss, C. M., & Staab, J. M. (2007). A preliminary examination of a theoretical model for researching educator beliefs. *Semiotica, 164*(1/4), 153–172.

Shewart, W. A. (1931). *Economic control of quality of manufactured product.* D. Van Nostrand Company, Inc.

Shortell, S. M., Blodgett, J. C., Rundall, T. G., & Kralovec, P. (2018). Use of lean and related transformational performance improvement systems in hospitals in the United States: Results from a national survey. *The Joint Commission Journal on Quality and Patient Safety, 44*(10), 574–582. https://doi.org/10.1016/j.jcjq.2018.03.002

Smith, I., Hicks, C., & McGovern, T. (2020). Adapting lean methods to facilitate stakeholder engagement and co-design in healthcare. *BMJ, 368*, m35. https://doi.org/10.1136/bmj.m35.

Sullivan, H., & Stewart, M. (2006). Who owns the theory of change? *Evaluation, 12*(2), 179–199. https://doi.org/10.1177/1356389006066971

Szucs, D., & Ioannidis, J. (2017). When null hypothesis significance testing is unsuitable for research: A reassessment. *Frontiers in Human Neuroscience, 11*, 390. https://doi.org/10.3389/fnhum.2017.00390

Trafimow, D., & MacDonald, J. A. (2017). Performing inferential statistics prior to data collection. *Educational and Psychological Measurement, 77*(2), 204–219. https://doi.org/10.1177/0013164416659745

Tversky, A., & Koehler, D. J. (1994). Support theory: A nonextensional representation of subjective probability. *Psychological Review, 101*, 547–567. https://doi.org/10.1037/0033-295X.101.4.547

Vogel, I. (2012). *Review of the use of 'Theory of Change' in international development.* UK: Department for International Development (DFID), 10. https://www.theoryofchange.org/pdf/DFID_ToC_Review_VogelV7.pdf

Weiss, C. H. (1995). Nothing as practical as good theory: Exploring theory-based evaluation for comprehensive community initiatives for children and families. In J. P. Connell, A. C. Kubisch, L. B. Schorr, & C. H. Weiss (Eds.), *New approaches to evaluating community initiatives: Concepts, methods, and contexts* (1, pp. 65–92). Aspen Institute.

FURTHER READING

Schreiber, J. B. (April, 2021). *William S. Gosset's Abductive reasoning to increase beer life at Guinness in the early 1900s.* To be presented at American Educational Research Association Virtual Meeting.

CHAPTER 12

Humility

CORE OBJECTIVE

■ Understand and explain the limitations of research

INTRODUCTION: REFOCUSING YOUR THOUGHTS

To our knowledge, a humility chapter has never been part of a statistical analysis book. Yet, it is an important topic for the data and analyses that are typically presented or published in quantitative research. The reason we have added this chapter is to remind researchers that the data they have used to make the claims they are making are not as strong as they are stating, especially in the discussion section. Therefore, a refocusing on the thoughts about the design, data, analysis, and results is important.

Why Your Results Are Probably Wrong

The results from the study being read or written up are probably wrong (Ioannidis, 2005) for a host of reasons. Now, we will add the caveat that wrong is actually a continuum in the way we are discussing being wrong. The two main reasons for the results being wrong are severe assumption violations and the nonrepresentativeness of the sample–not traditional power, which is what most researchers first think. Of these two, the sampling process used and the final implemented sample lead to incorrect parameter estimates (e.g., mean, standard deviation, beta coefficients) because the sample is not fully representative of the population and a different sample would lead to different or very different results and conclusions.

In **Figure 12.1**, the large (purple) distribution is the population, and the mean and standard deviation are 10 and 5, respectively. The distribution to the left (green) is a sample from the population and has a mean of 2 and standard deviation of 2. The distribution on the right (orange) has a mean of 15 and standard deviation of 2.5. Neither the left nor right distribution is fully representative of the population distribution. The inferences then made from either of these distributions are incorrect. This is related to the argument of Trafimow and MacDonald (2017) that the way to think about the sample size is to think

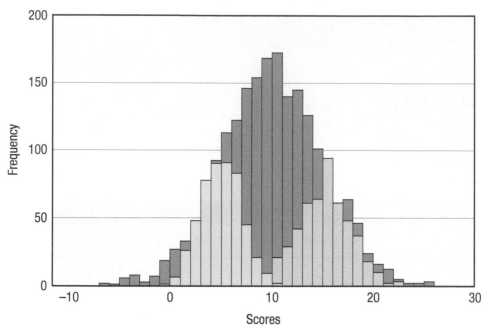

Figure 12.1. Population Example With Two Samples.

about how accurate the researchers want the estimates to be, which generally means you need a much larger sample size.

There are other issues that arise such as, poor measurement, levels of the manipulated variables in experiments (e.g., radically different drug dosages), and misspecified models. Measurement is always a concern because the data from survey instruments are not perfectly reliable, and that real error is propagated through the analysis and is generally not a part of the discussion at the end of the article. Studies can also lead to incorrect conclusions when one variable is manipulated, but the manipulations are very different. This is common across domains when the dosages that participants receive are different. For example, in health sciences, one group is a control, another group has a small dosage, and one group has a very large dosage. The large dose group typically performs best, or gets better faster, or learns more. That is not a very informative study and is probably wrong. If everyone was given a different dosage, and those dosages were closer together, the size of the dosage needed may not be the large dose. Finally, mis-specified models occur when key variables are not included in the analyses. This is most common with linear and logistic regression with variables that needed to be included but are not. There are other issues, such as the model needed an interaction included because previous research had shown the need for the interaction, or there is a curvilinear effect occurring and a squared variable is needed. Thus, it is wise to be humble and discuss all the ways your parameter estimates could be wrong.

Stats and the Assumption on Randomness

The designs and analyses discussed in this book within the Fisher/Frequentist framework assume the data were collected randomly, or random selection. This rarely occurs and possibly the most common sample is the convenience sample. Random selection is difficult and expensive, no doubt, and stratified samples have the same problems, cost and difficulty. Therefore, being a bit humbler in our results because of the sample researchers actually had along with the conclusions is warranted.

The assumption in a null hypothesis statistical test, is that the null hypothesis is true *and* an added assumption is the study is repeated an infinite number of times. And yes, science is supposed to work this way, repeating experiments to make sure you get the same result over and over and over, not the 1 in 20 chance Fisher talked about. Gosset wrote to Egon Pearson, "We have significant evidence that if farmers in general do this they will make money by it," but also "we have found it so in nineteen cases out of twenty and we are finding out why it doesn't work in the twentieth." To do that, you have to be as sure as possible which is the 20th—your real error must be small (Gosset to E. S. Pearson, 1937, in E. Pearson 1939, 244).

But this does not happen. Too many studies are one-offs that don't replicate and actually shouldn't under the frequentist framework. There is not a crises of replicability as many have said, the system is set up not to focus or reward replicability. The system gives you what it is designed to give you.

Finally, the (still) obsession with getting a *p*-value less than 0.05 has probably hurt science more than it has helped over the years. The focus should really be on the accuracy of the results through sampling processes and measurement and then analysis. Gosset termed this the low "real" error (Pearson, 1939). The system has rewarded *p*-values to the detriment of very exact and repeated measurements of a phenomenon. As Wasserstein et al. (2019) wrote, Don't believe you have something if the *p*-value is less than 0.05 and don't believe you have nothing if the *p*-value is more than 0.05.

ATOM MODEL OF ANALYSIS FROM THE AMERICAN STATISTICAL ASSOCIATION

One way to refocus the discussion of the data and results is to use the ATOM model from Wasserstein et al. (2019). ATOM stands for Accept uncertainty, be Thoughtful, be Open, be Modest. Each of these, along with their integration we believe will help improve the design, measurement, analysis, results, and the discussion of the results.

Accept Uncertainty

All research studies have varying levels of uncertainty, and researchers should embrace that uncertainty. This uncertainty is part of the error that is throughout a study. Gelman (2016) wrote about statistics that it is "often sold as a sort of alchemy that transmutes randomness into certainty, an 'uncertainty' laundering that begins with the data and concludes with success as measured by statistical significance." We clearly need to treat statistical results more incompletely than we do currently (Amrhein et al., 2019). And the uncertainty actually builds during the whole research process as subjective decisions are made from sampling processes, to slight design changes, to the data obtained from instruments used, changes in analyses and so on. Thus, we need to be cognizant of all the uncertainty that builds as a study unfolds.

Researchers also need to embrace uncertainty as part of the natural variation in the studies we run. As Wasserstein et al. noted, exact replication is exceedingly hard to accomplish. Researchers are generally doing SLI, "something like it," during a replication, and we should not be surprised in slightly or even very different results (natural variation). Balancing everything on being less than 0.05 creates more problems than it solves. The comparisons of studies in a replication should not be based on 0.05, but on the direction of association, effect sizes, sums of squares, and other pieces of evidence that can highlight similarities and differences across studies. And, as a byproduct, researchers can then focus on error (design, standard, measurement, sampling, etc.). This leads to researchers being forced to seek better tools to gather data, better designs, and more likely larger sample sizes as they move from "getting to 0.05" and focus on accuracy (Trafimow & MacDonald, 2017). This leads to the second point from Wasserstein et al., having to be more thoughtful.

Be Thoughtful

In the big picture, focus on producing "solid data" with a consideration of multitude of data analysis techniques. Locascio (2019) wrote that researchers should be ready to work in a new publishing world where the research is evaluated on the importance of the questions asked and the methods used to answer them and not on the results obtained. For many of us, in mid- to late-career, this is a welcomed statement. This change, though slow it may be, will cause researchers to be much more thoughtful about what they are doing. This is not to take away from exploratory research when you are trying to understand a phenomenon or testing something that leads to interesting discoveries. One never quite knows where a study will lead in the future. For example, during the testing of an electron microscope, Bangham and Horne added a negative stain to dry phospholipids and observed that the cell membrane was a bilary lipid structure (Bangham & Horne, 1964). This knowledge was then developed, and over time liposomes have become drug delivery devices for the mRNA vaccines, such as the ones for Sars-COV-2.

When we are being thoughtful, researchers are including their actual context and prior evidence related to the study. Statistical significance is the antithesis of this (Wasserstein et al.). Additionally, it completely ignores clinically meaningful results that can improve the lives of people. Specifically, researchers need to more fully acknowledge what we know and the level of uncertainty that we truly have. Too many studies are published with trivial effect sizes, for example, small R-squared values that are over interpreted when almost all of the variance is unexplained, that is, error. Researchers need to deeply include related prior evidence, the plausibility of the how it works, the exactness of the design, the real quality of the data, along with aspects that are specific to each domain, and not a singular focus or priority on p-values (McShane et al., 2019).

Ziliak's Guinnessonometrics

Stephen Ziliak has spent considerable amounts of time in the Guinness Archives in Dublin Ireland. Ziliak (2019) emerged with ten "*d*-values," which focused on trying to maximize the research and remove using *p*-values (Ziliak, 2019; Ziliak & MCloskey, 2008). Ziliak (2019) has a list of 10 *G*-values based on William S. Gosset's work at the brewery from 1899 to 1936 that increase the value of the study. Overall, Gosset focused on an economic approach to understanding uncertainty using balanced experimental designs in comparison to random designs. Ziliak is an economist and historian, and his 10 *G*-values have that flavor, but as a whole they are useful to help you think differently. We highlight a few of them here. The first is "Consider the purpose of the inquiry, and compare with best practice." Best practice is not looking for or designing for a specific *p*-value. The purpose should be to improve something or understand something. Relatedly, the purpose is not to reject a null, but to improve patient safety, for example. Thus, the researcher should focus on the purpose of the inquiry and design from there. Next, and a step past the first one is, "Estimate the Stakes." What is at stake with this hypothesis? What is the magnitude of the effect the researcher is expecting to see? Then, "Minimize the real error." By this Ziliak means, and we agree, Represent, Replicate, Reproduce. One and done studies, or failure to plan to replicate is not science. If you cannot replicate it, it is not science. Additionally, random error from sampling is not real error from measurement, design, and analysis. Repeating trials and controlling as much as possible leads to minimizing error. Then, "Visualize the data." Look at the effects across the distribution of the outcome data. Is the magnitude the same across the groups or does it vary by group or experimental groups? Researchers should be more heavily considering Priors and Posteriors because researchers do not enter a study with no knowledge or hypotheses—even those trying to do a complete Grounded Theory study. Researchers should consider moving to Bayes analyses, but even if that is not implemented, the researcher should discuss that prior knowledge in the context of the new knowledge to weigh it appropriately. Finally, "Cooperate up, down, and across networks." Guinness needed the cooperation of farmers; thus, it pays to cooperate. In return, Guinness funded a great deal of statistical theory development because he paid for employees to be on sabbatical (Ziliak & McCloskey, 2008). Cooperation will improve research because the conversations that occur during cooperation help improve the design and will keep the researcher from making expensive mistakes.

Openness

By openness, we are not talking about the larger transparency movement that is part of the replication problems. And in actuality, the way the system has evolved since the early 1930s, we are not surprised at the lack of replication because the system was not designed to value it. Openness is a full acceptance and declaration that researchers have made multiple subjective decisions during the design, implementation, and analysis phases. This includes all data analyses; even the artificial intelligence, machine learning, and predictive algorithms have subjective decisions events (O'Neill, 2016; Schreiber & London, 2019). For new researchers, this can be confusing because most statistical analyses are presented as perfectly objective, bordering on "truth," but that is simply not the case. Now, research is built on expert judgement and that is inherently subjective, but researchers are striving for objectivity (O'Hagan, 2019). Wasserstein and colleagues (2019) argue that being modest and being open will cause us to be more careful in our design phase and seek better data collection instruments.

If we are open to the fact we have made subjective decisions, there must also be an acknowledgement that the statistical models used *do not* remove the inherent ambiguity in the decisions and processes we have implemented and observed (Gelman, 2016; Wassersetein et al., 2019). We should focus on the fact the models illuminate the uncertainty and variability in the research observations. It is imperative that we learn to enjoy and work with that uncertainty and focus on reducing it.

The article by Wasserstein et al., is the first in a special issue in the American Statistician journal (e.g., Calin-Jageman & Cumming, 2019; Greenland, 2019; Kennedy-Shaffer, 2019). One article, in this openness idea, discusses the implementation of multiple statistical models focusing on trying to examine points of agreements and disagreement, which allow you to vary your confidence (Lavine, 2019). Jim and some colleagues recently implemented this in a response article (Yi et al., 2021). When a researcher tests multiple models, then the judgement and evaluations begin to focus on how well each model describes the data, not just trying to get to a p-value, and it causes the researcher to focus on the best argument and away from thinking trust has been observed. Other alternatives include an s-value based on Claude Shannon's information transformation of $s = -\log_2(p\text{-value})$ (Greenland, 2019; Shannon, 1948). Once the number, s, is calculated, it should be rounded. That value, now an integer, is the number of bits of information against the null. For example, if $p = 0.03$, from a study, the researcher would obtain a rounded s-value of 5, which would indicate 5 bits of information against the null. This can be thought of as tossing a fair coin and getting 5 heads in a row (Greenland, 2019). Benjamin and Berger (2019) created an upper-bounds data-based odds with $1 / (-e^p \ln p)$. Colquhoun (2019) argued that a calculation of the false positive risk needs to be completed and provides links to an online calculator. Johnson (2019) states that there should be a demand for basic transparency in the number of outcome variables that *were actually* analyzed and the number and values of all test statistics. There are many studies in our own research that should be reexamined and rethought based on the articles in this special issue.

Modesty

To us, being more modest about our results might be the most important of the four. Most of the quantitative studies we review are small, nonrepresentative convenience samples with measures that have accuracy problems. Additionally, the studies are not replicated, which increases the need to be modest about the results.

WHAT YOU CAN DO

There are many behaviors that researchers can begin to implement to improve the process. Following the ATOM model is one way to start. Even using Ableson's MAGIC model (Chapter 1) is a good place to begin. We provide some other starting points, next.

Importance of Theory Regardless of Sample Size

A strong theoretical model with a rich analysis of previous work provides a strong foundation and support for the current study and analysis regardless of sample size. For both of us, recently, theoretically developed models have been woefully inadequate in manuscripts we read. A main problem has been lack of discussion of the specific variables or analyses used later. For example, a theoretical model that argues for a mediated model where the main relationship changes with the addition of another, or more variables, must actually test that in the analysis. Not testing it creates a discontinuity between what is occurring theoretically and analytically. This is just one example of the problems we have seen in the theoretical model portion of manuscripts. Another common problem is retrofitting the theoretical framework to the project and not actually using it to guide the study. The theoretical concepts and assumptions should be clearly described, and the discussion of the methods should link back to the theoretical model, so the reader can easily see how it was used as a foundation for the project.

Probabilistic Causality

Probabilistic Causality, for our purposes here, is the move away from arguing exact causal arguments, for example, A causes B every single time, to A increases the probability of B (Eels, 2009; Hitchcock, 2021; Reichenbach, 1925/1978; Salmon, 2003; Spirtes et al., 2000; Suppes, 1970) This thinking is more in-line with most of the statistical analyses that are done and most of the theoretical frameworks used to justify the research being conducted.

A very common example of this is concerning dietary habits and health. The argument goes that a poor diet does not cause death, but a heart attack does. Therefore, it is helpful to discuss this in a probability way, that a poor diet increases the likelihood of having a fatal heart attack. Thus, we move from A causes B to A will probably lead to B.

Avoid Confirmation Bias

We like the idea of trying to break the research argument. We think it is important to not get swept up into confirmation bias trajectory. As Ioannidis (2019) points out there is a massive bias to only report what was "statistically significant" and publish that when other researchers actually need to see all of the analyses completed. Ioannidis (2019) also noted that even the information in the abstract is more positive than the full results section. Thus, research confirmation bias is even seen throughout a manuscript. This is also related to planning to replicate the work because one study is rarely enough (Wasserstein et al., 2019).

Replicate the Work

Ask or plan to have a colleague replicate your work and cooperate and help replicate their work. I know this reads as counterintuitive because so much of the value system is placed on winning the battle of ideas with your single authored research, but that will continue to lead to one-and-done studies that do not replicate. Single studies are similar to digging the foundation ground and laying the concrete. It is a great start but not anywhere near a livable house.

Interpret Within the Context of the Study

Every study has a context, and the desire to generalize outside of the sample and study is the tradition. But researchers need to interpret carefully the results within the context of the study and resist the desire to try to take it outside of that context or simply just put in a few sentences about "limitations." Within the context of the study, what appears clear? What has the most uncertainty? Where does it match or highlight previous knowledge? Where are the contradictions to previous work? We also note the caveat that if the study is a large representative sample, which is not common, then discussing outside of the context of the study would be more warranted.

Authors

For readers who are probably experiencing applied data analysis for the first time, there are several behaviors that can be implemented to improve research. We would recommend you read through the special issue in the American Statistician beginning with Wasserstein et al., (2019). There are more than 40 articles, but each will help you be better at quantitative research. The authors do not always agree on what should be done about p-values, but all have important points to understand.

p-values should be used descriptively and not as a conclusion. This includes not using the phrase "statistically significant" and any of the derivatives of that phrase. Relatedly, do not use an asterisk (*) to indicate the same thing in tables in the article. Include all analyses you completed not just those that fit your research hypotheses. This has been known as p-hacking or cherry picking the results (Gelman & Loken, 2013). This is, at the very least, problematic and at the most unethical, and, most importantly, it does not help a field advance.

There are other alternatives such as s-values that can be calculated along with Bayes factors, which could be implemented using a noninformative prior and running a Bayes based analysis. In addition to the alternatives to p-values, a focus on accuracy for sample sizes versus power (trying to get to $p < 0.05$) would drastically improve the quality of the studies.

In addition to the sample sizes, designing for replications at the early stages of study development and executing those replications would also quickly improve the quality of studies and knowledge produced.

Descriptive statistics and visualizations were limited to print space, but with the massive increase in supplemental digital space and open access, this is no longer a concern. Thus, we recommend researchers expand the descriptive statistics and visualizations of the data as supplemental material.

Detailed Measurement and Methods

We believe the method section needs to be much more detailed than currently available. The method and measurement components should be so rich that any researcher could replicate the process of the study. The level of detail we desire is very rare historically due to page space limitations, but this is not a serious limitation anymore. More detail can be accomplished for most research journals through the supplemental materials section and does not necessarily need to be within the text of the article. The first expansion needs to be on the actual sampling process. The sample is not an end state, but a process that occurred to get to the sample that was used in the study. For example, studies that used college students might state, "freshmen were recruited through introductory human development courses." Well, this statement could be an almost infinite number of processes to obtain the sample that was finally used in the study. One example of the process could be, "One of the researchers came to three classes of colleagues and recruited volunteers of which a subsection of students in each course agreed to be a part of the study."

The measurement section also needs more information than what is currently provided. A full description of the instruments used, the type of scaling, and a rich description of the reliability and validity work previously completed is necessary to increase the believability of the data that was obtained (Schreiber & Asner-Self, 2011). Finally, the reliability information from the study's data along with *why* valid inferences can be made from the data and the results.

Analyses completed, all analyses, should be specifically documented including all cleaning and related decisions that were completed. For example, whether to transform a continuous variable's distribution is a serious decision, and all the evidence used to transform or not transform should be discussed.

Finally, based on Wasserstein et al. article and their don'ts:

- Do not base your conclusions solely on whether an association or effect was found to be "statistically significant" (i.e., the p-value passed some arbitrary threshold such as $p < 0.05$).

- Do not believe that an association or effect exists just because it was statistically significant. Reminder, in the data you have, there appears to be an association. But you have one of infinitely many samples.

- Do not believe that an association or effect is absent just because it was not statistically significant.

- Do not believe that your *p*-value gives the probability that chance alone produced the observed association or effect or the probability that your test hypothesis is true.

- Do not conclude anything about scientific or practical importance based on statistical significance (or lack thereof).

- Follow the ATOM model and make that an explicit focus in your writing.

- Most importantly, implement and "be proud" of an *exhaustive* methods section because *p*-values are not stable as they should be.

SUMMARY

Statistical analysis has been presented as objective or truth, and that is simply not how the process unfolds during the design and analysis phases. Researchers as a group need to adjust how they view the results of their studies and be humbler about the conclusions of the study. We believe that implementing the ATOM model would be a large improvement to research along with the basic recommendations from Wasserstein et al. (2019). Finally, we also believe that researchers and funding agencies should be planning studies with a focus on replication.

END-OF-CHAPTER RESOURCES

REVIEW QUESTIONS

Answers and rationales for the review questions are located in the Appendix at the end of the book.

1. Discuss why the results obtained from the statistical analysis of a study's data may be incorrect.

2. Describe why a convenience sample is the most commonly used sample in research and why this is problematic.

3. Rather than focusing on obtaining "significant" *p*-values, where should investigators direct their efforts?

4. Discuss the various sources of error throughout a study that require researchers to accept the uncertainty of their findings.

5. Describe what it means to be thoughtful when we refocus the discussion of our data and project results.

6. An acute care DNP-prepared nurse practitioner implements a project to decrease the incidence of delirium in the ICU. His analysis suggests that the intervention was not effective at decreasing delirium because his results were not "statistically significant," $p = 0.09$. How should the nurse practitioner view his findings through the lens of openness and modesty?

7. Discuss what actions the acute care nurse practitioner can take to ensure he has a rigorous project with results that are as accurate as possible.

 A robust set of instructor resources designed to supplement this text is located at http://connect.springerpub.com/content/book/978-0-8261-6582-4. Qualifying instructors may request access by emailing textbook@springerpub.com.

REFERENCES

Amrhein, V., Trafimow, D., & Greenland, S. (2019). Inferential statistics as descriptive statistics: There is no replication crisis if we don't expect replication. *The American Statistician, 73*, 262–270. https://doi.org/10.1080/00031305.2018.1543137

Bangham, A. D., & Horne, R. W. (1964). Negative staining of phospholipids and their structural modification by surface-active agents as observed in the electron microscope. *Journal of Molecular Biology, 8*(5), 660–668. https://doi.org/10.1016/s0022-2836(64)80115-7

Benjamin, D., & Berger, J. (2019). Three recommendations for improving the use of p-values. *The American Statistician, 73*, 186–191. https://doi.org/10.1080/00031305.2018.1543135

Calin-Jageman, R., & Cumming, G. (2019). The new statistics for better science: Ask how much, how uncertain, and what else is known. *The American Statistician, 73*, 271–280. https://doi.org/10.1080/00031305.2018.1518266

Colquhoun, D. (2019). The false positive risk: A proposal concerning what to do about p-value. *The American Statistician, 73*, 192–201. https://doi.org/10.1080/00031305.2018.1529622

Eels, E. (1991). Probabilistic causality. In J. Williamson (ed.), *The Oxford handbook of causation*. Oxford University Press.

Gelman, A. (2016). The problems with p-values are not just with p-values. *The American Statistician, 70*, 1–2. (supplemental material to the ASA statement on p-values and statistical significance), 10.

Gelman, A., & Loken, E. (2013). The garden of forking paths: Why multiple comparisons can be a problem, even when there is no "fishing expedition" or "p-hacking" and the research hypothesis was posited ahead of time. *Department of Statistics, Columbia University, 348*.

Greenland, S. (2019). Valid p-values behave exactly as they should: Some misleading criticisms of p-values and their resolution with s-values. *The American Statistician, 73*, 106–114. https://doi.org/10.1080/00031305.2018.1529625

Hitchcock, C. (2021). Probabilistic causation. In E. N. Zalta (ed.), *The Stanford encyclopedia of philosophy* (Spring 2021 ed.). https://plato.stanford.edu/archives/spr2021/entries/causation-probabilistic/

Ioannidis, J. P. (2005). Why most published research findings are false. *PLoS Medicine, 2*(8), e124. https://doi.org/10.1371/journal.pmed.0020124

Ioannidis, J. P. (2019). What have we (not) learnt from millions of scientific papers with P values?. *The American Statistician, 73*(sup1), 20-25.

Johnson, V. (2019). Evidence from marginally significant t Statistics. *The American Statistician, 73*, 129–134. https://doi.org/10.1080/00031305.2018.1518788

Kennedy-Shaffer, L. (2019). Before p<0.05 to Beyond p<0.05: Using history to contextualize p-values and significance testing. *The American Statistician, 73*, 82–90. https://doi.org/10.1080/00031305.2018.1537891

Lavine, M. (2019). Frequentist, Bayes, or other? *The American Statistician, 73*, 312–318. https://doi.org/10.1080/00031305.2018.1459317

Locascio, J. J. (2019). The impact of results blind science publishing on statistical consultation and collaboration. *The American Statistician, 73*(sup 1), 346–351. https://doi.org/10.1080/00031305.2018.1505658

McShane, B., Gal, D., Gelman, A., Robert, C., & Tackett, J. (2019), Abandon statistical significance. *The American Statistician, 73*, 235–245. https://doi.org/10.1080/00031305.2018.1527253

O'Hagan, A. (2019). Expert knowledge elicitation: Subjective but scientific. *The American Statistician, 73*, 69–81.

O'Neill, C. (2016). *Weapons of math destruction: How big data increases inequality and threatens democracy.* Crown Publishing Group.

Pearson, E. S. (1939). "Student" as statistician. *Biometrika, 30*(3–4), 210–250.

Reichenbach, H. (1925/1978). Die Kausalstruktur der Welt und der Unterschied von Vergangenheit und Zukunft. *Sitzungsberichte der Bayerische Akademie der Wissenschaft*, November: 133–175. English translation "The causal structure of the world and the difference between past and future. In M. Reichenbach & R. S. Cohen (Eds.), *Hans Reichenbach: Selected writings, 1909–1953* (Vol. II, pp. 81–119). Reidel.

Salmon, M. H. (2003). Causal explanations of behavior. *Philosophy of Science, 70*(4), 720-738.

Schreiber, J., & Asner-Self, K. (2011). *Educational research: The interrelationship of questions, sampling, design, and analysis.* Wiley.

Schreiber, J. B., & London, A. (2019). *Considerations surrounding the data science world we are in* [Paper presentation]. Artificial Intelligence Conference: Thinking about law, law practice, and legal education, Pittsburgh, PA.

Shannon, C. E. (1948). A mathematical theory of communication. *Bell System Technical Journal, 27*, 379–423. https://doi.org/10.1002/j.1538-7305.1948.tb01338.x

Spirtes, P., Glymour, C., & Scheines, R. (2000). *Causation, prediction and search* (2nd ed.). MIT Press. First edition in 1993.

Suppes, P. (1970). *A probabilistic theory of causality.* North-Holland Publishing Company.

Trafimow, D., & MacDonald, J. A. (2017). Performing inferential statistics prior to data collection. *Educational and Psychological Measurement, 77*(2), 204-219.

Wasserstein, R. L., Schirm, A. L., & Lazar, N. A. (2019). Moving to a world "p<.05". *The American Statistician, 73*, 1–19. https://doi.org/10.1080/00031305.2019.1583913

Yi, Z., Schreiber, J. B., Paliliunas, D., Barron, B. F., & Dixon, M. R. (2021). P<. 05 is in the eye of the beholder: A response to Beaujean and Farmer (2020). *Journal of Behavioral Education, 30*, 1–23.

Ziliak, S. (2019). How large are your G-Values? Try Gosset's Guinnessometrics when a little 'P' is not enough. *The American Statistician, 73*, 281–290. https://doi.org/10.1080/00031305.2018.1514325

Ziliak, S., & McCloskey, D. N. (2008). *The cult of statistical significance: How the standard error costs us jobs, justice, and lives.* University of Michigan Press.

FURTHER READING

Abelson, R. P. (2012). *Statistics as principled argument.* Psychology Press.

Anderson, A. (2019). Assessing statistical results: Magnitude, precision and model uncertainty. *The American Statistician, 73*, 118–121. https://doi.org/10.1080/00031305.2018.1537889

Salmon, W. C. (1998). *Causality and explanation.* Oxford Press.

van Dongen, N. N. N., van Doorn, J. B., Gronau, Q., van Ravenzwaaij, D., Hoekstra, R., Haucke, M. N., Scheel, A. M., Sprenger, J., & Wagenmakers, E.-J. (2019). Multiple perspectives on inference for two simple statistical scenarios. *The American Statistician, 73*, 328–339.

Appendix: Review Question Answers and Rationales

CHAPTER I

1. Answer: TRUE

   RATIONALE: This is true because these are the aspects of applied statistics.

2. Answer: FALSE

   RATIONALE: This is false because the statement is not precise enough. Additional information should be given about how much of a difference there is between groups.

3. Answer: FALSE

   RATIONALE: This is false because most results are NOT very generalizable. Most samples are convenience samples and not randomly selected. Data may also contain a good bit of error due to the measurement tools used to collect it.

4. Answer: (d)

   RATIONALE: The Fisher (Frequentist) statistical approach with the associated p-value relies on comparing the test parameter using multiple replications of the results. Letter d conveys the best interpretation of the p-value.

5. Answer: (b)

   RATIONALE: In order to improve the quality of research and scholarly findings being produced and published, the concepts of accuracy and measurement precision are among the main emphases for this book.

6. Answer: Type II error

   RATIONALE: A type II error involves accepting a false null hypothesis (rejecting an alternate hypothesis when it is true).

7. Answer: (a)

   RATIONALE: Letter a is correct because the power of a study is directly affected by how many people or observations were a part of it (the larger the sample, the smaller the sampling error value, and the larger the power). Effect size is needed because a smaller effect is more difficult to detect and a larger sample is then needed.

8. Answer: A nonsignificant p-value using the convention of $p < 0.05$ does not provide much information to fully understand a study's results or what decisions should be made from its findings. The reader needs to closely examine the size of the sample of participants, how carefully the study was conducted, how precisely the variables were measured, and the size of the difference between the groups.

   RATIONALE: The rationale is provided in the response.

9. Answer: A nonspurious relationship must be demonstrated, meaning that the researcher needs to show that no other potential factor or variable could be the reason for the observed relationship between A and B.

   RATIONALE: The rationale is provided in the response; there are three main components to establishing causality. This is the third.

10. Answer: To conduct and interpret research well, one must first be a scholar who is immersed in the literature and has a deep understanding of the topic area. Being well-versed in the research conducted in the area of interest allows one to learn to write good research and evidence-based practice questions; plan robust sampling, data collection, measurement, and analysis methods; and understand how to design and carry out a rigorous study.

    RATIONALE: The rationale is provided in the response; these are essential components to conducting and interpreting research.

CHAPTER 2

1. Answer: Cronbach's alpha and 0.70

   RATIONALE: Because the tool's scores are continuous, Cronbach's alpha is an appropriate test for internal consistency, and 0.70 is a common minimally acceptable score.

2. Answer: TRUE

   RATIONALE: This is a true statement about the main difference between CCT and IRT.

3. Answer: TRUE

   RATIONALE: This is a true statement about the measurement concept of reliability.

4. Answer: TRUE

   RATIONALE: This is a true statement about the aspects of the measurement process that must be considered in order to come to the most accurate inferences and conclusions as possible.

5. Answer: FALSE

   RATIONALE: Test-retest reliability should only be calculated for stable variables that are not expected to change.

6. Answer: (c)

   RATIONALE: Criterion-related validity is supported by comparing a new tool to an established "gold-standard" tool.

7. Answer: Convergent validity

   RATIONALE: Convergent validity is a type of construct validity and refers to the degree to which two measurement tools that should be related theoretically are related.

8. Answer: (a)

   RATIONALE: Letter a is the only true statement. Research projects are performed to increase knowledge, not QI projects. Data from a QI project is only applicable to that setting, and research projects are intended to be generalizable, not QI projects.

9. Answer: (d)

   RATIONALE: Letter d is the only hypothesis that does not specify a direction for or difference in the relationship between the investigational drug and blood pressure, which is the key feature of a nondirectional hypothesis.

10. Answer: (b)

    RATIONALE: Gleason Grade is an example of ordinal data because there is a specific ordering of the categories; for example, grade 4 is worse than grade 3, which is worse than grade 2.

11. Answer: IVs: nutritional status, degree of subdural moisture, skin pigmentation

    DV: pressure ulcer development

    RATIONALE: Nutritional status, degree of subdural moisture, and skin pigmentation are the IVs because they are being examined for their effect on or association with the outcome variable (DV), pressure ulcer development.

CHAPTER 3

1. Answer: Examples: What is the mean score of the students at baseline?

   How many students were male?

   Is the overall shape of the clinical judgment scores normal after the end of the intervention?

RATIONALE: These research questions involve descriptive statistics such as the mean, proportion of males, and shape of the distribution of the dependent variable.

2. Answer: FALSE

RATIONALE: The mean and standard deviation are commonly reported; however, if the data are not normally distributed, it is more appropriate to report the mean and inter-quartile range.

3. Answer: TRUE

RATIONALE: Estimates are the results of a descriptive analysis of the variables.

4. Answer: TRUE

RATIONALE: This is the definition of the mean score.

5. Answer: 210

RATIONALE: You must first arrange the values in order. Since there are an odd number of values, you choose the exact middle value.

6. Answer: 59.502

RATIONALE: The mean (67.24) minus two times the standard deviation (3.869) is 59.502.

$67.24 - 2(3.869) = 59.502$

7. Answer: 4.005 (rounded)

RATIONALE: The standard deviation is calculated by taking the square root of the variance.

8. Answer: (c)

RATIONALE: A negatively skewed distribution is skewed to the left and has a long left tail.

9. Answer: (d)

RATIONALE: The direction of the correlation is negative because the coefficient has a negative value, and the magnitude of the correlation is weak because the value is close to 0.

10. Answer: (d)

RATIONALE: When data are missing at random (MAR), there is some level of relationship between the missing data and another variable (missing depression scores are among the participants who are younger than 50), and the researcher can account for the missingness.

11. Answer: The transformed variable should be examined and compared with the original variable to determine how the transformed variable has changed and how that affects interpretation; for example, the correlation between the transformed variable and the original variable, descriptive statistics of both variables.

    RATIONALE: When variables are transformed, the data are re-expressed mathematically, and proper interpretation of the results can be affected; thus, a careful comparison to the original variable is required.

12. Answer: FALSE

    RATIONALE: When conducting a correlation, only bivariate normality must be checked because there are only two variables involved.

CHAPTER 4

1. Answer: Visualizing the distribution of the data is essential for adequately understanding it, describing it, identifying outliers, and identifying the most appropriate analysis to conduct.

    RATIONALE: Explanation for why data visualization is important is provided in the response.

2. Answer: histogram: see the shape of the distribution

    bar charts: visually compare groups

    line chart or box plot: trend analysis

    scatterplot or heat map: see a relationship or connection

    pie chart or stacked bars: investigate part of something

    RATIONALE: Each of the different data visualization types has a slightly different goal, as provided in the response.

3. Answer: FALSE

    RATIONALE: Heat maps are used for multivariate visualization with continuous variables to highlight the range of the values along with other variables such as geographic location.

4. Answer: TRUE

    RATIONALE: The bell-shaped curve is the desired normal curve but it is rare, if not impossible, to see when working with real data.

5. Answer: TRUE

    RATIONALE: Box plots help the investigator to see outliers beyond the arms of the plot.

6. Answer: FALSE

   RATIONALE: It is essential to include the total sample size so that the viewer of the pie chart knows what actual numbers of participants or observations the proportions are reflecting.

7. Answer: (c)

   RATIONALE: The relationship between two variables is calculated using a correlation and visually displayed using a scatterplot.

8. Answer: Tightly clustered data points in the shape of an elliptical with the highest point in the upper right quadrant of the graph.

   RATIONALE: The visual representation for a strong positive relationship between two variables is that of a tightly clustered elliptical with the highest point in the upper right quadrant of the graph, as provided in the response.

9. Answer: (b)

   RATIONALE: Statistical software packages need to be told by the user how to handle missing variables. The default of the software may be to delete cases with missing variables, which may not be the approach to handling missing data that the investigator wishes to use.

10. Answer: (b, c, d)

    RATIONALE: Visualizing the data does not prevent the investigator from making errors and does not show where data are missing, but it does assist with revealing information that is not necessarily seen in descriptives, determining if transformations are needed, and evaluating if the underlying statistical assumptions are met.

CHAPTER 5

1. Answer: Both designs involve the manipulation of an independent variable and often assignment of participants to groups (e.g., control and experimental). In a quasi-experimental design, there is no random assignment of participants to groups.

   RATIONALE: See the description in the response. The key feature of an experimental design is the randomization of participants to groups. Quasi-experimental designs have no randomization.

2. Answer: In random assignment, participants are randomly placed in an experimental or control group using some predetermined system. This increases the chances that extraneous variables (e.g., confounding factors) that could impact the outcome are evenly distributed between the groups. In random selection, individuals are randomly chosen from the larger population to participate in the study. Random selection is more challenging to accomplish from a logistical perspective.

RATIONALE: See the description in the response. These two concepts are frequently confused, but randomization involves assignment to groups whereas random selection involves selection from the population.

3. Answer: FALSE

   RATIONALE: Because experimental designs use randomization, which is intended to disperse confounding variables between the groups, this design is considered stronger.

4. Answer: TRUE

   RATIONALE: These are the key features of a factorial design.

5. Answer: TRUE

   RATIONALE: This is a key feature of a cross-over design.

6. Answer: FALSE

   RATIONALE: Both the investigators and the participants do not know to which study group the participants belong in a double-blinded randomized controlled trial.

7. Answer: (c)

   RATIONALE: A prospective cohort design follows participants forward in time to look at the occurrence of outcomes of interest (e.g., heart disease) among participants with different levels of exposure or variables of interest (e.g., smokers vs. nonsmokers).

8. Answer: Selection history

   RATIONALE: In the selection history threat to internal validity, differences between the participants in the intervention and the comparison groups are exposed to differences in historical events that may impact the outcomes of interest.

9. Answer: (a)

   RATIONALE: A correlation analysis examines the relationship between two continuous variables, in this case, number of recruitment strategies and number of older adults enrolled.

10. Answer: (b)

    RATIONALE: Letter b is an example of compensatory rivalry because participants in the standard of care group try to compensate for the fact that they are not receiving the new therapy protocol (experimental intervention) by working harder on the outcome.

11. Answer: (b)

    RATIONALE: In the Hawthorne effect threat to external validity, participants change their behavior because they know they are being observed and/or evaluated.

12. Answer: (a, b)

    RATIONALE: Letters a and b are correct because measurement and sampling issues are key sources of error. The standard error of the mean represents how far sample means are likely to be from the population mean. Sample size is not a contributing source of error; larger samples tend to result in more precise parameter estimates.

CHAPTER 6

1. Answer: FALSE

   RATIONALE: Large variability would be demonstrated by a wide range in scores around the mean.

2. Answer: TRUE

   RATIONALE: This is the definition of *within group variability*.

3. Answer: FALSE

   RATIONALE: A dependent *t*-test looks at how much difference there is in the mean of one group from pre-test to post-test.

4. Answer: TRUE

   RATIONALE: This is how you calculate degrees of freedom for an independent *t*-test.

5. Answer: (c)

   RATIONALE: C is the only one with groups >2. The other options are associations, independent *t*-test, or paired *t*-test questions.

6. Answer: (b)

   RATIONALE: Letter b is an example of a question for an independent t-test because it is looking at differences in critical thinking skills between two groups—diploma graduates and BSN graduates.

7. Answer: Essential components of the description include 1) *t*-value, 2) the degrees of freedom, 3) the *p*-value, 4) the mean and standard deviation of the group, and 5) effect size.

   RATIONALE: These are the five essential components of a narrative description of a paired *t*-test analysis.

8. Answer: An effect size represents how meaningful the difference you have detected is, based on a standardized estimate that is not influenced by the scale used to measure the variable. Effect size is relevant because it reflects the practical or clinical significance of that difference. Common effect sizes for an independent t-test include Cohen's d, Hedge's g, and Glass's delta.

RATIONALE: The description of the effect size, its relevance, and common tests for it are in the answer provided.

9. Answer: (a)

RATIONALE: Letters B, C, and D can be used to assess normality. The Levene's test is a statistical test used to assess the equality of variances for a variable for two or more groups.

10. Answer: (a, b, d)

RATIONALE: Letters a, b, and d are parametric tests used with normally distributed data; letters c and e are nonparametric tests that can be used with data that are not normally distributed.

11. Answer: (b)

RATIONALE: The ANOVA F-test is known as an omnibus test that can tell you whether the means among three or more groups are different, but it does not tell you which groups are different from the others. The Bonferroni adjustment limits the possibility of getting a statistically significant result when testing multiple groups. This post hoc test is needed because the more tests you run, the more likely you are to get a significant finding.

12. Answer: (d)

RATIONALE: The Mann Whitney U test is a nonparametric test to compare outcomes between two independent groups.

CHAPTER 7

1. Answer: FALSE

RATIONALE: When there is an interaction effect, the researcher cannot just focus on the main effects of the two groups. The interaction indicates that the group effects are interacting with each other. Some have indicated the focus should be on the interaction, and that is often the case if the effect of the interaction is large; however, the discussion should include all three effects.

2. Answer: TRUE

RATIONALE: In a disordinal interaction, the effect between groups crosses over. This type of interaction indicates that a factor has one kind of effect under one condition and the opposite kind of effect under the other condition.

3. Answer: TRUE

RATIONALE: An interaction between the grouping variable and the time variable is possible; for example, one group changes more quickly than the other group.

4. Answer: (c)

RATIONALE: Letter c is correct because ANCOVA controls for a variable that may impact the outcome variable.

5. Answer: (d)

RATIONALE: Letter d is correct because factorial ANOVA is used with a 2x2 design as in this example. Letter a is repeated measures, letter b uses ANCOVA, and letter c is one-group repeated measures.

6. Answer: Treatment B has the larger effect size and, therefore, larger effect on the outcome.

RATIONALE: Partial eta^2 represents the percent of the total variance in the health outcome that is associated with the treatment, after controlling for the other variables in the model. For partial eta^2, 0.07 would be considered a medium effect, and 0.20 is a large effect.

7. Answer: Sphericity, or compound symmetry, is an assumption that is unique to repeated measures. It means that the variance of the differences between levels of the repeated variable (usually time) are equal. For example, when there are three time points, the variance scores between time 1 and time 2; time 1 and time 3; and time 2 and time 3 should be equal. Although far from ideal, Mauchly's Test of Sphericity is used to test the assumption of sphericity. Results of this test should not be statistically significant in order to support that sphericity is not violated.

RATIONALE: See the description in the response.

8. Answer: Smaller sample sizes are needed with a within-subjects repeated measures ANOVA because there is less error variance with one group, which reduces the amount of "noise" in the data, and power is gained with repeated measurements.

RATIONALE: See the description in the response.

9. Answer: (a), (c), (e), (f), and (h)

RATIONALE: Letters b, d, and g are incorrect because correlations between the repeated measures and Mauchly's Test of Sphericity are only reported for repeated measures analyses, and Levene's test for equal variances is not needed for within-group (repeated measures) ANOVA.

10. Answer: The covariate should not be affected by the treatment being examined. The treatment groups should not differ on the covariate at baseline. The covariate should have very low measurement error. Lastly, the more covariates included in the model, the larger the sample size you will need and the more contrasts and post hoc tests you will need to describe.

    RATIONALE: See the description in the response.

CHAPTER 8

1. Answer: FALSE

   RATIONALE: Although this is a strong positive relationship, as one variable increases, the other variable also increases.

2. Answer: TRUE

   RATIONALE: This is a true statement because cross-sectional data cannot establish causality.

3. Answer: (c)

   RATIONALE: Letter c reflects a linear regression analysis and the size of the variance in myocardial infarction that the three independent variables may account for in the model.

4. Answer: This is a small-to-medium size correlation, or relationship, between the variables.

   RATIONALE: According to Cohen (1988) correlations <0.10 are small, 0.30 are medium-sized, and ≥ 0.50 are large.

5. Answer: (b)

   RATIONALE: A scatter plot of the two variables allows the investigator to visually examine the directionality and linearity of the relationship between the two variables.

6. Answer: A Spearman rho rank-order correlation

   RATIONALE: A Spearman rho rank-order correlation is an appropriate analysis technique because it is used to look at bivariate relationships with continuous data that are not normally distributed.

7. Answer: Thirty five percent ($R^2 = 0.35$) of the variation in hemoglobin A1c is explained by the variables of age in years, BMI, and daily steps walked in the model.

   RATIONALE: The adjusted R^2 tells you the percentage of variation in the dependent variables that can be explained by the independent variables. It is better to use adjusted R^2 with multiple predictors in the regression model because R^2 (unadjusted) will always stay the same or increase with additional variables in the model.

8. Answer: Each 1-year increase in age is associated with a 0.54% increase in hemoglobin A1c.

   RATIONALE: The unstandardized beta (.54 here) is used to interpret the effect of the independent variable on the dependent variable. Because the unstandardized beta is positive, an increase in the IV is associated with an increase in the DV, and the beta value represents the amount of change in the DV associated with a one-unit change in that IV.

9. Answer: (a), (c), and (e)–(i)

   RATIONALE: Letter b is not an assumption, and it is the definition of *multicollinearity*. Letter d is a premise of logistic regression. The rest are assumptions of multiple linear regression.

10. Answer: In the *simultaneous model*, all predictors are included in the model at the same time and given equal weight. This approach is most appropriate when we have no practical or theoretical rationale for thinking that any one variable occurs prior to any other or is of any greater relevance than the others. In this method, the beta coefficients are estimating the unique relationship between the predictors and the DV.

    In the *hierarchical model*, the predictors are entered in "blocks" according to a specific hierarchy determined in advance. This approach is often used to control for variables that are known in the literature to affect the DV, and the new variables of interest are then included in a second block. For example, if age is known to affect the DV, it might be entered into the first block. Hierarchical linear regression may result in incorrect conclusions about the relationships of the new variables with the DV, however, because the first block has removed the overlapping relationships with the new variables.

    When using a *stepwise model* (either forward or backward), variables are added to or removed from the model based on meeting a statistical significance level, often $p < 0.05$ or $p < 0.10$. In the forward method, the predictor variables are added one by one until adding predictors does not add anything more to the model. In the backward method, all the predictor variables are added into the model. Then, variables that do not show a "significant" relationship with the DV are removed from the model one by one. We do not recommend stepwise entry, however, the backward method is generally preferred of the two, because the forward method results in suppressor effects which occur when predictors only turn out significant if another predictor is held constant.

    RATIONALE: See the description in the response.

CHAPTER 9

1. Answer: FALSE

    RATIONALE: Multinomial logistic regression must be used with more than two categories.

2. Answer: TRUE

    RATIONALE: Both types of IV can be used in logistic regression.

3. Answer: TRUE

    RATIONALE: The outcome variable is binary; thus, logistic regression can be used.

4. Answer: (c)

    RATIONALE: Phi-Coefficient reflects the size of the association and is interpreted like a correlation coefficient with values ranging from 0 to1.

5. Answer: (b)

    RATIONALE: This is interpreted as the odds ratio of being discharged in <7 days is 1.80 times greater if the patient is a nonsmoker compared to a smoker.

6. Answer: (d)

    RATIONALE: The Wald statistic is used to test the significance of individual predictors in the model. Cox & Snell R^2 and Nagelkerke R^2 are fit indices. The beta coefficient shows the expected change in the log odds of having the outcome per a unit change in the predictor, but it does not reveal significance.

7. ANSWER: x^2 with 1 degree of freedom = 4,855.3, which shows there is an overall difference between the cells

    RATIONALE:

    Compute expected frequency for each cell: 3740 / 6775 = 0.5520; slightly more than half would develop hypertension regardless of sodium intake.

    <2,000 gm expected = 0.5520 × 3195 = 1763.6 (<2,000 gm eaters expected to get hypertension)

    ≥2,000 gm expected = 0.5520 × 3580 = 1976.16 (≥2,000 gm eaters expected to get hypertension)

    Compute expected frequency for each cell: multiple row total by column total and divide by total sample size (noted in parentheses in the table).

Compute chi-square for each cell by squaring the difference between expected and observed frequencies and dividing by the expected frequency; then sum these values.

$$x^2 = \Sigma \; \frac{(\text{observed} - \text{expected})^2}{\text{expected}}$$

$$x^2 = + 1149.2 + 1416.4 + 1025.8 + 1263.9 = 4855.3$$

8. Answer:
   1. continuous variables must be checked for linearity with the logit of the DV
   2. error terms are not correlated; participants are independent of each other
   3. predictors are not correlated with each, i.e., no multicollinearity
   4. the sample of participants was randomly selected

   RATIONALE: These are the statistical assumptions underlying logistic regression analysis.

9. Answer: *Pseudo R^2* shows how well the model fits the data and how much variability in the outcome is explained by the model. Potential *pseudo R^2* tests include Cox & Snell R^2, Nagelkerke R^2, McFadden, and Tjur, to name a few.

   RATIONALE: The interpretation of the *pseudo R^2* value in logistic regression is essentially the same as the interpretation of R^2 in linear regression; the closer to 1 the *pseudo R^2* value is, the better the models fits.

10. Answer: Residuals are the difference between the observed values and the expected values, based on the model. Large residuals will result when the difference (or deviance) between the observed values in the data set and the predicted values is large. Residuals are important to examine because larger residuals indicate a poorly fitted model. Common options for residual analysis for logistic regression are Pearson, Dfbeta, C, Cbar, DIFDEV and DEFCHISQ, Cook's D, and Centered Leverage.

    RATIONALE: See the description in the response.

11. Answer: Sensitivity and specificity are statistical assessments of the performance of a logistic regression model in terms of how well it classifies participants into one outcome or the other.

    Sensitivity is also known as the true positive rate and measures the proportion of actual positives that are correctly identified as positive in the model (e.g., the percentage of people sick with COVID-19 who are correctly identified as having COVID-19). It is the complement to the false negative rate. *Sensitivity = true positives / (true positives + false negatives)*

Specificity is known as the true negative rate and measures the proportion of actual negatives that are correctly identified as negative (e.g., the percentage of healthy people who are correctly identified as not having COVID-19). It is the complement to the false positive rate.

Specificity = true negatives / (true negatives + false positives)

RATIONALE: See the description in the response.

12. Answer: The ROC curve provides a visualization of the predictive accuracy of logistic regression results for sensitivity and specificity. The closer the curve is to the top left corner of the graph, the better the sensitivity and specificity. A straight 45-degree line from the bottom left corner to top right corner represents the result occurring by chance alone.

RATIONALE: See the description in the response.

CHAPTER 10

1. Answer: The Bayesian approach is based on a formula that takes into consideration existing information together with the information at hand and keeps statistics in the domain of mathematical probability. Bayesian analysis uses the null and alternative hypotheses, does not assume a fixed probability but rather a distribution of possible outcomes, and has no need for repeated studies.

The Fisher approach uses only the data at hand, relies on a frequency definition of probability using long-run properties of repeated occurrences, and is based on the concept of the p-value, that is, rejecting the null hypothesis. Fisher analysis assumes the data are random and defined by the distribution of the population; thus, a different sample will result in different results.

RATIONALE: See the description in the response.

2. Answer: Three key features of a Bayesian analysis include the likelihood function, prior beliefs distribution, and the posterior distribution. The likelihood function represents the observed data, that is, the distribution of results the researcher assumes about her data. The prior beliefs distribution comes from previous research beliefs about the distribution of a phenomenon. The posterior distribution is the ultimate objective of the Bayesian analysis and is calculated by multiplying the likelihood function by the prior beliefs distribution. The posterior distribution shows us the uncertainty around a parameter using a distribution.

RATIONALE: See the description in the response.

3. Answer: The probability that a person with hypertension given there is chest pain is 0.80.

RATIONALE: Working through the components of the equation needed for $P(HTN|CP)$ using Bayes' Theorem:

$$P(HTN|CP) = \frac{P(HTN) \times P(CP|HTN)}{P(CP)}$$

- The probability of having HTN is $P(HTN) = 40 \div 100 = 0.40$
- The probability of having chest pain is $P(CP) = 25 \div 100 = 0.25$
- The probability that a someone with HTN has chest pain is $P(CP|HTN) = 20 \div 40 = 0.50$

$$P(HTN|CP) = \frac{0.40 \times 0.50}{0.25} = 0.80 \text{ OR } 20/25$$

4. Answer: TRUE

RATIONALE: Bayes factor gives us a numeric representation of the weight toward the null hypothesis or toward the alternative hypothesis. The p-value provides an inference for rejecting or not rejecting the null hypothesis. A $BF_{10} > 100$ is considered to provide extreme evidence for the alternative hypothesis.

5. Answer: FALSE

RATIONALE: These intervals are similar but not exactly the same. In the Fisher framework, the compatibility interval represents a range of values designed to include the true value of the parameter with a minimum probability (e.g., 90% or 95%). In the Bayesian framework, the data is seen as fixed while the parameters may vary.

6. Answer: TRUE

RATIONALE: Bayesian analysis incorporates prior data and ascribes to the philosophy that the data do not vary. The Fisher/Frequentist approach does not include prior data and assumes that the data are random; it also assumes repetition of studies that ultimately corrects differences from the population value.

CHAPTER 11

1. Answer: FALSE

RATIONALE: This is the definition of assignable causes not chance causes.

2. Answer: FALSE

RATIONALE: PDCA and PDSA often require several iterations. If the change did not result in improvement, the cycle is repeated.

3. Answer: TRUE

   RATIONALE: This is a frequent approach to using a Theory of Change to achieve the desired outcomes of a project.

4. Answer: (b)

   RATIONALE: The Charter is the first step in the PDSA cycle and answers the question, "What are we trying to accomplish?" together with the stakeholders who are involved in the work or the outcome of the project.

5. Answer: (d)

   RATIONALE: To help see the dynamic elements of a system, creating a flow chart of the people, materials and processes in the system is needed.

6. Answer: (c)

   RATIONALE: Balancing measures are used so that, as one measure improves, other measures do not indicate a reduced or negative performance.

7. Answer:
   - Recognize Cues: Identify the increased number of adverse event reports.
   - Generate Hypotheses: Brainstorm possible reasons for this increase.
   - Judge Hypotheses: Evaluate and rank the hypotheses based on how likely each is to explain the increase.
   - Take Action: Use a Theory of Change to determine behaviors needed to address the increase in falls and implement if behavior changes.
   - Evaluate Outcomes: Analyze data to determine of behavior changes resulted in a decrease in the number of falls on night shift.

   RATIONALE: These are the five steps of the NCRM as applied to the concern of increased patient falls.

8. Answer:
   - Understand Variation: Assess what is natural variation in the number of falls.
   - Appreciate the System: Know that the system is interdependent (e.g., what is happening on day shift could be impacting the falls on night shift).
   - Use a Theory of Change: Based on the theory chosen, changes in behavior can be predicted according to the relationships between theoretical concepts.
   - Psychology: Understand the people involved in the project to reduce the number of patient falls; know how they interact, how they learn, and what their intrinsic and extrinsic motivations are.

   RATIONALE: These are the four components of profound knowledge as applied to the project to decrease patient falls.

9. Answer:

- Define what is value-adding to patients: Patients want to be discharged in a timely manner.

- Map value streams (pathways that deliver care): Map out the processes taking place after the patient leaves the cath lab.

- Make value streams flow by reducing the waste, delay and duplication: Make these processes more efficient.

- Allow patients to "pull" value so their needs are met: Allow patients to report their satisfaction.

- Continually pursue perfection: Continually monitor processes and work to improve them.

RATIONALE: These are the components for following the Lean model.

CHAPTER 12

1. Answer: There are several common reasons results may be considered wrong. These reasons include:

   1. The study sample is a convenience sample that does not represent the population of interest.

   2. Violations of assumptions, such as the sample not being randomly selected

   3. Measurement of variables contains error.

   4. Very disparate manipulation of variables such that one condition differs greatly from the other(s)

   5. Statistical models are mis-specified and are missing important variables (e.g., confounders, or interactions).

   All of these reasons can lead to inaccurate parameter estimates and incorrect results.

   RATIONALE: See the description in the response.

2. Answer: Recruitment of participants is difficult, challenging from a geographic standpoint, time-consuming and expensive. So, recruiting the most available and convenient sample is most desirable. A convenience sample was not randomly selected to be in the study, however, which is an underlying assumption of the Fisher framework of analysis.

   RATIONALE: See the description in the response.

3. Answer: Researchers should focus on obtaining the most accurate results they can by conducting a well-designed study, including random sampling to achieve a sufficient size sample, measuring variables as precisely as possible, and using robust statistical analysis.

   RATIONALE: See the description in the response.

4. Answer: Error is pervasive in the entire research endeavor. Researchers make subjective decisions throughout the research process from who to include in the sample, to which design is most feasible, to which tools to use to measure the variables, to which statistical analyses to conduct. Also, exact replication of research is nearly impossible; thus, there will always be natural variation in results.

RATIONALE: See the description in the response.

5. Answer: Being thoughtful means providing the reader with the specific context of the study and the previous evidence in which it is situated. This includes discussing the findings within the existing body of evidence and how your results compare and contrast. It means carefully considering the strengths and weaknesses of the design and the true quality of the data collected. Collaborating with colleagues is also part of being thoughtful because it helps to enhance one's research by considering and incorporating diverse ideas.

RATIONALE: See the description in the response.

6. Answer: Openness entails acknowledging that subjective decision-making is present throughout the project from design, to implementation, to analysis, which affects the results we obtain, and statistical modeling cannot take out the uncertainty and error introduced by these decisions. By being Modest, we acknowledge the reality of this imperfection. We also must recognize that lack of statistical significance does not mean the results have no practical importance.

RATIONALE: See the description in the response.

7. Answer:
   1. Use a well-established theory as a framework to guide the project, the selection of variables, and the relationships examined.
   2. Consider probabilistic causality where the project's intervention increases the probability that delirium will decrease in the ICU.
   3. Avoid confirmation bias and work to publish the project's results despite "statistical nonsignificance" by reporting effect size and clinical significance of the outcome.
   4. Work with a colleague to replicate the project.
   5. Interpret the findings within the context of the specific project, for example, a small sample of elderly patients with several confounding factors impacting results.
   6. Include p-values as descriptive information only and focus on accuracy, project replication, and data visualization.

7. Include a detailed description of the project's methods and measurement of variables, including the sampling process used and the reliability and validity of the tools used to make inferences.

RATIONALE: These are additional behaviors investigators can take to improve the process of conducting and reporting their quality improvement and research projects.

Index